Nelson

Review of
Pediatrics

Nelson

Review of Pediatrics

Richard E. Behrman, M.D.
Director, Center for the Future of Children
The David and Lucile Packard Foundation
Clinical Professor of Pediatrics
Stanford University and
University of California, San Francisco
Attending Physician
Lucile Salter Packard Children's Hospital at Stanford
Stanford, California

Robert M. Kliegman, M.D.
Professor and Chairman
Department of Pediatrics
Medical College of Wisconsin
Pediatrician-in-Chief
Children's Hospital of Wisconsin
Milwaukee, Wisconsin

Ann M. Arvin, M.D.
Professor of Pediatrics and
Microbiology/Immunology
Associate Chair for Academic Affairs
Department of Pediatrics
Stanford University School of Medicine
Chief, Infectious Diseases
Lucile Salter Packard Children's Hospital at Stanford
Stanford, California

W.B. SAUNDERS COMPANY
A Division of Harcourt Brace & Company
Philadelphia   London   Toronto   Montreal   Sydney   Tokyo

W.B. SAUNDERS COMPANY
A Division of Harcourt Brace & Company

The Curtis Center
Independence Square West
Philadelphia, Pennsylvania 19106

Library of Congress Cataloging-in-Publication Data

Nelson review of pediatrics / Richard E. Behrman, Robert M. Kliegman, Ann M. Arvin.—1st ed.

p.   cm.

Review questions for: Nelson textbook of pediatrics. 15th ed. c 1996.

ISBN 0–7216–5579–3

1. Pediatrics—Examinations, questions, etc.   I. Kliegman, Robert M.
   II. Arvin, Ann M.   III. Nelson textbook of pediatrics.   IV. Title
   [DNLM: 1. Pediatrics—examination questions.   WS 18.2 B421n 1996]

RJ45.N4 1996 suppl   618.92′00076—dc20

DNLM/DLC   95-52571

NELSON REVIEW OF PEDIATRICS   ISBN 0–7216–5579–3

Printed in the United States of America.

Last digit is the print number: 9   8   7   6   5   4

This book is dedicated to Richard D. Krugman, M.D.,
who has been the author and editor of the previous four editions of
Review of Pediatrics. *Dr. Krugman is a world-renowned pediatrician*
who is currently the Dean of the University of Colorado School of Medicine.
Dr. Krugman's broad knowledge, insight, and wit have all contributed
to the education of child health care providers through this book
and through many other positive learning experiences.
We thank him for establishing the foundation for this book.

Preface

Publication of this review is highlighted by changes in authorship and organization, but at the same time, it maintains the original laudable educational principles and philosophies of previous editions. In keeping with the major reorganization of the 15th edition of *Nelson Textbook of Pediatrics,* this companion review has also undergone reformatting; both books are now divided into 34 dominant parts or topic areas. In addition, this volume is authored by the editors of *Nelson Textbook of Pediatrics.*

The goal of this review is to help the reader to continue to learn from the parent text, but in a different fashion. This work has been written in parallel with the concurrent edition of *Nelson Textbook of Pediatrics* and is thus a self-assessment guide to help reinforce what was learned from the parent text. Each question was written to continue the education of the reader. Case-based questions, multiple choice, or matching questions and the corresponding explanations help to reinforce knowledge of a broad spectrum of general pediatric facts.

Because learning occurs in many different settings, we anticipate that the questions in this review will help the reader to benefit from the knowledge in the parent text. We believe that this learning activity will help the reader in career advancement and will contribute to the ability to care for children. Past experience of previous readers has suggested that this work will also aid in the preparation for important steps for progression within the field of pediatrics. The majority of questions in this edition are new, but because of the excellent nature of some questions from the previous review, a few are repeated.

Finally, we encourage feedback from readers so that we may continue to create a reader-friendly study guide.

Richard E. Behrman, M.D.
Robert M. Kliegman, M.D.
Ann M. Arvin, M.D.

Contents

1 The Field of Pediatrics

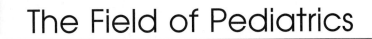

The broad field of pediatrics encompasses the art and science of medicine across the wide age range of 24-week-gestation immature neonates to 6-foot 8-inch adolescent football players. This *part* of the *Nelson Textbook of Pediatrics* covers the history of pediatrics in addition to providing information about the epidemiology and lives of children both in the United States and abroad. This *part* addresses the importance of understanding the cultural background of families in the context of disease prevention and therapy. Furthermore, it informs us about a useful ethical approach to patient care that enables us, as physicians, and our patients' families to make good medical decisions. The chapter on evaluating the medical literature helps readers gain better insight into interpreting clinical studies. In addition, this *part* emphasizes an essential aspect that distinguishes pediatrics as a specialty—that is, preventive pediatrics. Finally, an approach to the well child is developed for readers.

The questions for this *part* reinforce readers' learning on these basic topics. An understanding of these concepts creates an excellent foundation for pediatricians, child advocates, and epidemiologists.

1. Injuries, congenital anomalies, and malignancy are the three leading causes of death for which age group?

   A. 0 to 1 year

   B. 1 to 4 years

   C. 5 to 9 years

   D. 10 to 14 years

   E. 15 to 24 years

2. The three leading causes of death for 15- to 24-year-olds are

   A. injuries, malignancy, suicide

   B. injuries, malignancy, homicide

   C. injuries, anomalies, malignancy

   D. injuries, homicide, suicide

   E. injuries, malignancy, diseases of the heart

3. The sensitivity of a test is determined by

   A. $\dfrac{\text{true positives}}{\text{true + false positives}}$

   B. true positives $\times$ false negatives

   C. $\dfrac{\text{true positives}}{\text{true + false positives}}$

   D. true positives + false negatives

   E. $\dfrac{\text{true positives}}{\text{false positives}}$

4. The ability of a competent 18-year-old patient to refuse health care, even if the care will prevent death and provide excellent chances for a long and healthy life, is the principle of

   A. irrationality

   B. religious freedom

   C. paternalism

   D. autonomy

   E. nonmaleficence

5. In ethical principles, withholding futile medical treatment is no different from

   A. homicide

   B. battery

   C. beneficence

   D. withdrawing treatment

   E. paternalism

6. Examples of primary prevention include all of the following EXCEPT

   A. tetanus immunization

   B. chlorination of water

   C. fluoride treatment

   D. drug rehabilitation

   E. locking medicines in a cabinet

7. *Matching:*

   1. Measles vaccine
   2. Lead poisoning screening
   3. Anticipatory guidance by a pediatrician
   4. Scoliosis screening
   5. Speed limit

   A. Primary prevention

   B. Secondary prevention

   C. Tertiary prevention

6. Antibiotics for exacerbations of cystic fibrosis

7. Ortolani maneuver

8. Anticipatory guidance includes all of the following EXCEPT

   A. developmentally oriented advice

   B. removing small objects from the reach of toddlers

   C. explaining the decreased growth rate of 24- to 48-month-old children

   D. DPT immunization

   E. none of the above

9. *Matching:* Match the ethical principle with the example given in the statements below.

   1. A physician obtains a court order to permit an appendectomy on a child against the religious objections of the parents.

   2. Disclosure of biopsy result of a malignant tumor is withheld because no cure exists.

   3. A 13-year-old is asked to consent to chemotherapy.

   4. A physician is told by an adolescent that he is sexually involved with his 9-year-old sister.

   5. A physician does not report suspected abuse because she feels the family will be harmed.

   A. Autonomy
   B. Competence
   C. Beneficence
   D. Truth telling
   E. Confidentiality
   F. Conflict of interest

10. A study is undertaken to identify causes of diarrhea in children evaluated in the emergency department of a tertiary care children's hospital. Subjects included in the study are a convenience sample of patients evaluated by a single investigator whenever he was working. This investigator always vacations in a warm climate from January to April, and the study thus was interrupted during those months. This study will have problems with all of the following EXCEPT

    A. sampling bias

    B. external validity (generalizability)

    C. internal reliability

    D. precision

    E. accuracy

11. A study is performed to measure the effectiveness of inexpensive, old reliable drug A versus expensive, new drug B in the treatment of otitis media in children. The study finds no difference in outcome between the group of 15 children treated with drug A and the 15 treated with drug B. Questions you might want to consider when evaluating this trial include which of the following?

    A. Who paid for the study to be performed?

    B. How might bias in the selection of study subjects have altered the main result?

    C. How does the size of the study sample affect the outcome?

    D. All of the above

12. In a metropolitan area of 1,000,000 persons, there is an outbreak of diarrheal illness, and the following data are reported:

	Age <18 Years	Age 19–60 Years	Age >60 Years	Total
N	300,000	300,000	400,000	1,000,000
Diarrhea	150,000	50,000	300,000	500,000
Diarrheal deaths	10	40	50	100

Based on the foregoing data, which of the following statements is true?

    A. The case-fatality rate for diarrheal deaths is 100/1,000,000.

    B. The mortality rate for diarrheal deaths is 100/500,000.

    C. The relative risk of diarrhea in childhood compared with ages greater than 60 years is 0.67.

    D. The risk difference of diarrhea in childhood compared with ages 19 to 60 years is 100,000.

13. Of the following parts of a physical examination, which portion should usually be performed first on an infant or toddler?

    A. Abdominal examination

    B. Ear examination

    C. Extremity examination

    D. Cardiac examination

    E. Pharyngeal examination

14. Taking notes while obtaining a patient's history is controversial. Which of the following statements about this practice is true?

    A. All historical data must be recorded.

    B. Note taking is best done before observation.

    C. Note taking should cease if sensitive information is conveyed.

    D. Brief notations are superior to extensive notes.

    E. Notes should not be taken.

15. In a child younger than 2 years, observation is best done as the child

    A. sits in the parent's lap

    B. walks about the room

    C. lies on the examining table

    D. is sleeping

    E. is being weighed and measured

16. The data generated from observational assessment of a child's overall state of well-being are greatly influenced by the child's developmental stage. This is most importantly shown in which observational data?

    A. Hydration

    B. Skin color

    C. Visual response

    D. Respiratory effort

    E. Motor tone

17. Major portions of the well child evaluation, nutrition, accident prevention, and growth are best discussed with parents in the framework of

    A. modern pediatrics

    B. health care delivery

    C. social interactions

    D. child development

    E. family dynamics

18. The approach taken by a physician to eliciting data during a physical examination is linked to a child's stage of development. This is importantly demonstrated in the examination of

    A. the pharynx

    B. the ears

    C. arterial pulsations

    D. the chest

    E. the lumbrosacral spine

19. Global improvements in child mortality are primarily the result of

    A. antibiotics and improved distribution of essential drugs

    B. smallpox eradication and control of other vaccine-preventable illnesses

    C. oral rehydration therapy

    D. basic public health programs

20. International goals established at the United Nations World Summit for Children include all of the following EXCEPT

    A. halving of maternal mortality rates and child malnutrition

    B. universal availability of family planning and safe water

    C. control of major childhood diseases and a one-third reduction of child mortality

    D. basic education for all children

    E. establishing roads for emergency transport of ill children

21. In order to prevent malnutrition from developing in infants younger than 1 year, the best advice you should give a nursing mother in a developing country who discovers she is pregnant again is to

    A. continue nursing as long as possible and begin adding appropriate weaning food after 6 months of age

    B. consider an alternative to breast milk and wean as soon as possible to an appropriate weaning food

    C. discontinue the pregnancy and use family planning until the nursing child is 2 years old

    D. wean as soon as possible to an appropriate weaning food

22. All of the following statements about vitamin A are true EXCEPT that it

    A. stabilizes the structure and function of mucosal surfaces, is involved with T-cell function, and contributes to mucus production

    B. can decrease mortality from respiratory diseases in children after a single annual dose of an oral preparation

C. is recommended by the American Academy of Pediatrics for distribution for acute treatment of measles

D. is found in adequate amounts in breast milk until the child is 6 months old

E. enhances availability of vitamins K and D

23. Which of the following statements about diarrheal disease programs in developing countries is true?

A. Such programs have been most successful when pursued as selective initiatives.

B. U.S. health programs are being modeled after the successes of diarrheal disease programs abroad.

C. Oral rehydration therapy (ORT) solutions are standardized to include specific carbohydrates.

D. Nurses are the appropriate personnel to provide education about diarrheal disease prevention and treatment.

24. Of the following listed causes of death among children in the developing world, the most common is

A. plague

B. typhoid fever

C. diarrheal disease

D. malaria

E. Ebola virus

25. All of the following are appropriate individuals who may be used as language interpreters in a clinical setting EXCEPT

A. bilingual/bicultural designated interpreters

B. adult family members whom the patient has brought to the visit for the purpose of interpretation and who feel comfortable with the responsibility

C. bilingual children of the person who needs interpretation services

D. professional staff members who are bilingual and from a similar cultural and social background as the individual who needs the service

26. The mother of a 10-year-old asthmatic child with mild wheezing states that instead of administering the doctor-prescribed medications, she gave the child an herbal tea, which you determine to be nonharmful. The most sensitive approach to this situation with regard to patient/parent education is to

A. tell the mother to stop using the tea and give just the prescribed medicine the next time her child is wheezing

B. lecture the mother on the ineffectiveness of herbal teas in the management of asthma

C. refer the family to a child protective agency because of medical neglect

D. explain to the mother the importance of using the prescribed medication in addition to her home remedy

27. Culturally mediated health benefits may contribute to a patient's decision-making process for which of the following illnesses?

A. Asthma

B. *Mal de ojo* (evil eye)

C. Upper respiratory tract infections

D. Viral gastroenteritis

E. All of the above

28. Level of acculturation may provide insight into which patients may subscribe to cultural health beliefs and practices. All of the following informational items are helpful in assessing a patient's level of acculturation EXCEPT

A. the length of time the patient has lived away from his or her cultural areas of origin

B. the language preference of the patient

C. the level of formal education

D. the patient's surname

E. the number of generations the patient is removed from his or her cultural area of origin

29. In many clinical situations, the services of an interpreter are necessary. When conducting a patient interview through an interpreter, a physician should attempt to do all of the following EXCEPT

A. speak in short phrases

B. ask the patient if the interpreter is acceptable to him or her

C. maintain visual contact with the interpreter

D. consider using visual aids, such as charts and drawings

E. keep jargon to a minimum and use commonly understood terms

2 Growth and Development

This *part* of the *Nelson Textbook* is a broad but specific guide through the multiple developmental stages and normal physical and mental progression of a maturing child. The physical, emotional, social, neurodevelopmental, language, and intellectual aspects of normal and abnormal behavior are highlighted for each stage of development: the fetus, newborn, first year, second year, preschool, early school, and adolescent periods. Of even greater importance, this *part* helps readers assess normal and abnormal patterns of growth and development.

The study of growth and development is distinctive for pediatricians. Understanding the progression of organ system maturity is critical for the care of patients and for communication with them. Questions in this *part* focus on learning these skills in the context of patients and factual information.

1. *Matching:* Erikson stages of development

   1. 0 to 1 year of age
   2. 2 to 3 years of age
   3. 3 to 6 years of age
   4. 6 to 12 years of age
   5. 12 to 20 years of age

   A. Industry vs. inferiority
   B. Identity vs. identity diffusion
   C. Basic trust
   D. Initiative vs. guilt
   E. Autonomy vs. shame and doubt

2. A doula has been beneficial during a pregnant woman's labor and delivery. The effects of a doula include all of the following EXCEPT

   A. shorter labor
   B. fewer complications
   C. higher birth weight
   D. reduced length of hospital stay
   E. greater satisfaction

3. Behavioral states in the newborn period include

   A. quiet and active sleep
   B. drowsy and alert
   C. fussy and crying
   D. all of the above
   E. none of the above

4. The best formula to approximate average weight (kg) for a 4-year-old is

   A. $\dfrac{\text{Age (years)} \times 7 - 5}{2}$

   B. Age [years] $\times$ 2 + 8

   C. $\dfrac{\text{Age (months)} + 9}{2}$

   D. (age [years] $\times$ 5 + 17)

   E. (age [years] $\times$ 7 + 5)

5. A normal infant may cry for up to 3 hours a day during the developmental peak time of this behavior. The peak of crying is at about what age?

   A. 2 weeks
   B. 4 weeks
   C. 6 months
   D. 6 weeks
   E. 4 months

6. The best feeding protocol for a temperamentally irregular infant is

   A. a fixed schedule
   B. based on the parents' schedule
   C. every 1 to 2 hours
   D. on demand
   E. 60 minutes for each feeding

7. Object permanence is not present in a 2-month-old, whose response to dropping a ball is

   A. staring momentarily at the spot the ball was dropped from
   B. eyes descending as the ball descends
   C. crying when the ball hits the ground

D. smiling at the game of hide-and-seek

E. none of the above

8. Tooth eruption generally begins at what age?

A. 0 to 1 month

B. 2 to 4 months

C. 6 to 8 months

D. 10 to 14 months

E. 16 to 20 months

9. The ability to manipulate small objects with the pincer grasp is usually noted at what age?

A. 0 to 2 months

B. 3 to 5 months

C. 6 to 7 months

D. 8 to 9 months

E. 10 to 12 months

10. A developmentally normal child who is just able to run, build a tower of two cubes, pretend play with a doll, and speak in two-word sentences is what age?

A. 19 months

B. 15 months

C. 14 months

D. 24 months

E. None of the above

11. A developmentally normal child who is just able to sit without support, transfer objects from hand to hand, and speak in a monosyllabic babble is probably what age?

A. 3 months

B. 4 months

C. 9 months

D. 6 months

E. 11 months

12. Transitional objects are

A. training underwear

B. shoes without laces

C. cups with a special drinking spout

D. blankets and teddy bears

E. none of the above

13. A developmentally normal child who just hops on one foot, copies a cross and square,

tells a story, and goes to the toilet alone is probably what age?

A. 24 months

B. 36 months

C. 48 months

D. 60 months

E. 72 months

14. Handedness is usually determined by what age?

A. 2 to 4 months

B. 6 to 12 months

C. 15 to 18 months

D. 20 to 24 months

E. 36 to 48 months

15. Magical thinking is most common in preschool children and includes all of the following EXCEPT

A. animism

B. confusion of coincidence for causality

C. belief in the power of wishes

D. stating "the sun sets because it is tired"

E. paranoia

16. The best approach for parents to help a preschool child overcome monster fears is

A. to rationalize that monsters don't exist

B. to read books that do not have monsters in them

C. to have the pediatrician explain that monsters are make-believe

D. to use "great power" like monster spray to keep the monsters away

E. none of the above

17. All of the following are considered characteristics of temperament EXCEPT

A. intensity of a reaction

B. rhythmicity

C. distractibility

D. handedness

E. adaptability

F. attention span and persistence

18. Which one of the following tests best demonstrates that a newborn infant is capable of complex behavior?

A. Apgar score

B. Brazelton neonatal behavioral assessment scale

C. Denver Developmental Screening Test

D. Wechsler Intelligence Scale for Children

19. A mother brings her 6½-month-old circumcised boy to you for a "sick" visit. You saw the child 2 weeks earlier for health maintenance, including a DTP immunization, and the child appeared well. The mother's complaint is that the baby is waking up every night and is fussy during the day, especially when she leaves him. The child's history is otherwise normal, and physical examination reveals no problems. Which one of the following is most appropriate?

A. Perform urinalysis and obtain a complete blood count to rule out urinary tract infection.

B. Request that the mother feed the infant more.

C. Reassure the mother that the behavior is normal and will pass in time.

D. Reassure the mother that the behavior will pass because it is a reaction to the DTP shot.

20. The most rapid increase in height in boys is found in which Tanner SMR stage?

A. 1

B. 2

C. 3

D. 4

E. 5

21. The most rapid increase in height in girls is found in which Tanner SMR stage?

A. 1

B. 2

C. 3

D. 4

E. 5

22. Visual fixation by newborn infants is associated with which Prechtl behavioral state?

A. Drowsy

B. Quiet, alert

C. Awake, active

D. Crying

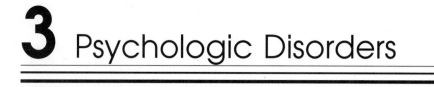

3 Psychologic Disorders

Mental health problems are frequent concerns of parents and result in common symptoms in childhood and adolescence. This *part* of the *Nelson Textbook* includes an extensive series of chapters that discuss the assessment and interviewing process in addition to psychosomatic illness; vegetative, habit, mood, and anxiety disorders; suicide; disruptive behavioral and attention deficit hyperactivity disorders; sexual behavior; psychoses; and treatment approaches to the many common mental health symptoms of children. This part of the book is a logical continuum from normal growth and development and helps readers gain a better understanding of what is a normal or an abnormal or pathologic manifestation of an underlying disorder.

The questions in this *part* do not prepare you for a psychiatry residency but do reinforce the important mental health principles that are discussed in greater detail in the *Nelson Textbook*. Because mental health issues directly or indirectly affect children so greatly, this *part* of the *Nelson Textbook* is critical to pediatricians.

---

1. Neuroleptic antipsychotic agents produce all of the following unwanted side effects EXCEPT

   A. bradykinesia

   B. hyperthermia

   C. tardive dyskinesia

   D. inappropriate ADH

   E. sedation

2. A 4-year-old boy is noted to have stereotypic body movements, poor verbal and nonverbal communication, and absent empathy. At daycare, he has not made any friends. The most likely diagnosis is

   A. attention deficit hyperactivity disorder

   B. dysthymic syndrome

   C. deaf-mutism

   D. autism

   E. cerebral palsy

3. *Matching:*

   1. Belief that one is a member of opposite gender
   2. Sense of self as either male or female
   3. Comfort with cultural expectations
   4. Cross-dressing

   A. Gender role
   B. Gender identity
   C. Transsexualism
   D. Transvestism

4. Therapy of attention deficit hyperactivity disorder (ADHD) is best initiated with

   A. methylphenidate (Ritalin)

   B. dietary sugar restriction

   C. avoidance of food additives

   D. megavitamins

   E. barbiturates

5. All of the following are diagnostic soft signs of ADHD EXCEPT

   A. mixed hand preference

   B. impaired balance

   C. dysdiadochokinesia

   D. astereognosis

   E. none of the above

6. Head banging, hair twirling, rocking, thumb sucking, teeth grinding, and nail biting, all are

   A. habit disorders that probably relieve tension

   B. easy to cure in children

   C. evidence of insecurity in the majority of children and of poor parenting by their parents

   D. tics

7. Which is the most likely diagnosis in an 8-year-old boy with findings of an early history of colic, poor academic performance, impaired peer relations, excessive dawdling over homework, and oppositionalism?

   A. Autism

   B. Conduct disorder

C. Petit mal epilepsy

D. Attention deficit hyperactivity disorder

E. Separation anxiety disorder

8. Which of the following statements about depression in childhood and adolescence is true?

A. It is rarely encountered in clinical practice.

B. In a large majority of cases, it is accurately diagnosed by using the dexamethasone suppression test.

C. It can be successfully treated with stimulant medications in about half of the cases.

D. It is associated with dysphoria, anhedonia, and elation in about half of the cases.

E. It has a much higher concordance rate between monozygotic twins than between dizygotic twins.

9. Which of the following statements about Gilles de la Tourette syndrome is true?

A. It is characterized by tics and coprolalia.

B. It is characterized by tics and encopresis.

C. It is treated with haloperidol and methylphenidate.

D. It is a common disorder of childhood.

E. It affects girls more often than boys.

10. Night terrors are associated with

A. REM sleep

B. overeating after 7:00 P.M.

C. the use of antipsychotic medication

D. inception in preschool years and sometimes with somnambulism

E. anger within the family

11. Which of the following statements about current views on the etiology of autism is most likely to be correct?

A. Autism is caused by inadequate and hostile parenting.

B. Autism is of unknown cause.

C. Autism is caused by intrauterine trauma.

D. Autism is caused by malfunction of the immune system.

E. Autism is caused by a viral agent.

12. Separation anxiety disorder is most likely to be associated with

A. aggressive behaviors

B. poor academic performance

C. school refusal

D. increased risk of schizophrenic outcome

E. maternal neglect

13. Nocturnal enuresis in an 8-year-old boy is most likely to be associated with

A. genitourinary structural abnormalities

B. familial history of enuresis

C. genitourinary tract infections

D. childhood psychosis

E. attention deficit hyperactivity disorder

14. Which of the following statements about carbamazepine is false?

A. It is used to treat anxiety.

B. It can cause aplastic anemia secondary to a diminution of white blood cells.

C. Therapeutic blood levels are measured to monitor clinical response.

D. It is used to treat self-injurious behavior in organically impaired children and adolescents.

E. It has the structure of a tricyclic antidepressant.

15. All of the medicines listed below have shown efficacy in treating attention deficit hyperactivity disorder (ADHD) EXCEPT

A. methylphenidate

B. thiothixene

C. clonidine

D. desipramine

E. dextroamphetamine

16. Conduct disorder in childhood and adolescence is associated with all of the following EXCEPT

A. antisocial behavior

B. criminality in the father

C. physical abuse

D. marital discord within the home

E. mental retardation

17. Encopresis is associated with all of the following EXCEPT

A. more common occurrence in boys than in girls

B. low socioeconomic background

C. unconscious or conscious anger

D. highly achieving children

E. poor hygiene skills

18. Completed suicides in childhood and adolescence can be associated with all of the following EXCEPT

    A. previous suicide attempts

    B. alcohol or drug abuse

    C. a history of depression and suicide within the family

    D. easy access to firearms

    E. perfectionism within the classroom

19. Which of the following findings is most likely to be encountered in a student with poor active working memory?

    A. Delayed spelling

    B. Difficulty interpreting language

    C. Problems in mathematics and writing

    D. Trouble studying for tests

    E. Poor recall of prior knowledge

20. A 9-year-old boy is chronically rejected by peers. No one ever wants to sit near him. He is never invited to birthday parties. He often alienates his peers with his aggressive behaviors. He makes "weird" comments and tells jokes that no one else laughs at. He often boasts and becomes aggressive when he has a conflict with a peer. Which of the following forms of management is most likely to be effective with this child?

    A. Social skill training

    B. Methylphenidate

    C. Psychotherapy

    D. Behavior modification

    E. Summer camp

21. A child in the third grade has problems with spelling and reading. She appears very quiet and confused in class. Her teacher has noticed that this girl has trouble following directions. Her mind seems to wander whenever the teacher tells a story or explains something complicated. She is skilled in art and so far has performed very well in arithmetic. Which of the following diagnostic procedures is most likely to yield useful findings in this child?

    A. An attention deficit questionnaire

    B. An intelligence test

    C. A language evaluation

    D. A psychiatric assessment to rule out depression

    E. A neurologic examination

22. Which of the following statements correctly describes children with attentional dysfunction?

    A. They are always hyperactive.

    B. Their problems are mainly behavioral.

    C. They often have additional neurodevelopmental dysfunctions.

    D. They all respond to treatment with methylphenidate.

    E. Their difficulties lessen significantly after puberty.

23. An 11-year-old child has excellent ideas in a class discussion, but what she records on paper is primitive and unsophisticated. She can spell well in isolation and understands rules of punctuation and capitalization, but in her own writing she makes multiple errors and mistakes in punctuation and capitalization. Her handwriting is legible, but writing is painfully slow. This girl most likely is having problems with

    A. expressive language

    B. graphomotor production

    C. ideation

    D. attention

    E. simultaneous retrieval memory

24. An 8-year-old child is significantly delayed in acquiring reading decoding skills. Which of the following is the most likely explanation?

    A. Visual perceptual problems

    B. Phonologic weaknesses

    C. Retrieval memory dysfunction

    D. Temporal-sequential disorganization

    E. Attentional dysfunction

25. *Matching:*

1. Projective	A. Stanford-Binet
2. Parent-child interaction	B. Peabody Picture Vocabulary
3. Intelligence	C. Rorschach
4. Screening	D. Nursing child assessment feeding and teaching scale

26. Somatoform disorders, as part of psychosomatic illness, include all of the following EXCEPT

A. conversion reaction

B. asthma

C. hypochondriasis

D. pain disorders

E. none of the above

27. Munchausen by proxy syndrome is characterized by all of the following EXCEPT

A. recurrent illness that cannot be explained

B. experienced pediatricians' stating that they have never seen such a case

C. symptoms that disappear with the parent present

D. an attentive parent caregiver who never goes home

E. an unworried parent caregiver

F. poor response to therapy

G. doctor shopping

28. Enuresis is associated with

A. increased bladder capacity

B. tight underwear

C. urinary tract infection

D. bicycle riding

E. none of the above

29. *Matching:*

1. Sleep paralysis	A. Narcolepsy
2. REM sleep	B. Nightmares
3. Non-REM sleep	C. Night terrors
4. Somnambulism	
5. Daytime naps	
6. Memory of episode	
7. Autonomic activity	

30. Major depression is characterized by all of the following EXCEPT

A. insomnia

B. hypersomnia

C. anhedonia

D. dysphoria

E. excessive physical activity

31. Dysthymic disorder is associated with all of the following EXCEPT

A. delusions

B. chronic dysphoria

C. periods of normal mood

D. anxiety disorder

E. social maladjustment

32. Common methods of suicide attempts in preadolescent children include all of the following EXCEPT

A. jumping from heights

B. carbon monoxide

C. hanging

D. drug overdose

E. firearms

33. Lying in 2- to 4-year-old children is often

A. malicious

B. oppositionalism

C. testing parental reaction

D. impulsiveness

E. a precursor to sociopathic behavior

34. Truancy is considered developmentally normal if it is associated with

A. lying

B. fear of school failure

C. fear of peer ridicule

D. depression

E. none of the above

35. *Matching:*

1. Chronic stealing	A. Conduct disorder
2. Continuous arguing	B. Oppositional defiant disorder
3. Fire setting	
4. Obscene language	C. Neither
5. Rape	D. Both
6. Property destruction	
7. Poor school performance	
8. Sibling rivalry as the cause	

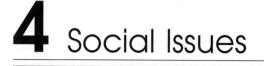

4 Social Issues

In an ever-changing socioeconomic climate, social issues have direct or indirect effects on the mental and physical health of children. Societal and personal issues such as adoption, foster care, a mobile family, childcare, separation from and death of loved ones, violence, and neglect and abuse of children all create problems for the children we care for and thus require physicians to be aware of the adverse circumstances associated with these issues. In addition, it is important for physicians to help children and families to adjust and to cope with these issues.

Questions related to this *part* of the *Nelson Textbook* help to build on the basic principles discussed in the individual chapters on each topic. This reinforcement is essential as more and more of our children encounter challenging social issues each day.

1. In genital specimens or serum from a 10-year-old girl, all of the following are considered laboratory evidence of sexual abuse EXCEPT

   A. *Chlamydia*

   B. syphilis

   C. gonorrhea

   D. herpes simplex type 1

   E. sperm

   F. HIV seroconversion

2. Which of the following are true about pedophiles?

   A. Stepfathers are more often perpetrators than fathers.

   B. They choose vulnerable children.

   C. They begin in their adolescence.

   D. They are found in all cultures and socioeconomic levels.

   E. They use pornography to initiate contact.

   F. All of the above.

   G. None of the above.

3. A 6-month-old boy is brought to the emergency room and is afebrile but responds poorly to tactile and auditory stimuli. He becomes apneic and unresponsive after a generalized seizure. The parents state that he was perfectly well in the car on the way to the hospital and that they only brought him to the emergency room because of constipation. He requires 10 minutes of cardiopulmonary resuscitation, after which he is noticed to have a bulging fontanel and bilateral retinal hemorrhages. A chest x-ray reveals two posterior rib fractures. The most likely diagnosis is

   A. CPR-induced retinal hemorrhages and rib fractures

   B. hemorrhagic shock and encephalopathy

   C. hemophilia

   D. status epilepticus

   E. child abuse—shaken baby syndrome

4. *Matching:* Differential diagnosis of child abuse

1. Multiple fractures	A. *Candida* diaper rash
2. Ecchymosis	B. Osteogenesis imperfecta
3. Perineal burns	C. Thrombocytopenia
4. Bruises (old)	D. Impetigo
5. Cigarette burn	E. Mongolian spots

5. Child abuse should be suspected for all of the following EXCEPT

   A. delay in seeking care

   B. an implausible history

   C. chip fracture of a long bone

   D. spiral fracture of the femur

   E. tibial fracture in a toddler

6. *Matching:* Bruise discoloration

Age of Bruise (days)	Bruise Appearance
1. 1 to 2	A. Resolved
2. 4 to 5	B. Green

3. 6 to 7   C. Red-blue

4. 8 to 10   D. Yellow-brown

5. 20 to 28   E. Blue-purple

7. All of the following are associated with child abuse and neglect EXCEPT

   A. living on a military base

   B. parental drug misuse

   C. spousal abuse

   D. parental psychosis

   E. parent experiencing abuse as a child

   F. child being mentally retarded

8. A prevalent concern among school-age children is that they may

   A. become hungry

   B. miss a favorite TV show

   C. have a toy stolen

   D. lose a loved one to violence

   E. never get married

9. A young child's response to the death of a parent often is characterized by

   A. depression and weight loss

   B. denial and magical wishing

   C. anger and crying

   D. wishes of death for himself or herself

   E. none of the above

10. The effect that statements such as "stop it or you'll give me a headache" have on young children is to

    A. teach children to behave

    B. give children a pattern of headaches

    C. create guilt and unrealistic fault

D. provide parents with a way to cope

E. prepare children for separation

11. When should adopted children be told of their adoption?

    A. By the age of 3 to 4 years

    B. By the age of 10 to 12 years

    C. By Tanner stage 5

    D. Before entering college

    E. Never

12. Childcare has been shown to influence children's development. Which of the following is an accurate statement about the impact of childcare on children's development?

    A. Most infants in childcare are insecurely attached to their mothers.

    B. For disadvantaged children, childcare experiences make them less sociable and more aggressive than their peers.

    C. Children attending daycare during infancy display long-term emotional insecurity.

    D. Children with childcare experience are more self-confident and interactive with peers.

13. During her 4-month-old infant's child health supervision visit, a mother informs you of her plans to return to work and place her son in childcare. From a developmental standpoint, which of the following is the ideal type of childcare for this infant?

    A. Licensed family daycare

    B. Not-for-profit daycare center

    C. In-home care by a relative or nonrelative

    D. Proprietary daycare center

    E. Care by a relative or nonrelative in the caregiver's home

5 Children with Special Health Needs

I t is stated that at least 10% of all children may have a chronic illness. Furthermore, a small percentage of children use the vast majority of our health care resources. In addition, although chronic illness or disability may interfere with some function, it is important to recognize the positive aspects of the child and to focus on strengths and ways to maximize these strengths as well as to reduce dysfunction or disability. Many curriculums have weaknesses in this area of pediatrics; this is an unfortunate circumstance for trainees and their future patients.

Questions in this *part* of the book focus on children with special health needs related to failure to thrive, chronic illnesses, and developmental disabilities. Questions on the care of children with a fatal illness and children at special risk are also included.

1. A mentally retarded child with microphthalmia, microcephaly, chorioretinitis, and a history of a neonatal petechial rash most likely has

   A. chromosomal syndrome

   B. TORCH infection

   C. fetal alcohol syndrome

   D. galactosemia

   E. hyperammonemia

2. All of the following are valid and reliable tests to diagnose mental retardation EXCEPT

   A. the Bayley scale

   B. the Denver developmental test

   C. the Stanford-Binet test

   D. the Wechsler scale

3. Common causes of mental retardation include all of the following EXCEPT

   A. fragile X syndrome

   B. chromosomal trisomies

   C. fetal alcohol syndrome

   D. hypoxic-ischemic brain injury

   E. congenital rubella syndrome

4. Frequent problems of children with common chronic illnesses include all of the following EXCEPT

   A. unpredictability

   B. pain

   C. expense

   D. multiple providers

   E. failure to graduate high school

   F. isolation

   G. psychologic or behavioral problems

5. The five leading causes of chronic childhood conditions in the United States include all of the following EXCEPT

   A. congenital heart disease

   B. arthritis

   C. seizure disorders

   D. asthma

   E. cystic fibrosis

   F. diabetes mellitus

6. An infant with multiple grotesque congenital anomalies dies on the third day of life. Her mother has not had an opportunity to see her before death, owing to postpartum complications. When informed of the baby's death, she says she wants to see her. She cannot be moved from where she is receiving intensive care. The best response to her request is to

   A. tell her that she is too sick to see the baby

   B. tell her she will be able to see the baby later

   C. take the baby to her bedside

   D. tell her she won't want to see the baby

   E. tell her that it is too late for her to see the baby

7. You have made the diagnosis of a fatal illness

in John, a 10-year-old boy who has siblings 2 and 6 years old. The parents ask how they should deal with the siblings. Among the following, your best response would be,

A. "Tell them Johnnie is sick and that they should treat him nicely."

B. "Tell them that Johnnie is sick and going to die."

C. "Tell them nothing. They will find out soon enough."

D. "Tell them that Johnnie is sick and that they had nothing to do with his illness."

8. A 10-year-old girl who is in the terminal phase of leukemia, after several remissions and relapses, asks you, "Am I going to die?" Among the following, your best response is likely to be

A. "No. We expect you to have another remission in a few days."

B. "It's discouraging, isn't it?"

C. "Why do you ask that just now?"

D. "Not for a long time."

9. Which of the following is the LEAST likely response of parents who hear for the first time that their child has a fatal illness?

A. Disbelief

B. Anger

C. Guilt

D. Fear

E. Resignation

10. The parents of a 10-year-old girl with mental retardation are seeking information on what to expect for her future. The youngster is in a mainstreamed educational program, is just beginning to master simple reading skills, and has one close friend. Recognizing the difficulty of long-term prognostication, which of the following is a possible life goal for this child?

A. Holding a regular job

B. Getting married

C. Having children

D. All of the above

11. A preschooler with Down syndrome is seen for a routine health supervision visit. A knowledgeable clinician will pay particular attention to screening for problems that are known to occur with increased frequency in children with this condition. Which of the following conditions would be LEAST likely to be found?

A. Atlantoaxial instability

B. Neurogenic bladder

C. Hypothyroidism

D. Conductive hearing loss

12. A 3-year-old boy with a limited vocabulary is referred for formal psychometric testing and is found to have an IQ of 60. Physical examination is essentially unremarkable except for mild hypotonia. Appropriate initial laboratory studies would include all of the following EXCEPT

A. karyotype, including test for fragile X

B. audiologic evaluation

C. cranial CT scan

D. formal speech and language evaluation

13. Children develop understanding of illness mechanism in a predictable developmental sequence. By what grade level should children of normal intelligence understand physiologic interaction of body parts (e.g., heart and lungs)?

A. Grade 2

B. Grade 4

C. Grade 6

D. Grade 8

E. Grade 10

14. Pediatricians working with families whose children have chronic conditions must often work with other community agencies to help families obtain needed services. All of the following agencies provide services especially for children with chronic health conditions EXCEPT

A. early intervention programs

B. maternal and child health programs

C. Social Security Administration Supplemental Security Income Program

D. Women's, Infants, and Children (WIC) nutrition programs

E. special education programs

15. Adolescents with chronic illness face several common problems regardless of the specific

illness they have. Which of the following statements is accurate?

A. Most adolescents with chronic illness have significant psychologic problems associated with their condition.

B. Most adolescents with chronic illness require special education services.

C. Most adolescents with chronic illness survive to adulthood.

D. Most adolescents with chronic conditions require personal attendant services.

16. Many chronic health conditions affect children and adolescents. Among the more common are all of the following EXCEPT

A. diabetes mellitus

B. seizure disorders

C. congenital heart disease

D. hypertension

E. arthritis

F. asthma

17. The general approach to psychosocial failure to thrive includes all of the following EXCEPT

A. keeping meal time brief

B. offering solid foods before liquids

C. forcing the child to eat

D. minimizing environmental distractions

E. minimizing the intake of water and juice

18. Indications for hospitalization for failure to thrive include all of the following EXCEPT

A. third-degree malnutrition

B. minor infection

C. evaluation of parent-child feeding interaction

D. further diagnostic and laboratory evaluation

E. lack of catch-up growth

19. All of the following are routine laboratory tests that should be included when evaluating children for failure to thrive EXCEPT

A. CBC

B. lead level evaluation

C. urinalysis

D. electrolyte determinations

E. amino acid screen

6 Nutrition

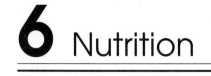

Nutrition, once a major component of medical education, unfortunately is often an undertaught topic. Students and residents may not be able to identify a specific "nutrition department" or curriculum in their formal education and often have difficulty in recognizing nutritional disorders. Nutrition is an essential topic, not just because of the occasional patient (in the United States) with an identifiable nutritional deficiency (much more common in developing countries) but because of the great influence that appropriate nutrition has on supporting normal growth and development. In addition, parents are increasingly aware of nutritional issues and constantly bring nutrition questions to the pediatrician to answer.

Questions in this *part* address normal and abnormal states of water, energy, nutrient, and vitamin intake. Normal feeding practices are addressed as well.

1. The breast-fed infant of a strict vegan may develop which vitamin deficiency if the mother is not receiving supplements of this vitamin?

   A. K

   B. B_6

   C. B_{12}

   D. Folate

   E. Biotin

2. A 10-year-old boy weighing 95 kg manifests daytime somnolence, polycythemia, congestive heart failure, and cyanosis. The most likely diagnosis is

   A. drug abuse

   B. pickwickian syndrome

   C. severe scoliosis

   D. cardiomyopathy

   E. primary pulmonary hypertension

3. The most effective therapy for the condition described in the preceding question is

   A. continuous positive airway pressure

   B. nocturnal oxygen

   C. weight loss

   D. tracheotomy

   E. theophylline

4. *Matching:* Vitamin deficiencies

   1. Xerosis conjunctivae
   2. Tender nerves
   3. Photosensitivity
   4. Seizures
   5. Bitot spots
   6. Diarrhea
   7. Cheilosis
   8. Alopecia
   9. Subperiosteal hemorrhage
   10. Craniotabes
   11. Cerebellar ataxia

   A. B_1 (thiamine)
   B. Riboflavin
   C. A
   D. Niacin
   E. B_6
   F. Biotin
   G. C (ascorbic acid)
   H. D
   I. E

5. *Matching:* Mineral deficiencies

   1. Zinc
   2. Selenium
   3. Phosphorus
   4. Iron
   5. Iodine
   6. Calcium
   7. Fluoride
   8. Manganese
   9. Chloride

   A. Rickets
   B. Dwarfism
   C. Microcytic anemia
   D. Cardiomyopathy
   E. Caries
   F. Goiter
   G. Metabolic alkalosis
   H. None known

6. *Matching:* Vitamin excess

   1. D
   2. C
   3. B_6
   4. A
   5. B_{12}

   A. Neuropathy
   B. Hypercalcemia
   C. Pseudotumor cerebri
   D. Oxaluria
   E. Unknown

7. There are relatively few contraindications for breast-feeding. Which of the following is a

contraindication for breast-feeding in the United States?

A. Mastitis

B. Maternal autoimmune disease (SLE)

C. Maternal Dilantin therapy

D. HIV-positive mother

E. None of the above

8. *Matching:* For each symptom of the deficiency disease, select the appropriate vitamin.

1. Seizures, neuropathy

2. Pseudoparalysis

3. Craniotabes, enlarged costochondral junctions

4. Dermatitis, diarrhea, dementia

A. Vitamin A

B. Vitamin B_1 (thiamine)

C. Niacin

D. Vitamin B_6 (pyridoxine)

E. Vitamin C

F. Vitamin D

9. *Matching:*

1. Contains approximately 20 calories per ounce

2. Gastrointestinal allergy less common

3. Free of bacterial contamination

4. Contains secretory IgA antibodies

5. Associated with increased mortality rates in underdeveloped countries

6. Associated with decreased incidence of colic and eczema

7. Associated with prolonged unconjugated hyperbilirubinemia

8. Higher carbohydrate concentration but lower protein concentration

A. Breast milk only

B. Formula only

C. Both breast milk and formula

D. Neither breast milk nor formula

10. The best source of iron for 1-month-old infants is

A. iron fortified cereals

B. yellow vegetables

C. fruits

D. breast milk

E. 2% low-fat cow's milk

11. *Matching:* For each disorder, select the appropriate vitamin deficiency.

1. Beriberi

2. Scurvy

3. Rickets

4. Pellagra

5. Night blindness

A. Vitamin A

B. Riboflavin

C. Vitamin B_1 (thiamine)

D. Niacin

E. Vitamin C

F. Vitamin D

12. A 4-month-old with vitamin D–deficient rickets would be expected to show all of the following EXCEPT

A. craniotabes

B. bowlegs

C. rosary

D. low serum phosphate levels

E. high alkaline phosphatase levels

13. Which of the following does NOT have recognized anti-infectious properties?

A. Vitamin A

B. Vitamin D

C. Iron

D. Zinc

14. Which of the following vitamins is in higher concentration in cow's milk than in human milk?

A. A

B. C

C. E

D. K

E. B_6

7 Pathophysiology of Body Fluids and Fluid Therapy

A "Peanuts" cartoon once depicted a dehydrated Charlie Brown being graciously treated by Sally with a statement that all he needed was a little salt and water. If only this were as easy in all of our nonfictional patients. Normal and abnormal states of water, minerals, and acid-base balance often perplex the most intelligent pediatrician. This *part* covers the various states of fluid, electrolyte, and acid-base disturbances. In addition, specific diseases are addressed in more detail.

Questions in this *part* help readers better understand the issues of acid-base abnormalities, dehydration, and electrolyte disturbances. As is always needed in this topic, the questions reinforce the basic principles of pathophysiology, diagnosis, and therapy.

1. Diabetes insipidus may be due to all of the following EXCEPT

   A. pituitary adenoma
   B. renal epithelial ADH reception deficit
   C. hypokalemia
   D. hypercalcemia
   E. adrenal deficiency

2. The normal fractional excretion of sodium in children older than 1 year on a diet containing regular amounts of sodium is

   A. 1%
   B. 7%
   C. 10%
   D. 15%
   E. 25%

3. A 1-month-old boy presents with severe failure to thrive, emesis, and a temperature of 41°C. Serum electrolyte measurements reveal a sodium level of 185 mEq/L, and the urine specific gravity is 1001. The most likely diagnosis is

   A. adrenal insufficiency
   B. salt poisoning
   C. hypernatremic dehydration
   D. malignant hyperthermia
   E. nephrogenic diabetes insipidus

4. A well-grown 6-month-old presents with a tonic-clonic seizure lasting 30 minutes. The child is found to be hypothermic and remains lethargic. The diet history reveals that the mother is a participant in the WIC program, but because it is the end of the month, she has begun to dilute the remaining formula with water because there is not enough to last until she receives her next allotment of formula next week. The most likely diagnosis is

   A. hypocalcemia
   B. hyponatremia
   C. hypoglycemia
   D. hypernatremia
   E. hypokalemia

5. Hyperkalemia in patients with shock may be due to all of the following EXCEPT

   A. transcellular K^+ shifts secondary to acidosis
   B. renal failure
   C. rhabdomyolysis
   D. hypoglycemia
   E. none of the above

6. Hyperkalemia may be associated with all of the following EXCEPT

   A. succinylcholine use
   B. burns
   C. trauma
   D. chemotherapy
   E. metabolic alkalosis
   F. digitalis toxicity
   G. uremia

7. Hypokalemia is associated with all of the following EXCEPT

A. rhabdomyolysis

B. muscle weakness

C. prolonged QT interval

D. hypertension

E. aciduria

F. digitalis toxicity

G. ileus

8. A normal anion gap acidosis is most likely due to

A. diabetes mellitus

B. renal tubular acidosis

C. nephrotic syndrome

D. uremia

E. shock

9. Increased intestinal calcium absorption occurs most often in

A. oxalosis

B. short gut syndrome

C. nephrotic syndrome

D. sarcoidosis

E. none of the above

10. Hypercalcemia is noted in all of the following EXCEPT

A. hyperparathyroidism

B. poor phosphate intake

C. hyperthyroidism

D. supravalvular aortic stenosis

E. trisomy 21

F. thiazide diuretic use

11. An early sign of hypermagnesemia is

A. hyporeflexia

B. coma

C. ileus

D. apnea

E. none of the above

12. A 10-month-old patient with vomiting and diarrhea, tachycardia, normal blood pressure, dry mucous membranes, a capillary refill time of 2 seconds, deep respirations, and irritability is what percent dehydrated?

A. 0% to 3%

B. 3% to 5%

C. 6% to 9%

D. 10% to 12%

E. 12% to 15%

13. A serious complication of the treatment of hypernatremic dehydration is

A. cerebral thrombosis

B. cerebral edema

C. hyperchloremia

D. hypoglycemia

E. none of the above

14. An 18-year-old presents with a crouplike voice and painful flexion of the wrists with extended fingers. The most likely diagnosis is

A. hypocalcemia

B. hypoglycemia

C. hyponatremia

D. adrenal crisis

E. none of the above

15. Which of the following is considered an insensible water loss?

A. Pulmonary loss

B. Stool loss in normal nondiarrheal stools

C. Sweat

D. Urinary loss to excrete obligatory solutes

E. None of the above

16. Poor urine output during rehydration of hypernatremic dehydration may be due to

A. acute tubular necrosis

B. persistent ADH secretion

C. persistent hypovolemia

D. all of the above

E. none of the above

17. The best method to reduce the potassium level during hyperkalemia, by reducing the body burden of potassium, is

A. sodium bicarbonate infusion

B. glucose and insulin infusion

C. calcium infusion

D. albuterol aerosol

E. Kayexalate enema

18. All of the following can be used acutely to

lower serum potassium levels during hyperkalemia EXCEPT

A. glucose with insulin intravenously

B. albuterol aerosol

C. sodium bicarbonate infusion

D. captopril

E. none of the above

19. All of the following may be encountered in hypernatremic dehydration EXCEPT

A. hyperglycemia

B. azotemia

C. metabolic acidosis

D. severe signs of dehydration out of proportion to the degree of weight loss

E. none of the above

20. The finding of marked metabolic alkalosis with acidic urine indicates

A. marked sodium depletion

B. marked potassium depletion

C. hyperventilation

D. diabetes mellitus

E. laboratory error

21. Respiratory alkalosis occurs in which one of the following conditions?

A. Pickwickian syndrome

B. Hyperventilation syndrome

C. Kyphoscoliosis

D. Guillain-Barré syndrome

22. A 12-month-old infant is admitted to the hospital because of dehydration and diarrhea of 3 days' duration. The infant weighed 10 kg at a well visit 1 week ago. She has had 10 to 12 stools per day for the past few days and a temperature of 39°C. She has not urinated for the past 18 hours. Physical examination reveals sunken eyes and dry, tenting skin. Which of the following would you do first?

A. Order a complete blood count and blood cultures.

B. Obtain a urine specimen for culture, electrolytes, and specific gravity.

C. Begin lactated Ringer solution, 20 mL/kg intravenously, after obtaining blood for electrolytes and blood urea nitrogen.

D. Obtain stool for fats, reducing subtances, and culture.

23. If the child in Question 22 had been receiving only Kool-Aid for two days as clear fluid therapy, which electrolyte picture would you expect?

	Sodium (mEq/L)	Potassium (mEq/L)	Chloride (mEq/L)	Bicarbonate (mEq/L)
A.	142	4.5	100	26
B.	154	3.4	112	10
C.	124	3.6	94	10
D.	102	6.9	119	20

24. Had the mother in Question 22 given the child only boiled skimmed milk for the preceding 48 hours, which serum sodium level would you expect before therapy?

A. 142 mEq/L

B. 154 mEq/L

C. 124 mEq/L

D. 102 mEq/L

25. Assuming 10% dehydration, the best way to monitor initial improvement in the child in Question 22 is by measuring

A. weight gain

B. urinary output

C. central venous pressure

D. blood pressure

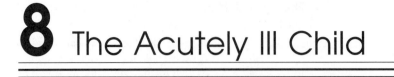

8 The Acutely Ill Child

owhere else in pediatrics are the basic physiologic principles that are taught in the first 2 years of medical school more important to apply than in the care of acutely ill children. In addition, the principles of prevention, acute stabilization, and pharmacology all apply to these children. Discussion of acutely ill children includes topics such as injury control, evaluation, emergency services, critical care medicine, coma, resuscitation, shock, drowning, burns, hypothermia, acute (adult) respiratory distress syndrome, pain management, and principles of drug therapy. Whenever possible, prevention is emphasized.

Questions in this *part* work closely with the related chapters in the *Nelson Textbook* to help readers identify, prioritize, stabilize, and treat acutely ill children. Specific diseases are discussed in other *parts* of the *Nelson Textbook,* but the basic principles of multiple system organ dysfunction such as that occurring in shock are included in this *part.*

1. Indications for admission to the hospital after a burn injury include all of the following EXCEPT

   A. suspected child abuse

   B. electric burns through an extremity

   C. perineum burns

   D. poor follow-up

   E. unimmunized for tetanus

   F. inhalation injury

2. Which of the following statements about the neonatal pain experience (compared with the adult) is true?

   A. Neonates have a higher pain threshold.

   B. Perception is reduced because of immaturity.

   C. Unmyelinated C fibers transmit nociceptive signals.

   D. Narcotics are dangerous and produce addiction.

   E. The stress hormone response is markedly attenuated.

3. Components of the pediatric trauma score include all of the following EXCEPT

   A. decerebrate posture

   B. closed fractures

   C. weight less than 10 kg

   D. tachycardia

   E. hypotension

4. A poor prognosis following a near-drowning is associated with all of the following EXCEPT

   A. initial Glasgow Coma Scale score of less than 5

   B. no brainstem activity at 24 hours

   C. no purposeful movement at 24 hours

   D. submersion greater than 10 minutes

   E. age

5. A 10-year-old has a Glasgow Coma Scale score of 4 and develops irregular respirations after head trauma. The next important step in the care of this patient is to

   A. perform endotracheal intubation

   B. administer 20 mL/kg of lactated Ringer solution

   C. administer naloxone

   D. administer mannitol

   E. obtain a head CT scan

6. The patient described in Question 5 is successfully intubated but then reveals a blood pressure of 150/100 and a pulse of 50. The next step should be to

   A. induce hyperventilation

   B. administer dexamethasone

   C. obtain a head CT scan

   D. administer furosemide

   E. increase the PEEP

7. After hyperventilation, the vital signs of the patient described in Question 5 normalize. The next step is to perform

A. lumbar puncture

B. head CT scan

C. skeletal survey

D. coagulation profile

E. type and crossmatch

8. A 10-year-old trauma victim with eye opening in response to pain, inappropriate words in response to verbal stimuli, and extension in response to pain has a Glasgow Coma Scale score of

A. 3

B. 7

C. 5

D. 12

E. 15

9. *Matching:* Cold injuries

1. Persistent sweating, pain hypersensitivity
2. Stinging, aching skin
3. Erythematous, vesicular, ulcerative lesions
4. Clumsiness, confusion
5. Purple, papular-nodular lesions

A. Frostbite

B. Chilblain

C. Hypothermia

D. Panniculitis

E. Trench foot

10. Which of the following augurs the poorest prognosis for the acute (adult) respiratory distress syndrome?

A. Whiteout on chest radiograph

B. PEEP >6 cm H_2O and FIO_2 >0.5

C. Hypercarbia >60 mm Hg

D. Multisystem organ dysfunction

E. Systemic inflammatory response syndrome

11. Bradycardia during anesthesia is most likely due to

A. undiagnosed rheumatic fever

B. maternal lupus erythematosus

C. atropine overdose

D. hypoxia

E. increased intraocular pressure

12. *Matching:* Anesthetic risks

1. Asthma
2. Sleep apnea

A. Chest crisis

B. Pneumothorax

3. Sickle cell anemia
4. Malignancy
5. Diabetes mellitus
6. Ventricular septal defect
7. Hepatic disease

C. Postoperative airway obstruction

D. Endocarditis

E. Oxygen-exacerbated drug toxicity

F. Reduced drug metabolism

G. Silent hypoglycemia

13. Epinephrine is useful in cardiopulmonary arrest for all of the following EXCEPT

A. bradycardia

B. asystole

C. apnea

D. hypotension

E. anaphylaxis

14. A respiratory disorder characterized by decreased tidal volume and tachypnea is most likely due to

A. abnormal neuromuscular control

B. obstructive disease

C. hypoxia

D. restrictive disease

E. hypercarbia

15. The leading cause of death among children between 4 and 15 years of age is

A. malignancy

B. AIDS

C. motor vehicle accidents

D. burns

E. drowning

16. *Matching:*

1. High suicide rate
2. Air bags
3. Seat belts
4. Covered pick-up truck
5. Bicycle helmets

A. Passive injury prevention

B. Carbon monoxide poisoning

C. Active injury prevention

D. Native Americans

E. ANSI testing

17. Which of the following statements about firearm injuries is FALSE?

A. Nonintentional injury usually occurs at school.

B. Firearm use has caused an increase in fatal suicides.

C. Firearms make homicide the leading cause of death in black adolescent males.

D. Home ownership of a handgun is more dangerous to the family than to an intruder.

E. A significant number of students bring guns to school.

18. Which of the following statements about cardiopulmonary resuscitation is FALSE?

    A. Most episodes start as respiratory arrests.

    B. Half of children who suffer arrest are infants.

    C. The carotid pulse is checked in neonates.

    D. The Heimlich maneuver is effective in a conscious patient with complete airway obstruction due to a foreign body.

    E. A rate of five compressions to one ventilation is appropriate for one- or two-person resuscitation.

19. A 10-year-old boy sustained significant trauma and hemorrhage in a motor vehicle accident. After 15 minutes of resuscitation, you are unable to find a peripheral vein for cannulation. You should now

    A. place a Swan-Ganz catheter

    B. perform a femoral cutdown

    C. administer fluid by nasogastric tube

    D. place an intraosseous line

    E. give intratracheal medications

20. A 10-year-old patient falls to the ground from a third-story balcony. He is unconscious, tachypneic, and cyanotic. He has abrasions over the chest wall and decreased breath sounds and resonance over the left side of his chest. The point of maximal cardiac impulse is palpated at the left sternal border. The most likely diagnosis is

    A. hemothorax

    B. ruptured diaphragm

    C. chylothorax

    D. tension pneumothorax

    E. esophageal rupture

21. All of the following are common sites of childhood drowning EXCEPT

A. buckets

B. bathtubs

C. camp pools

D. home pools

E. lakes

22. A 3-year-old presents with coma after a near-drowning episode. The blood glucose level is 250 mg/dL. The most appropriate management of the hyperglycemia is to administer

    A. normal saline

    B. insulin

    C. 2½% dextrose in water

    D. 5% dextrose in water

    E. oral sulfonylurea agents

23. All of the following are observation items on the acute illness observational scale EXCEPT

    A. sobbing

    B. crying in response to parents' playing

    C. cyanosis

    D. a bulging fontanel

    E. doughy skin

    F. an anxious facial look

24. *Matching:*

    1. Pulmonary aspiration
    2. Inactivates surfactant
    3. Washes out surfactant
    4. Ventilation-perfusion mismatch
    5. Tracheitis
    6. Hypothermia
    7. Hemolysis

    A. Seawater drowning
    B. Freshwater drowning
    C. Both
    D. Neither

25. Which of the following statements about home ownership of firearms is true?

    A. It has not been shown to appreciably increase the risk of suicide in teens.

    B. It does not increase the risk of homicide.

    C. It poses a risk to adolescents even if guns are kept unloaded and locked.

    D. It has been shown to be safe if children are properly educated about gun safety.

    E. It is inappropriate to bring up in a discussion at well child visits.

26. The most common burn injury resulting in hospitalization in young children is due to

A. house fires

B. clothing ignition

C. hot food or drinks

D. hot tap water

E. fireworks

27. All of the following are effective in decreasing the high rate of motor vehicle injuries among teenage drivers EXCEPT

    A. nighttime curfews

    B. driver education programs

    C. raising the legal age for purchase of alcohol

    D. air bags

    E. driving a large car

28. The most effective methods of injury control focus on

    A. modification of the product or environment to make it less hazardous

    B. identification and special precautions for accident-prone children

    C. education of parents about injury risks and ways to prevent them

    D. decreasing the cost of devices such as car seats and bike helmets

    E. legislation increasing the penalties for drunk driving

29. Which of the following statements about the incidence of injuries is FALSE?

    A. Pedestrian injuries have the highest incidence in the 5- to 9-year-old age group.

    B. Approximately 20% to 25% of children are treated for an injury each year.

    C. Suicide rates among teens have decreased in recent years, thanks to crisis hotlines.

    D. Homicide is now the leading cause of death among African-American teenage males.

    E. The incidence of drowning is highest in the toddler age group.

30. Peripheral perfusion (warm versus cool extremities) is a poor indicator of the severity of shock in which of the following?

    A. Anaphylaxis

    B. Shock due to blood loss secondary to trauma

C. Cold septic shock

D. Shock secondary to vomiting and diarrhea

E. None of the above

31. A child presents with hypotension and poor peripheral perfusion due to severe hypovolemic shock. You have sent off samples for an arterial blood gas determination, a complete blood count, and electrolyte evaluation. While you await the results, which of the following would be part of the therapy?

    A. Volume resuscitation with half normal saline, then change to normal saline if the sodium level is normal or low

    B. Oxygen administration

    C. Epinephrine infusion at 0.2 μg/kg/min

    D. Isoproterenol infusion at 0.2 μg/kg/min

    E. None of the above

32. Physiologic parameters present in cold septic shock include

    A. increased cardiac index (CI) and increased systemic vascular resistance (SVR)

    B. increased CI and increased CVP

    C. increased CI and decreased CVP

    D. decreased CI and decreased SVR

    E. decreased CI and increased SVR

33. In anaphylactic shock, all of the following therapeutic approaches are appropriate EXCEPT

    A. volume resuscitation

    B. epinephrine infusion

    C. isoproterenol infusion

    D. diphenhydramine administration

    E. oxygen administration

34. All of the following are indications for hospitalization for burn injury EXCEPT

    A. burn covering greater than 15% of body surface area

    B. electric burn of the corner of the mouth (chewing through cord)

    C. inadequate home situation

    D. high-tension electric burn

35. Adequate fluid resuscitation in a burn patient is best monitored by which of the following?

A. Serial hematocrit determinations during the first 24 hours

B. Direct (Swan-Ganz catheter) measurement of cardiac filling pressure

C. Serial measurements of serum albumin levels

D. Hourly urine volume determination

E. Serial serum sodium levels

36. Which of the following burn patterns is suggestive of child abuse?

A. Scald burn on side of face, neck, and shoulder

B. Burn on palm of hand

C. Glove distribution burns on both hands and wrists

D. Burn on calf and thigh of one leg

37. Parent should be instructed to call 911 if (may select more than one)

A. their child is blue

B. they don't have transportation to get to an ER

C. their child is vomiting

D. their child is lethargic after a fall

E. their child has a temperature of 105°F

38. The best time to transfer critically injured pediatric patients to a regional referral center is

A. as quickly as possible

B. when they develop complications of therapy

C. immediately after stabilization

D. when they need rehabilitation

39. You are called to the emergency department to evaluate a child with fever, purpura, and a heart rate of 180. Your first priority in the resuscitation is to

A. determine blood pressure

B. establish an IV line

C. administer ceftriaxone

D. supply supplemental oxygen

E. perform endotracheal intubation

40. Indications for immobilization of the cervical spine in a pediatric trauma patient include all of the following EXCEPT

A. head injury

B. first rib fracture

C. neck pain

D. multiple system injury

E. midface fractures

F. fall from 15 feet

G. bathtub drowning

41. A 10-year-old child with a history of asthma presents to your office sleepy, with a respiratory rate of 40, marked intercostal retractions, and few wheezes. Of the following, which is the best mode of transport to the local emergency department, which is 10 minutes away?

A. BLS ambulance

B. ALS ambulance

C. The mother's car

D. Your car

E. Aeromedical helicopter transport

42. Despite three attempts, the resuscitation team has been unable to secure an intravenous line in a 1-year-old near-drowning victim. Which of the following statements about intraosseous infusion is FALSE?

A. Resuscitation medications may be administered through an intraosseous line.

B. Intraosseous infusion may be attempted in the flat, medial surface of the proximal tibia below the tibial tubercle.

C. Intraosseous infusion is contraindicated in a fractured bone.

D. During intraosseous needle insertion, the needle penetrates the entire bone and punctures the opposite cortex. The needle is removed. A second attempt may be performed on the same bone proximal to the site of the first attempt.

E. Intraosseous infusion is considered a more effective method of medication delivery than endotracheal administration.

43. A 2-month-old infant is brought to the emergency department in full cardiopulmonary arrest. The paramedics have successfully intubated the child and administered the first dose of epinephrine into an intraosseous infusion catheter. It is now 4 minutes since the epinephrine dose. The second dose should be

A. 0.01 mg/kg (0.1 mL/kg) of 1:10,000 epinephrine intratracheally

B. 0.1 mg/kg (0.1 mL/kg) of 1:1000 epinephrine intratracheally

C. 0.01 mg/kg (0.1 mL/kg) of 1:10,000 epinephrine intraosseously

D. 0.1 mg/kg (0.1 mL/kg) of 1:1000 epinephrine intraosseously

E. none of the above

44. A child with a seizure disorder is having recurrent seizures. She is currently arousable and is spontaneously breathing but has gurgling upper airway sounds. Appropriate measures would include all of the following EXCEPT

A. insertion of an oropharyngeal airway

B. providing oxygen with a facemask

C. positioning of the airway with the chin-lift maneuver

D. suctioning of the oropharynx

E. monitoring of oxygen saturation

45. Which of the following statements about basic life support measures is FALSE?

A. Chest compressions are performed a fingerbreadth below the intermamillary line in infants.

B. The ratio of compressions to ventilations during CPR is five to one for infants and children.

C. The chin lift is the desired method for opening the airway in traumatized children.

D. Effective chest compressions should result in a palpable central pulse.

E. Efficacy of ventilation is determined by watching for adequate chest rise.

46. Repeating portions of the clinical examination after a febrile child is made more comfortable by antipyresis and by feeding is an example of which phenomenon?

A. The Hawthorne effect

B. Clinical probability, a priori

C. Paradoxic irritability

D. Regression to the mean

E. Clinical probability, a posteriori

47. Most observational data that a pediatrician gathers during an acute illness should focus on assessing a child's

A. color

B. hydration

C. respiratory effort

D. response to stimuli

E. muscle tone

48. Which of the following is the most common serious illness documented in febrile children in the first 36 months of life?

A. Pneumonia

B. Meningitis

C. Cellulitis

D. Bacterial diarrhea

E. Arthritis (bacterial)

49. In the first 2 months of life, a febrile, previously full-term infant is more likely than an older febrile child to have

A. Sepsis caused by *Streptococcus pyogenes*

B. Pharyngitis caused by group A streptococci

C. Meningitis caused by *Neisseria meningitidis*

D. Urinary tract infection caused by *Staphylococcus epidermidis*

E. Sepsis caused by group B streptococci

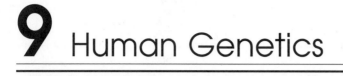

9 Human Genetics

The past decade, even the past year, has seen a massive expansion in our understanding of human genetics. Indeed, now identified are inheritance patterns such as mitochondrial inheritance or parental disomy, which were undiscovered only 10 to 20 years ago. Furthermore, our ability to locate genes on human chromosomes and then isolate the actual gene and identify the gene's product has greatly enhanced our knowledge of diseases and is leading to the development of specific and novel forms of therapy.

Questions in this *part* are directed at clinical physicians and not at molecular biologists. Nonetheless, a basic understanding of this wonderful new science is essential for all pediatricians. Because genetic disturbances of all kinds are quite common in children and influence development, growth, and susceptibility to diseases such as cancer, readers should pay particular attention to this growing area of pediatrics.

1. A mentally retarded 15-year-old boy is found to have macro-orchidism and large, prominent ears. He most likely has

   A. cerebral giantism

   B. acromegaly

   C. hypothyroidism

   D. trisomy 21

   E. fragile X syndrome

2. Patients with Turner syndrome should have a careful analysis of their chromosomes for Y chromosome material because they may

   A. become masculinized

   B. grow tall

   C. become pregnant

   D. develop gonadoblastoma

   E. none of the above

3. The partial karyotype in the top row of Figure 9–1 is that of the mother. If she mates with a

genotypically normal male, what is her risk for having a child with trisomy 21?

   A. 10%

   B. 20%

   C. 30%

   D. 50%

   E. 100%

4. **Matching:** Trisomies

1. Cleft lip	A.	Trisomy 13
2. Rocker-bottom feet	B.	Trisomy 18
3. Hypoplastic ribs	C.	Trisomy 21
4. Risk of abortion	D.	All of the above
5. Brushfield spots	E.	None of the above
6. Meiotic nondysjunction		
7. Duodenal atresia		
8. Normal intelligence		
9. Epicanthal folds		
10. Hypotonia		

5. In patients with Prader-Willi syndrome without an obvious chromosomal deletion, the most likely explanation is

   A. uniparental disomy

   B. anticipation

   C. CCG repeat expansion

   D. mitochondrial inheritance

   E. pleiotropism

6. Kearns-Sayre syndrome and Leber hereditary

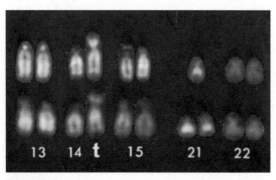

Figure 9–1

optic neuropathy are noted in both males and females but are inherited only through the mother. These are examples of

A. uniparental disomy

B. mitochondrial inheritance

C. anticipation

D. X-linked recessive inheritance

E. X-linked dominant inheritance

7. *Matching:* Chromosomes-genes

1. Chromosome 7
2. X chromosome
3. Chromosome 11
4. Chromosome 13
5. Chromosome 15

A. Duchenne muscular dystrophy

B. Cystic fibrosis

C. α-Thalassemia

D. Sickle cell anemia

E. Retinoblastoma

8. *Matching:* Genetics

1. Expanded CGG trinucleotide repeat
2. Nonsense mutation
3. Successive increase in trinucleotide repeat expansion in each generation
4. Translocation
5. Expanded CAG trinucleotide repeat

A. Huntington disease

B. Fragile X syndrome

C. Duchenne muscular dystrophy

D. Anticipation

E. Chronic myelogenous leukemia

9. Approximately what percent of newborn infants have a hereditary malformation?

A. 0.1% to 0.3%

B. 0.5% to 0.8%

C. 1% to 2%

D. 3% to 5%

10. Which of the following most accurately defines an allele?

A. Two genes at homologous loci on their respective chromosomes

B. A specific gene at a specific point on a single chromosome

C. A gene having a specific effect on a heterozygous individual

D. A gene having no effect on a heterozygous individual

11. *Matching:* For each of the following diseases, select the appropriate pattern of inheritance.

1. Achondroplasia
2. Sickle cell disease
3. Phenylketonuria
4. Bruton hypogammaglobulinemia
5. Color blindness
6. Polycystic kidney (adult type)
7. Vitamin D–resistant rickets
8. Tuberous sclerosis
9. Hurler syndrome
10. Hemophilia A (factor VIII deficiency)
11. Hemophilia B (factor IX deficiency)
12. Duchenne muscular dystrophy

A. Autosomal recessive

B. Autosomal dominant

C. X-linked recessive

D. X-linked dominant

10 Metabolic Diseases

Welcome back to biochemistry, metabolic pathways, unusual odors in urine samples, and now the potential for cure, successful management, or palliation of what is traditionally called inborn errors of metabolism. This *part* of the *Nelson Textbook* includes chapters on defects in the metabolism of amino acids, carbohydrates, lipids, mucopolysaccharides, purines, pyrimidines, and porphyrins. It also includes excellent chapters on hypoglycemia and on the approach to inborn errors of metabolism. Individually, each inborn error of metabolism is relatively rare, but together all of these disorders at one time or another can keep a house officer busy and up all night when an affected patient becomes ill or presents in a metabolic crisis.

Questions in this *part* may jog your biochemistry memory but are more likely to help reinforce important aspects about the recognition and management of inborn errors of metabolism.

1. **Matching:** For each inborn error of amino acid metabolism, select the correct urine odor.

   1. Glutaric acidemia (type II)
   2. Phenylketonuria
   3. Methionine malabsorption
   4. Trimethylaminuria
   5. Oasthouse disease
   6. Hawkinsinuria

   A. Cabbage
   B. Hoplike
   C. Sweaty feet
   D. Rotting fish
   E. Mousy
   F. Swimming pool
   G. Maple syrup

2. Hepatomegaly and liver disease are presenting factors of all of the following EXCEPT

   A. glycogen storage disease
   B. Wilson disease
   C. propionic acidemia
   D. tyrosinemia
   E. galactosemia

3. Self-destructive behavior is a component of

   A. xanthinuria
   B. Lesch-Nyhan syndrome
   C. orotic aciduria
   D. adenosine deaminase deficiency

4. A 9-day-old full-term infant is admitted to the hospital with lethargy, fever, and increasing jaundice. Physical examination also reveals hepatomegaly. Laboratory results reveal a blood glucose value of 10 mg/dL, total and direct bilirubin values of 15 and 7 mg/dL, respectively, and liver enzyme test results of AST = 700 and ALT = 650. The next day, the blood culture is positive for a gram-negative rod. The most likely diagnosis is

   A. necrotizing enterocolitis
   B. galactosemia
   C. neonatal hepatitis
   D. glycogen storage disease
   E. biliary atresia

5. A previously healthy 6-month-old presents with hepatomegaly, lethargy, increasing jaundice, and severe emesis. The child appears dehydrated; the urine also has a positive reaction for reducing substances. The child's diet had been solely breast milk until 5 months of age, when fruit juices and baby food were added to the diet. The most likely diagnosis is

   A. galactosemia
   B. glycogen storage disease
   C. benign fructosuria
   D. hereditary fructose intolerance
   E. pyruvate carboxylase deficiency

6. A 2-month-old presents with failure to thrive, emesis, alopecia, skin rash, and a chronic metabolic acidosis. An older sibling died at 3 months of age with hypotonia and chronic lactic acidosis. One important diagnostic study should be determination of

   A. blood galactose level
   B. serum lactate dehydrogenase level
   C. serum biotinidase level
   D. plasma triglyceride levels
   E. serum calcium and magnesium levels

7. ***Matching:*** Glycogen storage diseases—glycogenoses

1. Glycogen storage disease Ia	A. Doll face
2. Glycogen storage disease Ib	B. Marked CNS symptoms
3. Glycogen storage disease IIa	C. Vitamin D–resistant rickets
4. Glycogen storage disease V	D. Neutropenia
5. Glycogen storage disease VIII	E. Hypotonia, cardiomegaly, macroglossia
6. Glycogen storage disease VI	F. Postexercise muscle cramps

8. A previously healthy 4-month-old now manifests increasing hypotonia and poor feeding. Physical examination reveals macroglossia, a gallop rhythm and tachycardia, marked flaccidity, but normal mental status. Laboratory studies reveal a blood glucose level of 85 mg/dL and sinus tachycardia with a shortened PR interval on an electrocardiogram. The most helpful diagnostic study would be

A. MRI of the spine

B. glucagon infusion test

C. skin biopsy

D. muscle biopsy

E. lumbar puncture

9. A 2-year-old girl with severe developmental delay has height and weight at the 25th percentile and head circumference greater than 95%. She cannot support her head. She is hypotonic and cannot sit or stand, although she smiles and interacts. Eye examination shows some degree of optic atrophy. No organomegaly is found. MRI of the brain shows diffuse white matter disease. Urine organic acid analysis reveals elevated *N*-acetylaspartic acid (NAA) values. The diagnosis is

A. metachromatic leukodystrophy (MLD)

B. glutaric acidemia I

C. Tay-Sachs disease

D. Canavan disease

E. Hurler disease

10. A 3-year-old boy is referred because of developmental delay. Physical examination reveals some coarseness of the facial features, clear corneas, and hepatosplenomegaly. This child has an umbilical hernia 3×3 cm. Muscle tone and reflexes are normal, but the joint movement seems limited. Family history reveals two maternal uncles who died early in life with an unknown diagnosis, but they resembled the patient. The report of the skeletal survey indicates dysostosis multiplex. The most likely diagnosis is

A. Hunter disease

B. Sanfilippo A

C. Farber disease

D. Fabry disease

E. Maroteaux-Lamy disease

11. ***Matching:*** Match the disease with its enzyme.

1. Alpha-galactosidase	A. Hurler
2. Iduronidase	B. Gaucher
3. Sphingomyelinase	C. Tay-Sachs
4. β-Hexosaminidase A	D. Niemann-Pick A
5. β-Glucosidase	E. Fabry

12. A 1-year-old patient who is developmentally delayed presents with chronic rhinitis, noisy breathing, corneal clouding, hepatomegaly, and gibbus. The most likely diagnosis is

A. Gaucher disease

B. Tay-Sachs disease

C. Krabbe disease

D. Morquio disease

E. Hurler disease

13. A 15-year-old Ashkenazi Jewish girl is seen because of chronic fatigue. On examination, she seems pale and thin and has a somewhat large abdomen. Her spleen is felt in the iliac fossa. She is mentally alert and has a history of normal development and normal school performance. Her blood count shows hemoglobin of 9.0 g/dL and a white blood cell count of 3000 with normal differential and no abnormal cells. Platelet count is 60,000. The likely diagnosis is

A. Tay-Sachs disease

B. Niemann-Pick A disease

C. Gaucher type I disease

D. Mucolipidosis IV

E. Canavan disease

14. A patient with Gaucher type I disease is referred to you for treatment. What is considered the treatment of choice?

    A. Blood transfusion

    B. Enzyme therapy with glucocerebrosidase

    C. Steroid therapy

    D. Splenectomy

    E. Bone marrow transplant

15. Patients with medium-chain acyl-CoA dehydrogenase deficiency, the most common inherited disorder of fatty acid oxidation, usually do not become symptomatic in the first 3 to 6 months of life. The most likely explanation for this observation is that

    A. carnitine is present in breast milk

    B. nighttime feedings are usually given until this age

    C. the percentage of fat in the diet is low in newborns

    D. sucrose replaces lactose as the major dietary sugar

    E. infants become more active physically after they can roll over

16. A 13-month-old infant is found comatose in bed after sleeping later than usual. On physical examination, the infant is afebrile and of normal size, and the liver is palpated 4 cm below the costal margin. The plasma glucose level is 15 mg/dL, the bicarbonate level is 20 mEq/L, BUN is 35 mg/dL, ammonia is 295 μmol/L, AST is 320 U/L, ALT is 425 U/L, and bilirubin is normal. Urinalysis is negative for glucose, ketones, protein, and reducing substances. Which of the following is the most likely diagnosis?

    A. Medium-chain acyl-CoA dehydrogenase deficiency

    B. Glucose-6-phosphatase deficiency (type I glycogenosis)

    C. Congenital hyperinsulinism

    D. Growth hormone deficiency

    E. Isovaleric acidemia

17. In which of the following porphyrias would results of a *urine* porphyrin screen appear normal?

    A. Porphyria cutanea tarda

    B. Erythropoietic protoporphyria

    C. Acute intermittent porphyria

    D. Variegate porphyria

    E. Congenital erythropoietic porphyria

18. Which porphyria is characteristically associated with immediate onset of burning and stinging of the skin with sun exposure?

    A. Porphyria cutanea tarda

    B. Erythropoietic protoporphyria

    C. Acute intermittent porphyria

    D. Variegate porphyria

    E. Congenital erythropoietic porphyria

19. Which of the following porphyrias is inherited in an exclusively autosomal recessive fashion?

    A. Porphyria cutanea tarda

    B. Erythropoietic protoporphyria

    C. Acute intermittent porphyria

    D. Variegate porphyria

    E. Congenital erythropoietic porphyria

20. Which of the following porphyrias is NOT associated with cutaneous manifestations?

    A. Porphyria cutanea tarda

    B. Erythropoietic protoporphyria

    C. Acute intermittent porphyria

    D. Variegate porphyria

    E. Congenital erythropoietic porphyria

21. A child with the biochemical defect of adrenoleukodystrophy (ALD) has an HLA-identical unaffected sibling. His plasma C26:0 level has been normalized by dietary therapy. Under what circumstances is bone marrow transplantation recommended most strongly?

    A. Results of neurologic and neuropsychologic examination and brain MRI are normal.

    B. Results of neurologic and neuropsychologic examination are normal, but brain MRI shows abnormalities consistent with ALD.

    C. Neurologic and/or neuropsychologic examination shows early changes, and brain MRI shows abnormalities consistent with ALD.

    D. Results of neurologic examination are normal, IQ is less than 75, and brain MRI shows abnormalities consistent with ALD.

    E. There are significant motor and visual

abnormalities, and brain MRI shows changes consistent with ALD.

22. In which of the following disorders is peroxisome structure intact?

    A. Zellweger syndrome

    B. Neonatal adrenoleukodystrophy

    C. X-linked leukodystrophy

    D. Infantile Refsum disease

    E. Hyperpipecolic acidemia

23. Peroxisomal disorders in the neonatal period are most commonly manifested by

    A. hypotonia and seizures

    B. adrenal insufficiency

    C. renal cysts

    D. multiple congenital malformations

    E. enlarged liver

24. The diagnosis of adrenomyeloneuropathy is established in a 50-year-old man who previously had been misdiagnosed as having multiple sclerosis. Which of the following is FALSE?

    A. All of his daughters are carriers of ALD.

    B. If other members of his family also have ALD, they will probably also have the milder adult form of the disease rather than the severe childhood cerebral form.

    C. His sons cannot inherit the illness from him.

    D. His daughters' children have a 50% risk of carrying the ALD gene.

    E. His adrenal function may be normal.

25. The most reliable test for the diagnosis of males with X-linked adrenoleukodystrophy is

    A. brain MRI

    B. plasma ACTH level

    C. plasma assay of very long-chain fatty acids

    D. electroencephalogram

    E. brain biopsy

26. Plasma very long-chain fatty acids are elevated in all of the following peroxisomal disorders EXCEPT

    A. Zellweger syndrome

    B. rhizomelic chondrodysplasia punctata

    C. pseudo-Zellweger syndrome

    D. neonatal adrenoleukodystrophy

    E. infantile Refsum disease

27. The most common first manifestation of X-linked childhood cerebral adrenoleukodystrophy is

    A. paresis or incoordination

    B. nausea or vomiting

    C. deteriorating school performance

    D. seizure

    E. hyponatremia

28. The step I or the Prudent diet contains

    A. 30% of total calories as fat and less than 10% of calories as saturated fat

    B. 27% of total calories as fat and 7% of calories as saturated fat

    C. less than 10% of total calories as saturated fat and no total fat restriction

    D. less than 300 mg of cholesterol per day, less than 10% of total calories as saturated fat, and no total fat restriction

    E. 25% of total calories as fat

29. The 35-year-old father of a 9-month-old girl has a massive myocardial infarction. The parents place the child on skim milk and seek to limit the child's fat intake significantly. As their pediatrician, you advise them that

    A. because heart disease has its roots in childhood, it is important to start dietary intervention as soon as possible

    B. placing the child on a low-fat diet at this age will encourage compliance when the child grows older because she will have no taste preference for fat

    C. low-fat diets are not recommended for children younger than 2 years because of their rapid growth and the rapid development of their central nervous system

    D. such early heart disease is most likely genetic; therefore, dietary change will not be effective

    E. cow's milk is not recommended for children older than 12 months

30. Lipoprotein lipase deficiency is a rare autosomal recessive condition that is associated with massively elevated plasma triglyceride levels from soon after birth. This

condition can be life threatening because of the development of

A. biliary cirrhosis

B. renal failure secondary to renal tubular dysfunction

C. recurrent episodes of pancreatitis

D. cerebral edema

E. pulmonary fibrosis

31. Which of the following dominantly inherited hyperlipidemias associated with premature coronary heart disease is expressed most commonly in children?

A. Familial hypercholesterolemia

B. Familial defective apoB-100

C. Familial combined hyperlipidemia

D. Familial dysbetalipoproteinemia

E. Familial hypertriglyceridemia

32. Of the following physical findings found in some patients with hyperlipidemia, which one is most likely to be found in a 17-year-old boy with heterozygous familial hypercholesterolemia?

A. Arcus corneae

B. Xanthelasma

C. Cutaneous xanthomas over the buttocks

D. Tuberous xanthomas causing Achilles tendinitis

E. Tuberous xanthomas over the elbow

33. A 7-year-old boy with a family history of premature coronary heart disease has a total cholesterol determination in your office on fingerstick blood. The result is 195 mg/dL. You order a lipid profile on fasting venous blood from the local hospital laboratory. The results are

$$\text{Total cholesterol (TC)} = 188 \text{ mg/dL}$$
$$\text{HDL cholesterol (HDL-C)} = 62 \text{ mg/dL}$$
$$\text{Triglyceride (TG)} = 50 \text{ mg/dL}$$

The laboratory uses the following formula to calculate the LDL cholesterol (LDL-C):

$$\text{LDL-C} = \text{TC} - \left[(\text{HDL-C}) + \frac{\text{TG}}{5} \right]$$

You determine that this boy has

A. low HDL-C levels

B. moderately elevated LDL-C levels

C. elevated triglyceride levels

D. significantly elevated LDL-C levels

E. normal plasma lipid levels

11 The Fetus and Neonatal Infant

The good news is that the infant mortality rate is falling. The bad news is that the low-birth-weight rate has not declined in more than a decade. This means that past readers of this *part* of the *Nelson Textbook* have learned their lessons well and have mastered the technology, physiology, science, and art of neonatal intensive care. We are increasingly called on to care for less mature infants; many of these immature neonates develop the diseases or complications discussed in the chapters in this *part* of the *Nelson Textbook*. Other neonatal problems are discussed in the organ system–specific *parts* of the *Nelson Textbook* or in the infectious disease *part*.

You do not need to be a neonatologist to correctly identify the answers to these questions. The questions are directed at what a general pediatrician needs to know about high-risk neonates, their stabilization, initial management, and prognosis.

1. *Matching:* Malformations

   1. Deletion of elastin allele
   2. Microdeletion 16p13.3
   3. Deletion of band q11-12 chromosome 15
   4. Endocardial Cushing defects
   5. Mandibular hypoplasia
   6. Tracheoesophageal fistula
   7. Anal atresia
   8. Radial hypoplasia

   A. Rubinstein-Taybi syndrome
   B. Trisomy 21
   C. Williams syndrome
   D. Pierre Robin syndrome
   E. Prader-Willi syndrome
   F. VATER syndrome
   G. None of the above

2. *Matching:* Dysmorphology

   1. Error in morphogenesis
   2. Digital amputation
   3. Porencephaly
   4. Multifactorial recurrence risk of 2% to 5%
   5. Congenital hip dislocation
   6. Talipes foot disorder

   A. Malformation
   B. Deformation
   C. Disruption

3. An infant has the following findings at 5 minutes of life: pulse 130 per minute, cyanotic hands and feet, good muscle tone, and a strong cry and grimace. This infant's Apgar score is

   A. 7
   B. 8
   C. 9
   D. 10

4. The Apt test takes advantage of the biochemical fact that

   A. adult hemoglobin is alkali resistant
   B. fetal hemoglobin is alkali resistant
   C. sickle hemoglobin is alkali resistant
   D. Rh-sensitized cells are alkali resistant

5. A newborn is noted to have a right parietal cephalohematoma. Which suture lines does the swelling obliterate?

   A. Sagittal
   B. Parietal
   C. Occipital
   D. Coronal
   E. None of the above

6. Newborns (term or premature) should be given all of the following prophylactic measures EXCEPT

   A. daily hexachlorophene baths
   B. triple dye on the cord
   C. silver nitrate in the eyes
   D. vitamin K intramuscularly

35

7. An infant in the delivery room is noted to have respiratory movements, but no air is entering the lungs with the mouth closed. The most likely diagnosis is

 A. narcosis

 B. choanal atresia

 C. diaphragmatic hernia

 D. pulmonary hypoplasia

 E. congenital heart disease

8. Which of the following statements is true regarding extracorporeal membrane oxygenation (ECMO)?

 A. It is available routinely for infants with severe hyaline membrane disease.

 B. Infants weighing less than 2.0 kg can be safely treated.

 C. If treated, 85% to 90% of infants with persistent fetal circulation survive.

 D. Ventilator therapy must be continued at approximately the same rate, pressure, and oxygenation.

9. Jaundice is most likely to be physiologic in a term infant in which one of the following situations?

 A. Jaundice at 12 hours of age

 B. Serum bilirubin level increasing less than 5 mg/dL/24 hours in the first 2 to 4 days

 C. Direct (conjugated) serum bilirubin greater than 1 mg/dL

 D. Jaundice at 12 days of age

10. Which of the following is most appropriate for treating hyperbilirubinemia (11.2 mg/dL) in a 3-week-old, breast-fed infant with normal growth and development?

 A. Phototherapy

 B. Exchange transfusion

 C. Phenobarbital

 D. None of the above

11. A 2-week-old infant is brought to the emergency room in coma with retinal hemorrhages and severe pallor. He was born at home and was first seen by a physician at 10 days of age and placed on amoxicillin for otitis media. His diet is breast milk. The day before admission, his parents took him in a 4-wheel-drive vehicle over a rough road in the mountains. Seizures began 8 hours later, and

he steadily deteriorated for the next 16 hours. He oozes blood from all venipuncture sites. Diagnostic tests should include all of the following EXCEPT

 A. coagulation studies

 B. skeletal survey

 C. CT scan

 D. complete blood count

 E. lumbar puncture

12. Immediate therapy for the infant described in Question 11 should include administration of vitamin

 A. A

 B. B_6 (pyridoxine)

 C. C

 D. E

 E. K

13. The diagnosis for the child described in Question 11 is most likely

 A. pyridoxine deficiency

 B. severe scurvy

 C. hemorrhagic disease of the newborn

 D. child abuse

 E. hypervitaminosis A

14. The death of the infant described in Question 11 could have been prevented by which one of the following measures?

 A. AquaMEPHYTON (vitamin K) at birth

 B. Home-visitor services

 C. Discontinuance of antibiotics

 D. Proper use of an infant seat

15. The second infant of a twin gestation in a primiparous mother weighed 1500 g at 36 weeks' gestation. Both twins were breast-fed and maintained in a neutral thermal environment. On the third day of life, the infant was noted to be hypotonic and to respond poorly to stimuli. The most likely diagnosis is

 A. polycythemia

 B. twin-twin transfusion syndrome

 C. kernicterus

 D. hypoglycemia

 E. renal vein thrombosis

16. You are called to the delivery of a boy at 42 weeks' gestational age with thick meconium stained fluid and type II decelerations. The obstetrician rapidly delivers the infant and hands him to you for care. The boy is hypotonic, cyanotic, apneic, and bradycardic. The most appropriate next step is to

    A. stimulate the infant to breathe

    B. administer epinephrine

    C. provide positive-pressure bag-and-mask ventilation

    D. intubate the trachea and provide positive-pressure ventilation

    E. intubate the trachea and apply negative-pressure suction

17. A 900-g infant of 27 weeks' gestational age developed respiratory distress syndrome and required endotracheal intubation on the first day of life. At 36 hours of age, the infant developed hypotension, bradycardia, cyanosis, and a tense anterior fontanel. The most appropriate diagnostic test is

    A. electroencephalography

    B. echocardiography

    C. serum coagulation profile

    D. ultrasonography of the head

    E. complete blood count with platelet determination

18. A 1700-g infant is born at 36 weeks' gestation complicated by severe oligohydramnios. The Apgar scores are 3 at 1 minute and 5 at 5 minutes. The infant requires endotracheal tube placement as part of the resuscitation and continued mechanical ventilation to improve the arterial blood gases. At 1 hour of age, the infant shows acute deterioration with cyanosis, bradycardia, and hypotension. The most likely diagnosis for this acute change is

    A. patent ductus arteriosus

    B. intraventricular hemorrhage

    C. hypoglycemia

    D. pneumothorax

    E. respiratory distress syndrome

19. A 42-week-gestational-age, 3600-g, breast-fed, white female is noted to have persistent hyperbilirubinemia at 2 weeks of age. On physical examination, the infant has not gained weight since birth and has decreased tone, an umbilical hernia, and an anterior fontanel measuring 4×6 cm. The most likely diagnosis is

    A. Crigler-Najjar syndrome

    B. Gilbert disease

    C. biliary atresia

    D. hypothyroidism

    E. galactosemia

20. A 4-week-old, A-positive, African-American, former 40-week-gestational-age infant was born to an O-positive mother and developed hyperbilirubinemia requiring 2 days of phototherapy in the newborn nursery after birth. The infant appears apathetic and demonstrates pallor, a grade 2/6 systolic ejection murmur, and a heart rate of 175. The most likely diagnosis is

    A. anemia of chronic disease

    B. cholestasis secondary to neonatal hepatitis

    C. hereditary spherocytosis

    D. sickle cell anemia hemolytic crisis

    E. ABO incompatibility with continued hemolysis

21. A 3-day-old, 28-week-gestational-age infant was weaning from the respirator during the course of moderate to severe respiratory distress syndrome. Intravenous fluids had been increased to 175 mL/kg/24 hours. Today the infant developed mild hypoxia and hypercarbia necessitating higher ventilator settings to maintain normal blood gas values. On physical examination, the precordium is active, the pulse pressure is wide, and a grade 2/6 systolic ejection murmur is auscultated at the upper left sternal border with no radiation. After 24 hours of fluid restriction and diuretic therapy, the respiratory status has not improved. The most appropriate diagnostic test is

    A. renal ultrasonography

    B. echocardiography

    C. a renal perfusion scan

    D. an electrocardiogram

    E. cardiac catheterization

22. A 1-hour-old, 32-week-gestational-age infant develops progressive cyanosis, grunting, flaring, and retractions. The chest radiograph reveals a ground glass–air bronchogram pattern. The infant now requires endotracheal tube intubation and mechanical ventilation

with 40% oxygen. Antibiotics are administered after drawing blood for culture, but the infant continues to require 40% to 50% oxygen to maintain adequate oxygenation. The most appropriate therapeutic intervention would be to administer

A. oral indomethacin

B. intravenous dexamethasone

C. intramuscular vitamin E

D. endotracheal surfactant

E. intravenous sodium bicarbonate

23. A term infant is born with Apgar scores of 5 at 1 minute and 7 at 5 minutes. The infant has a heart rate of 170 and demonstrates pallor with hepatosplenomegaly. A Kleihauer-Betke test on maternal blood has positive results. The most likely diagnosis is

A. erythroblastosis fetalis

B. hereditary spherocytosis

C. chronic fetal-maternal hemorrhage

D. ABO incompatibility

E. Blackfan-Diamond syndrome

24. A 24-week-gestation fetus of an Rh-negative, antibody-positive (sensitized) mother is noted on fetal ultrasonography to have bilateral pleural effusions, ascites, and scalp edema. The most effective way to evaluate this fetus is to perform

A. amniocentesis

B. percutaneous umbilical blood sampling

C. fetal real-time ultrasonography

D. maternal serum α-fetoprotein determination

E. an oxytocin challenge test

25. A 30-hour-old, 4300-g infant of a gestational diabetic mother has been feeding well but has become jittery during the past 30 minutes. Fifteen minutes later, the infant has a tonic-clonic seizure. The most likely diagnosis is

A. hypoglycemia

B. hypocalcemia

C. hypomagnesemia

D. hyponatremia

E. hyperviscosity

26. A newborn female has a ventricular septal defect, cleft lip and palate, and imperforate anus. All of the following laboratory tests would be appropriate EXCEPT

A. a karyotype analysis

B. TORCH titer

C. renal ultrasonography

D. ultrasonography of the brain

27. A newborn female has a tracheoesophageal fistula. All of the following would be appropriate EXCEPT

A. renal ultrasonography

B. cardiac ultrasonography

C. brainstem auditory evoked response testing

D. evaluation for anal atresia

E. vertebral radiographs

28. A newborn male has a cleft lip on his left side. A careful physical examination reveals that he is otherwise completely normal. Neither of his parents has a cleft lip. The recurrence risk is

A. zero, based on the defect being secondary to a fresh gene mutation

B. 2% to 5%

C. 25%

D. 50%

29. A newborn infant has clinical features of the Down syndrome. Her karyotype reveals a 21/21 translocation. Her mother has had two previous spontaneous abortions. She has no other living children. The most appropriate approach is to

A. quote the family a 1% recurrence risk for the Down syndrome

B. obtain blood from the father for karyotype testing

C. obtain blood from both parents for karyotype testing

D. obtain blood from the mother for karyotype testing

12 Infections in the Neonatal Infant

Infectious diseases in the newborn period are difficult to identify and even more difficult to distinguish from common neonatal disorders such as respiratory distress syndrome. Furthermore, at times it is equally arduous to differentiate bacterial from viral causes of infection. In addition, the spectrum of intrauterine infection has been extended so that TORCH is no longer an all-inclusive term and is being replaced by STORCH or TORCHES.

Nonetheless, the good news is that our ever-growing technologic diagnostic advances, such as polymerase chain reaction, have helped identify difficult-to-diagnose infectious diseases. Finally, our treatment options for the therapy of in utero and postnatal infections have improved.

The goal of the questions in this *part* is to make pediatricians aware of the presentations and treatments of common neonatal pathogens.

1. A 21-day-old infant born at 27 weeks' gestational age is recovering from RDS and a grade IV intraventricular hemorrhage. She now manifests increasing apnea and bradycardia, a tense fontanel, lethargy, and split sutures. A sepsis evaluation reveals a normal complete blood count (CBC), and analysis of the cerebrospinal fluid (CSF) reveals a protein value of 290 mg/dL, glucose level of 10 mg/dL, and 159 leukocytes. The Gram stain is negative for bacteria. The most likely diagnosis is

   A. bacterial meningitis

   B. HSV encephalitis

   C. tuberculous meningitis

   D. posthemorrhagic hydrocephalus

   E. *Citrobacter* brain abscess

2. *Matching:* Congenital infections

   1. Megaesophagus
   2. Patent ductus arteriosus
   3. Cerebral periventricular calcifications
   4. Limb hypoplasia
   5. Myocarditis
   6. Fetal anemia
   7. Hydrocephalus

   A. CMV
   B. Varicella
   C. Enteroviruses
   D. Rubella
   E. Parvovirus
   F. Toxoplasmosis
   G. *Trypanosoma cruzi*

3. Cephalosporins (second or third generation) as single therapy for neonatal sepsis are inappropriate initial therapy because of all of the following EXCEPT

   A. *Listeria* are resistant

   B. enterococci are resistant

   C. *Staphylococcus aureus* is moderately sensitive

   D. *Escherichia coli* may be resistant

   E. they penetrate the CSF poorly

4. Late-onset neonatal sepsis in full-term infants is associated with which of the following?

   A. 75% rate of meningitis

   B. Osteoarticular infections

   C. Group B streptococci

   D. *Escherichia coli*

   E. Onset as late as 60 days of life

   F. All of the above

5. All of the following pathogens are a likely cause of early-onset neonatal sepsis EXCEPT

   A. group B streptococcus

   B. *Listeria monocytogenes*

   C. *Escherichia coli*

   D. *Staphylococcus epidermidis*

   E. *Haemophilus influenzae*

   F. pneumococci

6. A 2700-g 36-week-gestational-age white male is born after 22 hours of premature rupture of the amniotic membranes. The Apgar scores are 3 and 5. He immediately develops respiratory distress and cyanosis requiring endotracheal intubation and mechanical ventilation with 100% oxygen. Vital signs are temperature 35.7°C, heart rate 195, and mean

blood pressure 22 mm Hg. Laboratory tests reveal a white blood cell count of 1500 and 59,000 platelets. The next most appropriate treatment for this child is to administer

A. surfactant by aerosol

B. intravenous ampicillin and gentamicin

C. intravenous immunoglobulin

D. intravenous acyclovir

E. oscillator ventilation

7. The patient described in Question 6 is most likely suffering from

A. respiratory distress syndrome

B. diaphragmatic hernia

C. congenital pneumonia with sepsis

D. pneumothorax

E. TORCH infection

8. All of the following are true about neonatal herpes simplex infections EXCEPT

A. herpes simplex virus type 2 (HSV-2) represents 99% of cases

B. the encephalitic form appears later than the disseminated or local (skin, eye, mouth) form

C. primary maternal genital HSV infection at the time of birth has a neonatal transmission rate of 40% to 45%

D. recurrent maternal genital HSV infection at the time of birth has a neonatal transmission rate of 3%

E. acyclovir is the treatment of choice for all forms of neonatal infection

9. The best method of preventing neonatal HSV infection in a mother who was seronegative at the start of her pregnancy is to

A. examine her genitourinary tract in early labor with intact membranes and if lesions are noted perform a cesarean section

B. treat the mother with a symptomatic primary HSV infection with acyclovir

C. monitor serial IgG titers to HSV-2

D. treat all infants born to mothers with genital lesions with acyclovir after birth

E. do none of the above

10. The blueberry muffin appearance in infants with TORCH infections most likely represents

A. palpable purpura

B. dermal erythropoiesis

C. metastatic hepatic tissue

D. viral lesions

E. none of the above

11. The most common manifestation of congenital cytomegalovirus (CMV) infection at birth is

A. asymptomatic viruria

B. deafness

C. microcephaly

D. intrauterine growth retardation

E. retinitis

F. hepatosplenomegaly

12. Conditions that may mimic neonatal sepsis include all of the following EXCEPT

A. hypoglycemia

B. methylmalonicacidemia

C. urea cycle defects

D. hyperthyroidism

E. Hurler syndrome

F. galactosemia

13. Neonatal infections that are partially or completely preventable include all of the following EXCEPT

A. cytomegalovirus

B. group B streptococci

C. rubella

D. syphilis

E. tetanus

F. toxoplasmosis

14. Microorganisms that commonly cause chronic intrauterine infections include all of the following EXCEPT

A. *Toxoplasma gondii*

B. *Treponema pallidum*

C. rubella virus

D. cytomegalovirus

E. herpes simplex virus

15. The most common cause of late-onset infections in infants weighing less than 1500 g is

A. *Candida albicans*

B. coagulase-negative staphylococci

C. *E. coli*

D. group B streptococci

E. *Pseudomonas*

16. The most common focus of infection of group B streptococcal early-onset disease of the newborn is the

    A. skin

    B. lungs

    C. meninges

    D. urinary tract

    E. bone

17. A full-term male, product of a normal spontaneous vaginal delivery, appeared well until 3 weeks of age, when he developed fever, irritability, and poor feeding. Twelve hours later, the examination revealed a pale, lethargic infant with poor suck and fair muscle tone. His temperature was 40°C, pulse was 180, and respiratory rate was 60. His fontanel was firm, his chest was clear, his abdomen was not distended, and no organs or masses were palpable. His skin showed normal turgor with capillary refill less than 3 seconds. White blood cell (WBC) count was 2.8, with 13% segmented cells and 12% bands. The most appropriate next step in diagnosis is

    A. blood culture

    B. urine culture

    C. chest radiography

    D. head ultrasonography

    E. spinal fluid analysis

18. A 3200-g infant was born on August 15, 1996, at 40 weeks' gestation, to a rubella-immune, STS-negative woman whose membranes ruptured 2 hours before delivery. The mother had reported a temperature of 38.5°C and diarrhea 1 hour before delivery. Apgar scores were 9/9. The infant appeared well and was discharged at 48 hours. Because of poor feeding and a temperature of 38.3°C, the infant was readmitted, cultured, and treated with cefotaxime and gentamicin. Two days later, the infant developed pallor, ecchymoses, bleeding from puncture wounds, hepatomegaly, and lethargy. Laboratory studies showed hemoglobin, 10 g/dL; WBCs, 14,000; platelets, 18,000; fibrinogen, 65 mg/dL; PTT, 25 seconds (control 11 seconds); and SGPT, 1200. The most likely cause of this infant's sepsis is

    A. toxoplasmosis

    B. group B streptococcus

    C. cytomegalovirus

    D. rubella

    E. enterovirus

13 Special Health Problems During Adolescence

Since antiquity (or even before), teenagers have held a special place in our hearts and our minds as physicians, as parents, and as former adolescents. Many diseases affect the physical and mental health of adolescents. Specific organ-related problems are often discussed in other *parts* of the *Nelson Textbook*. This *part* addresses adolescent epidemiology, depression, suicide, substance mis-use, sleep and eating disorders, pregnancy, contraception, sexually transmitted diseases (STDs), menstrual problems, and disorders of the skin, breast, or bone.

Questions in this *part* are fairly straightforward and helpful in following and reinforcing the adolescent curriculum as discussed in the respective *part* and chapters in the *Nelson Textbook*.

1. Oral contraceptive agents are associated with all of the following risks EXCEPT
   A. thrombophlebitis
   B. carbohydrate intolerance
   C. high levels of high-density lipoproteins
   D. premature epiphyseal closure
   E. none of the above

2. *Matching:*

   1. Pregnancy rate 0.8% per year
   2. Norgestrel, two pills after coitus and two more in 12 hours
   3. Administered every 3 months
   4. Spermicidal
   5. Administered every 5 years

   A. Depo-Provera
   B. Norplant
   C. Oral contraception
   D. Morning-after pill
   E. Nonoxynol-9

3. Risks associated with an intrauterine device (IUD) include all of the following EXCEPT
   A. ectopic pregnancy
   B. dysmenorrhea
   C. congenital malformations
   D. pelvic infection
   E. menstrual bleeding

4. An 18-year-old white sexually active woman presents with fever, rash, and malaise for 2 weeks. One of her sexual partners was recently given an intramuscular antibiotic for "VD." Your patient is noted to have a positive Venereal Disease Research Laboratories (VDRL) test result. The next step to take is to
   A. administer ceftriaxone
   B. culture for gonorrhea and *Chlamydia*
   C. discuss the use of condoms
   D. perform an ANA
   E. perform a specific treponemal antibody test

5. False-positive VDRL test results would most likely occur in
   A. mononucleosis
   B. systemic lupus erythematosus
   C. endocarditis
   D. intravenous drug misuse
   E. tuberculosis
   F. all of the above

6. The appropriate serologic response to adequately treated early syphilis is
   A. persistent VDRL, declining FTA-IgG
   B. declining VDRL, persistent FTA-IgG
   C. persistent VDRL, persistent FTA-IgG
   D. declining VDRL, declining FTA-IgG
   E. none of the above

7. False-positive treponemal antibody test results occur in all of the following EXCEPT
   A. rat-bite fever
   B. Lyme disease

C. leptospirosis

D. yaws

E. mononucleosis

8. A foul-smelling vaginal discharge that emits a fishy odor with 10% potassium hydroxide and that demonstrates clue cells on the wet preparation is most likely due to

A. gonorrhea

B. *Chlamydia*

C. chancroids

D. *Gardnerella vaginalis*

E. *Candida*

9. Causes of secondary amenorrhea include all of the following EXCEPT

A. phenothiazine use

B. opiate misuse

C. pregnancy

D. testicular feminization syndrome

E. anorexia nervosa

F. none of the above

10. A 19-year-old man presents in an unresponsive state with miosis, slow respirations, and pulmonary edema. He has hypertrophic lesions over the dorsum of the left hand and the antecubital fossa. The most effective therapy is

A. intravenous glucose

B. flumazenil

C. disulfiram

D. Narcan

E. intravenous calcium

11. Toluene (glue, solvents) misuse is associated with

A. hallucinations

B. tolerance

C. pulmonary edema

D. peripheral neuropathy

E. rhabdomyolysis

F. all of the above

12. Anabolic steroid use is associated with all of the following EXCEPT

A. enhanced school performance

B. testicular atrophy

C. aggressive behavior

D. cholestasis

E. increased low-density lipoprotein levels

13. **Matching:** Eating disorders

1. Increasing in frequency

2. Primarily males

3. Most common disorder

4. "Feels fat" when emaciated

5. Amenorrhea

6. Binge eating with fear of not being able to stop

7. Bradycardia

8. Parotid swelling

9. Leukopenia

10. Hypothermia

11. Hyperthyroidism

12. Esophagitis

A. Anorexia nervosa

B. Bulimia

C. Both

D. Neither

14. The most common cause of a breast mass in an adolescent girl is

A. fibroadenoma

B. cystosarcoma phylloides

C. abscess

D. carcinoma

15. **Matching:** For each of the following symptoms or signs, select the appropriate disorder.

1. Recurrent episodes of binge eating

2. Weight loss of at least 25%

3. Frequent weight fluctuations

4. Amenorrhea

5. Females more affected than males

6. Onset at puberty

7. Esophagitis

8. Constipation

9. Increased susceptibility to infection

A. Anorexia nervosa

B. Bulimia

C. Both anorexia nervosa and bulimia

D. Neither anorexia nervosa nor bulimia

16. The leading listed cause of mortality in adolescence is

    A. violence

    B. neoplasms

    C. infectious diseases

    D. congenital anomalies

    E. sexually transmitted diseases

17. The best contraceptive for a 16-year-old with a history of two pregnancies while on combination estrogen-progestin oral contraceptives and a steady sexual partner is

    A. an intrauterine device

    B. an all-progestin oral contraceptive

    C. condoms

    D. Norplant

    E. a cervical cap

18. Routine immunizations for a 15-year-old girl who has been sexually active with four different partners in the past 6 months and who has not received any immunizations since entry into elementary school should include all of the following EXCEPT

    A. MMR

    B. dT

    C. hepatitis B

    D. BCG

19. A 15-year-old girl has experienced loss of 30 pounds during the past 6 months and has developed amenorrhea. She denies vomiting, diarrhea, and abdominal pain and claims to feel well. Physical examination reveals cachexia and a pulse of 40 per minute. Electrolyte determination reveals a serum potassium level of 3.0 and bicarbonate of 30. Hematocrit is 30, and erythrocyte sedimentation rate is 3 mm/hour. The most likely cause of this patient's condition is

    A. inflammatory bowel disease

    B. anorexia nervosa

    C. bulimia nervosa

    D. Addison disease

    E. pituitary adenoma

20. A 12-year-old who had been in excellent health experiences profuse, painless vaginal bleeding with her first menstrual period. She is brought to the emergency department in shock. She has no history of sexual intercourse or vaginal discharge before this. Physical examination, with the exception of rapid, faint pulse and low blood pressure, is unremarkable. What is the most likely cause of this condition?

    A. Threatened abortion

    B. Dysfunctional uterine bleeding

    C. Von Willebrand disease

    D. Aplastic anemia

    E. Aspirin sensitivity

14 The Immunologic System and Disorders

lthough acquired immunodeficiency syndrome (AIDS) is a common cause of immunodeficiency, its differential diagnoses could include many of the diseases discussed in the chapters in this *part* of the *Nelson Textbook*. The chapters have been completely updated and include topics such as B-cell, T-cell, and combined B- and T-cell disorders in addition to diseases of the complement system and the leukocytes. Finally, the treatment of some of these disorders, bone marrow transplantation, is discussed in a separate and detailed chapter.

Questions in this *part* are related to the approach to children with recurrent infections. The questions help distinguish the many different disorders based on the nature and extent of the infectious complications.

1. A 9-year-old male presents with pallor and petechiae. The complete blood count (CBC) reveals a platelet count of 7000, an absolute neutrophil count of 200, and a hematocrit of 25% with a reticulocyte count of 1%. The most likely diagnosis is

   A. transient erythroblastopenia of childhood

   B. Blackfan-Diamond disease

   C. aplastic anemia

   D. osteopetrosis

   E. none of the above

2. The least likely next step as part of the treatment of the boy described in Question 1 is

   A. bone marrow examination

   B. packed red blood cell transfusion

   C. HLA match siblings

   D. psychosocial evaluation

   E. none of the above

3. The factor that most likely contributes to improved outcome in patients who have leukemia and who are treated with bone marrow transplantation is

   A. the degree of neutropenia

   B. graft-versus-host disease

   C. the number of blasts in the peripheral blood count

   D. thrombocytopenia

   E. none of the above

4. A 12-year-old child underwent a bone marrow transplant for leukemia 1 month ago. The absolute neutrophil count has steadily increased, indicating engraftment. Today the patient has a maculopapular rash over 35% of the body, jaundice (bilirubin 4.5 mg/dL), and 1000 mL of diarrhea per 24 hours. This child most likely has

   A. recurrent leukemia

   B. acute stage 2 graft-versus-host disease

   C. acute stage 4 graft-versus-host disease

   D. chronic stage 2 graft-versus-host disease

   E. chronic stage 4 graft-versus-host disease

5. All of the following are associated with chronic granulomatous disease (CGD) EXCEPT

   A. autosomal recessive inheritance

   B. pyloric outlet obstruction

   C. *Aspergillus* pneumonia

   D. perianal abscess

   E. hypogammaglobulinemia

6. A 5-year-old boy presents with his third episode of painful cervical lymphadenitis. Each was treated with incision and drainage and grew *Staphylococcus aureus*. At the age of 2 years, he required surgical aspiration of a liver abscess. The most important laboratory test is

   A. PCR for ADA deficiency

   B. nitroblue tetrazolium

   C. MAC-1 assay

   D. neutrophil count

   E. bone marrow aspiration

7. The most likely diagnosis in the patient described in Question 6 is

   A. Bruton agammaglobulinemia

   B. AIDS

   C. chronic granulomatous disease

   D. Kostmann disease

   E. cyclic neutropenia

8. Long-term effective therapy for the patient described in Question 6 is best accomplished with

   A. intravenous immunoglobulin

   B. interferon-γ

   C. G-CSF

   D. bone marrow transplantation

   E. granulocyte transfusions

9. The findings of marked leukocytosis in the presence of severe recurrent necrotizing bacterial infections in a child with a history of delayed separation of the umbilical cord most likely suggests

   A. a leukocyte adhesion defect

   B. chronic granulomatous disease

   C. Shwachman-Diamond syndrome

   D. Kostmann disease

   E. agammaglobulinemia

10. Cyclic neutropenia is usually associated with all of the following EXCEPT

    A. oral ulcerations

    B. periodontal disease

    C. cyclic reticulocytosis

    D. septicemia

    E. cellulitis

11. A 6-month-old presents with recurrent cellulitis and bacteremias due to *Streptococcus pyogenes* or *Staphylococcus aureus*. The white blood cell count is 2500 with 5% neutrophils, 10% eosinophils, 35% monocytes, and 50% lymphocytes. The platelet count is 650,000. A brother and a female cousin died at the age of 18 months and 2 years, respectively. The most likely diagnosis is

    A. AIDS

    B. severe combined immunodeficiency

    C. Kostmann disease

    D. cyclic neutropenia

    E. chronic granulomatous disease

12. Long-term treatment of the disease described in Question 11 is best accomplished with

    A. prophylactic antibiotics

    B. intravenous immunoglobulin

    C. interferon

    D. G-CSF

    E. bone marrow transplant

13. Neutropenia is noted in children in all of the following EXCEPT

    A. Kostmann disease

    B. viral infections

    C. maternal preeclampsia

    D. Hunter syndrome

    E. Shwachman-Diamond syndrome

    F. glycogen storage disease type Ib

    G. neonatal alloimmune processes

14. Secondary complement deficiency is associated with all of the following EXCEPT

    A. cardiopulmonary bypass

    B. burns

    C. chronic membranoproliferative glomerulonephritis

    D. rheumatic fever

    E. severe combined immunodeficiency disease

15. *Matching:* Complement deficiency

    1. Lupus-like syndrome   A. C5, 6, 7, 8, 9

    2. Recurrent neisserial infection   B. C3

         C. C1q

    3. Severe, recurrent pneumococcal infection   D. C1 inhibitor

    4. Fatal meningococcal infection in males   E. Properdin

    5. Nonpitting edema

16. A 14-month-old boy presents with a high fever, bilateral otitis media, and a right lower lobe pneumonia. He has a history of chronic atopic dermatitis and recurrent otitis media. Laboratory studies reveal a platelet count of 59,000. A brother died of lymphoma at the age of 15 years. The most likely diagnosis is

    A. AIDS

B. Bruton agammaglobulinemia

C. ADA deficiency

D. Omenn syndrome

E. Wiskott-Aldrich syndrome

17. The long-term treatment of Wiskott-Aldrich syndrome is

A. intravenous immunoglobulin

B. interferon

C. tumor necrosis factor

D. bone marrow transplantation

E. prophylactic chemotherapy

18. The complete DiGeorge syndrome is associated with all of the following EXCEPT

A. neonatal hypocalcemia

B. aortic atresia

C. graft-versus-host disease after blood transfusion

D. chromosomal deletion at 22q11

E. onset after 12 months of age

F. micrognathia

19. Possible complications of intravenous immunoglobulin therapy include all of the following EXCEPT

A. hepatitis C

B. anaphylaxis

C. fluid overload

D. AIDS

E. pain at sites of infection

F. aseptic meningitis

20. A 3-year-old boy presents with fever, cough, and tachypnea of 1 week's duration. In addition, the physical examination demonstrates small to absent tonsils and no palpable lymph nodes. A chest radiograph demonstrates a right lower lobe pneumonia. The white blood cell count is 2500, and the blood culture reveals pneumococci. The past medical history reveals multiple episodes of pneumonia and otitis media; at age 10 months, he had an episode of *Haemophilus influenzae* type b bacteremia. Before 6 months of age he was well. A brother died at the age of 12 months with an unspecified febrile illness. The most likely diagnosis is

A. AIDS

B. Bruton agammaglobulinemia

C. cyclic neutropenia

D. selective IgA deficiency

E. DiGeorge syndrome

21. The most appropriate long-term therapy for patients with Bruton agammaglobulinemia is

A. suppressive oral antibiotics

B. interferon-γ

C. intravenous immunoglobulin

D. bone marrow transplant

E. none of the above

22. *Matching:* Immunodeficiency

1. Fatal echovirus encephalitis

2. Splenomegaly

3. Chromosome 2q12

4. Mandibular hypoplasia

5. May be confused with AIDS

6. Most severe of congenital immuno-deficiencies

7. High frequency of autoimmune disorders

8. Rib cage anomalies

9. Lymphopenia plus severe neutropenia

10. Elevated IgE levels and eosinophilia

A. DiGeorge syndrome

B. Bruton syndrome

C. Common variable immunodeficiency

D. Hyper IgM

E. CD8 lymphocytopenia

F. Nezelof syndrome

G. SCID

H. Omenn syndrome

I. Reticular dysgenesis

J. Adenosine deaminase (ADA) deficiency

23. An infant with eczema, thrombocytopenia, and recurrent otitis media is most likely to have which one of the following disorders?

A. DiGeorge syndrome

B. Bruton disease

C. Graft-versus-host disease

D. Wiskott-Aldrich syndrome

E. Nezelof syndrome

24. Which of the following is characterized by unusual susceptibility to staphylococcal

infections, chronic skin lesions, and "cold" abscesses?

A. Chédiak-Higashi syndrome

B. Kartagener syndrome

C. Anchor disease

D. Shwachman syndrome

E. Job syndrome

25. In chronic granulomatous disease, the neutrophils are

A. markedly decreased in number

B. unable to increase their numbers in response to a bacterial infection

C. incapable of intracellular killing of certain bacteria

D. leukemoid in number

E. able to reduce nitroblue tetrazolium (NBT) dye

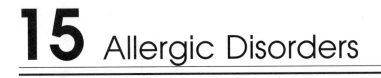

15 Allergic Disorders

It must be an "allergy"! This seems to be many patients' or parents' belief about many signs and symptoms. Allergies may be relatively benign but annoying problems, such as allergic rhinitis; however, allergy-related immune problems such as asthma may create life-threatening crises. Furthermore, the prevalence of all allergies may be increasing, including the prevalence and possibly the severity of asthma. This *part* of the *Nelson Textbook* also discusses serum sickness, atopic dermatitis, urticaria, angioedema, insect and ocular allergies, and adverse food reactions. Finally, the treatments for these disorders are discussed in detail with current data.

Being able to answer the questions in this *part* will help readers identify and manage common, uncomplicated allergic problems in children.

1. The skin of patients with atopic dermatitis exhibits all of the following EXCEPT

   A. papule formation after intradermal injection of an allergen

   B. white dermographism

   C. abnormal rates of cooling

   D. blanching after intradermal histamine injection

   E. reduced threshold for skin infections

2. The lesions of atopic dermatitis are most often produced by

   A. cold climate

   B. wool clothing

   C. perfumes

   D. scratching

   E. none of the above

3. *Matching:*

   1. Begins on scalp   A. Eczema
   2. Weepy, crusty lesions   B. Seborrhea
   3. Responds more rapidly   C. Neither
   4. Greasy lesions   D. Both
   5. Dry skin
   6. Pruritus
   7. Keratoconus
   8. Stomatitis
   9. Scales

4. A 12-year-old with repeated episodes of streptococcal pharyngitis develops another episode of sore throat. The rapid strep test is positive, and oral ampicillin is started, with the first dose given in the office. One hour later, she develops a funny feeling and a tingling sensation around her mouth. Next she becomes apprehensive, has difficulty swallowing, and develops a hoarse voice. On arrival at the emergency room, she has giant urticaria and the following vital signs: pulse 130, respiratory rate 32, blood pressure 70/30, and temperature 37.2°C. The most appropriate therapy is

   A. epinephrine

   B. prednisone

   C. Benadryl

   D. cimetidine

   E. lactated Ringer solution

5. The most likely diagnosis for the condition described in Question 4 is

   A. streptococcal toxic shock

   B. scarlet fever

   C. infectious mononucleosis

   D. anaphylaxis

   E. serum sickness

6. A patient with stable asthma is being treated with theophylline and inhaled steroids. Three days before admission, she developed otitis media. Because she is also allergic to penicillin, the physician prescribed Pediazole. Today she manifests nausea, vomiting, and hematemesis. The next step in evaluating the patient is to

   A. perform tympanocentesis

   B. obtain a theophylline level

   C. order an upper GI series

D. begin cisapride

E. administer albuterol

7. For the patient described in Question 6, both theophylline and Pediazole therapies are stopped. The next appropriate step in the treatment of this patient is to administer

A. activated charcoal

B. ipecac

C. diazepam to prevent seizures

D. lidocaine to prevent ventricular tachycardia

E. none of the above

8. A 14-year-old white female with the diagnosis of severe recurrent reactive airway disease since age 1 year comes to the emergency room with fever and cough for 2 weeks. The child has purulent sputum, bilateral wheezing, and rales but is not "tight." Her weight is below the fifth percentile, she has no secondary sex characteristics, and mild digital clubbing is noted. The most likely diagnosis is

A. steroid-dependent asthma

B. cystic fibrosis

C. allergic bronchopulmonary aspergillosis

D. tuberculosis

E. celiac disease

F. foreign body aspiration

9. Eosinophilia is observed in all of the following EXCEPT

A. *Giardia* infection

B. *Toxocara* infection

C. drug hypersensitivity

D. periarteritis nodosa

E. allergy

10. Allergy to peanuts should be managed in the long term by

A. avoidance

B. nonsedating antihistamines (daily)

C. desensitization

D. prednisone after exposure

E. none of the above

11. All of the following are of use in the management of house dust mite allergy EXCEPT

A. using airtight mattress and pillow covers

B. removing carpeting in the bedroom

C. weekly vacuuming the bedroom

D. high humidity

E. use of benzyl benzoate in the carpet

F. weekly washing the sheets and blankets in hot water

12. All of the following may increase plasma levels of theophylline EXCEPT

A. cimetidine

B. erythromycin

C. influenza vaccine

D. smoking marijuana

E. ketoconazole

13. Associated epidemiologic facts about asthma include all of the following EXCEPT

A. another name could be chronic desquamating eosinophilic bronchitis

B. a child with two affected parents has a 50% risk of asthma

C. asthma is universally present in monozygotic twins

D. asthma is transferred with lung transplantation

E. both large and small airways are affected

14. Risk factors for asthma include all of the following EXCEPT

A. black race

B. dust mite exposure in infancy

C. maternal smoking

D. neonatal respiratory distress syndrome

E. frequent respiratory infections in infancy

15. Risk factors for fatal asthma include all of the following EXCEPT

A. sudden severe obstruction

B. an allergic component

C. underuse of steroids

D. underestimation of the severity

E. poor compliance

F. sedation

16. Clinical facts associated with asthma include all of the following EXCEPT

A. aspirin may exacerbate asthma

B. cough may be a manifestation

C. wheezing may not be present during an active asthma attack

D. a silent chest is a good sign

E. a pulsus paradoxus exceeding 20 mm Hg is a sign of severe disease

17. Severe asthma is predicted by

A. speaking in single-word sentences

B. cyanosis

C. P_{CO_2} greater than 40

D. peak expiratory flow rate less than 50% of baseline

E. all of the above

18. A 12-year-old presents with sneezing, clear rhinorrhea, and nasal itching. Physical examination reveals boggy, pale nasal edema with a clear discharge. The most likely diagnosis is

A. foreign body

B. vasomotor rhinitis

C. neutrophilic rhinitis

D. nasal mastocytosis

E. allergic rhinitis

19. Two weeks later, the patient described in Question 18 complains of headache, poor nasal airflow (mouth breathing), fever, and a change in the nature of the nasal discharge; it is now mucopurulent. The most likely diagnosis is

A. sinusitis

B. foreign body

C. rhinitis medicamentosa

D. choanal stenosis

E. ciliary dyskinesia

20. Immunotherapy provides symptomatic improvement in all of the following EXCEPT

A. ragweed allergy

B. local reaction to bee sting

C. tree pollen allergy

D. house dust mite allergy

E. anaphylaxis to a wasp sting

21. A 4-year-old boy experienced facial urticaria at a birthday party during vigorous activity after eating ice cream and chocolate cake with red and white frosting. You notice his face is almost as red as his balloon. The LEAST likely cause of the reaction is

A. milk

B. egg

C. red dye

D. the balloon

E. exercise

22. An 8-year-old boy experienced generalized urticaria immediately after a honeybee sting 2 months ago. He had no other symptoms except for a large local reaction at the site of the sting. Skin testing with honeybee venom has been strongly positive at a weak concentration. Appropriate recommendations include all of the following EXCEPT

A. immunotherapy

B. an Epi-Pen for administration if stung again

C. wearing shoes when outdoors

D. a Medic-Alert bracelet

E. wearing long pants

23. A 10-year-old girl with acute streptococcal pharyngitis had an urticarial eruption during treatment with penicillin 3 years ago and after trimethoprim-sulfamethoxazole 4 years ago. Prick skin testing with Pre-Pen has elicited a wheal 8 mm in diameter with erythema 11 mm in diameter. All of the following are true EXCEPT that

A. she has no risk of allergy to erythromycin

B. her risk of allergy to a cephalosporin is probably less than 10%

C. her mother's allergy to penicillin increased the child's risk for development of drug allergy

D. she is not certain to be allergic to amoxicillin

E. administration of penicillin is very likely to cause an allergic reaction

24. The mother of an 8-year-old boy with acute streptococcal tonsillitis calls to report that within 15 minutes after the first dose of penicillin V you prescribed, he is complaining of itching and has developed hives. You should recommend

A. oral Benadryl and call again if not improved within 30 minutes

B. immediate return to your office or the nearest emergency room

C. return to your office or the nearest emergency room if he becomes short of breath or loses consciousness

D. that they go to the laboratory for determination of serum tryptase level

E. substitution of erythromycin for penicillin

25. Risk factors for death due to asthma include all of the following EXCEPT

A. late administration of corticosteroids

B. inappropriate use of metered dose inhalation agents

C. psychosocial dysfunction

D. previous admission to an intensive care unit

E. onset of asthma at an early age

26. Risk factors for asthma include all of the following EXCEPT

A. family history of asthma

B. eczema

C. smoking in the family

D. rural housing

E. allergen exposure

27. A 3-year-old boy has had persistent nasal congestion, clear nasal discharge, and sneezing for the past 18 months. Allergy skin testing has confirmed allergy to house dust mites. Although the parents are very concerned about their son's symptoms and agree to most precautions to reduce exposure to mites, they are reluctant to remove the carpet from his bedroom. You should

A. insist on removal of the carpet

B. recommend rush immunotherapy to mites

C. suggest Acarosan

D. recommend a central electronic filter

E. suggest waiting a few months to see whether he outgrows the allergy

28. A 17-year-old boy who has seasonal allergic rhinitis has been incapacitated by sneezing and nasal discharge the past few days. Intranasal cromolyn and intranasal steroids have caused

him frequent epistaxis in the recent past. His SATs (college entrance examinations) are scheduled 4 days from now. What should you recommend?

A. Another intranasal steroid

B. Hydroxyzine

C. Loratadine

D. Chlorpheniramine

E. Rescheduling the examination

29. A 4-year-old boy with asthma has had mild wheezing only four times since you began treating him 6 months ago with Slo-bid Gyrocaps twice each day. He previously had coughing and wheezing at least three times each week. (A peak serum theophylline concentration 5 months ago was 16 μg/mL.) For the past 4 days, he has again had mild coughing and wheezing responsive to inhaled albuterol. Two days ago, an emergency room physician began treatment with Pediazole for otitis media. This morning the youngster began vomiting. You should consider the likely cause of vomiting to be

A. provocation by coughing

B. infection

C. theophylline toxicity

D. albuterol toxicity

E. Pediazole intolerance

30. A 12-year-old girl has had a history of frequent nasal congestion, nasal discharge, and sneezing from March through September for the past 3 years and three episodes of acute sinusitis responsive to antibiotics. Treatment with Hismanal and an intranasal steroid has afforded only partial relief of symptoms. An allergy consultant reports no evidence of allergy from allergy skin testing 1 week after discontinuation of Hismanal. The most likely explanation for the negative skin tests is

A. lack of allergy

B. failure to test with the relevant allergens

C. suppression of skin reactivity by Hismanal

D. improper testing technique

E. suppression of skin reactivity by intranasal steroids

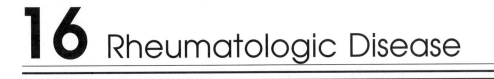

16 Rheumatologic Disease

Rheumatic, autoimmune, connective tissue, and collagen vascular diseases are common, often difficult to distinguish from one another, difficult to manage, and rarely curable. This *part* teaches you to avoid the old statement, "When in doubt of a diagnosis with multiple organ involvement, say SLE." Indeed this *part* has individual chapters on juvenile rheumatoid arthritis (JRA), the spondyloarthropathies, systemic lupus erythemato-sus (SLE), vasculitis syndromes (Henoch-Schönlein purpura, Kawasaki disease), dermatomyositis, scleroderma, mixed connective tissue disease, and many more. Included are excellent tables that are useful in differentiating one disease from the other.

Readers will find these questions educationally rewarding as they reiterate important concepts and points from the *Nelson Textbook*.

1. A child has abdominal pain, arthritis, microscopic hematuria, and a purpuric rash only on the lower extremities. Which of the following is the most likely diagnosis?

    A. Meningococcemia

    B. Varicella

    C. Henoch-Schönlein vasculitis

    D. Poststreptococcal glomerulonephritis

    E. Infectious mononucleosis

2. A 5-year-old boy develops severe abdominal pain of 3 days' duration. He is unable to eat and has occasional emesis. Physical examination reveals an anxious, acutely ill child with generalized abdominal tenderness, voluntary guarding of the anterior abdominal muscles, and normal findings on rectal examination. A surgical consultant believes the child has an acute abdomen, possibly appendicitis. Before the child is sent to the operating room, the urinalysis reveals 3 + hematuria and 1 + proteinuria. You should

    A. perform coagulation studies

    B. obtain a complete blood count

    C. perform renal ultrasonography

    D. proceed with the operation

    E. cancel the operation

3. On repeat physical examination, the patient described in Question 2 now has petechiae over the dorsal surfaces of the feet and hands and over the buttocks. His platelet count is 350,000. The most likely diagnosis is

    A. Kawasaki syndrome

    B. Henoch-Schönlein purpura

    C. Rocky Mountain spotted fever

    D. meningococcemia

    E. appendicitis with gram-negative sepsis

4. All of the following are part of the revised diagnostic criteria for SLE EXCEPT

    A. nonerosive arthritis

    B. lymphopenia

    C. Raynaud phenomenon

    D. discoid rash

    E. oral ulcers

    F. pleuritis

5. A 7-year-old white male presents with malaise, chest pain, high spiking fevers, and chills for 3 weeks. He has had no ill contacts, and he has missed school during the last week of the illness. Physical examination reveals an acutely ill child with a heart rate of 125, a temperature of 40.5°C, a fine but faint macular red-pink rash on the trunk and proximal extremities, lymphadenopathy, a liver 4 cm below the right costal margin, and a palpable spleen tip. Laboratory studies reveal a hemoglobin of 9.7 g/dL, a total white blood cell count of 26,000, and a platelet count of 650,000. The most important step in evaluating this patient would be to order

    A. an erythrocyte sedimentation rate (ESR)

    B. Lyme titers

    C. a chest radiograph

    D. an echocardiogram

    E. bone marrow aspiration

6. On further evaluation, the patient described in

Question 5 has no evidence of pericardial tamponade or reduced cardiac function. His pulse normalizes when he defervesces. The approach to the management of this patient's pericardial effusion is to

A. perform pericardiocentesis

B. begin digitalization

C. improve preload with fluids

D. begin an oral nonsteroidal anti-inflammatory agent

E. begin methotrexate

7. The most likely diagnosis for the patient described in Question 5 is

A. systemic-onset juvenile rheumatoid arthritis

B. uremia

C. systemic lupus erythematosus

D. scleroderma

E. rheumatic fever

8. *Matching:*

1. High spiking fevers	A. Pauciarticular JRA type I
2. Chronic iridocyclitis	B. Pauciarticular JRA type II
3. Spondylo-arthropathy	C. Systemic-onset JRA
4. Ninety percent females	D. Polyarticular rheumatoid factor positive
5. Most severe sequela of arthritis	E. Polyarticular rheumatoid factor negative

9. Rheumatoid factor may be positive in all of the following disease states EXCEPT

A. congenital infections (TORCH)

B. bacterial endocarditis

C. *Toxocara canis* infection

D. eosinophilic granuloma

E. systemic lupus erythematosus

F. chronic active hepatitis

10. *Matching:*

1. Wegener granulomatosis	A. Antibody to double-stranded DNA
2. Neonatal lupus	B. Anti Ro (SSA)
3. Antiphospholipid antibody	C. Antibody to ribonuclear protein
4. Mixed connective tissue disease	D. False-positive VDRL result
5. Specific for SLE	E. HLA-B27
6. Spondylo-arthropathies	F. Antineutrophil cytoplasmic antibodies

11. A 9-year-old female notices she has difficulty combing her hair and walking up stairs for approximately 1 month. Physical examination reveals a positive Gower sign and a faint maculopapular rash over the metacarpophalangeal joints. The most appropriate laboratory study to order is

A. erythrocyte sedimentation rate

B. serum creatine phosphokinase

C. rheumatoid factor

D. motor nerve conduction study

E. antinuclear antibodies

12. The most likely diagnosis for the patient described in Question 11 is

A. muscular dystrophy

B. dermatomyositis

C. periarteritis nodosa

D. systemic lupus erythematosus

E. myotonic dystrophy

13. The most appropriate initial therapy for the patient described in Question 11 is

A. aspirin

B. intravenous immunoglobulin

C. plasmapheresis

D. prednisone

E. cyclosporine

14. All of the following are diagnostic features of Kawasaki disease EXCEPT

A. generalized lymphadenopathy

B. fever for at least 5 days

C. nonpurulent conjunctivitis

D. desquamation of the fingers

E. polymorphous rash

15. During the acute phase (1 to 10 days) of Kawasaki disease, mortality is related to

A. febrile seizures

B. aspirin intoxication

C. myocardial ischemia

D. coronary artery aneurysm

E. myocarditis

16. An 18-year-old male develops a swollen right wrist and left ankle with bilateral pain over both Achilles tendons. Two weeks before this he received an antibiotic for a urethral discharge; his girlfriend was also treated. Physical examination reveals tenderness over both Achilles tendons, swollen painful joints (right wrist, left ankle), and limited forward bending at the waist. The most likely course of treatment would be

A. ceftriaxone

B. doxycycline

C. prednisone

D. nonsteroidal anti-inflammatory agents

E. intravenous immunoglobulin

17. On further evaluation, the patient described in Question 16 has sterile pyuria and iritis. The most likely diagnosis is

A. disseminated gonococcemia

B. *Chlamydia* infection

C. Behçet disease

D. systemic lupus erythematosus

E. Reiter syndrome

18. *Matching:*

1. Antibody to ribonuclear protein

2. Tuberculosis

3. Eosinophilia

4. Painful red nodules on the thighs

5. Recurrent and chronic "croup"

6. Uveitis

7. Xerostomia

A. Fasciitis

B. Relapsing panniculitis

C. Behçet syndrome

D. Mixed connective tissue disease

E. Erythema nodosum

F. Relapsing polychondritis

G. Sjögren's syndrome

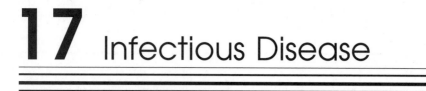

17 Infectious Disease

Talk about a "play within a play"—this mega *part* is a book within a book. The *part* is divided into eight sections with a total of more than 100 chapters and subchapters. The sections include an overview in addition to clinical syndromes caused by various infectious agents (fever, sepsis, meningitis, pneumonia, gastroenteritis, and others); there are sections on bacterial, viral, mycotic, rickettsial, and parasitic infections as well as one on prevention. Because infections are common pediatric problems at all ages of development, this *part* of the *Nelson Textbook* has been extensively updated by many new and authoritative contributors.

Readers should enjoy working on the questions in this *part* of the book. You will not become an immediate infectious disease consultant, but you should be more knowledgeable about the common and occasionally the uncommon infectious diseases of children. By the way—beware of the uncommon. If one of the physician contributors can encounter malaria and typhoid fever in Wisconsin, then almost anything may appear in your own clinic, emergency room, hospital ward, or intensive care unit.

1. A 2-year-old male comes to your office with profuse watery diarrhea. His father just returned from a trip to St. Petersburg, Russia, and has been suffering from diarrhea for more than a week. His physician diagnosed *Cryptosporidium* infection on stool examination. Which of the following steps would be appropriate?

   A. Begin the patient on sulfamethoxazole.

   B. Discuss aggressive oral rehydration with the child's mother to prevent dehydration.

   C. Send off three stool specimens for culture.

   D. Arrange for endoscopy and biopsy.

   E. Request an infectious disease consultation.

2. You are asked to investigate an outbreak among children with profuse watery diarrhea in a daycare center. Likely etiologic agents that you should consider include all of the following EXCEPT

   A. *Cryptosporidium*

   B. *Giardia*

   C. *Rotavirus*

   D. *Ascaris lumbricoides*

3. Therapy of human herpesvirus 6 (HHV-6) infection is associated with all of the statements EXCEPT

   A. therapy is generally symptomatic with antipyretics

   B. therapy may involve anticonvulsants for recurrent febrile seizures

   C. in life-threatening cases, in vitro data would suggest a trial of ganciclovir

   D. there are no controlled trials of treatment of HHV-6 in immunocompromised persons

   E. Oral acyclovir is indicated to shorten the duration and prevent complications of roseola

4. In a 15-year-old patient 1 month after a bone marrow transplantation, HHV-6 is associated with all of the following EXCEPT

   A. idiopathic interstitial pneumonitis

   B. bone marrow suppression

   C. frequent finding of HHV-6 antigen in peripheral blood cells by polymerase chain reaction (PCR)

   D. a roseola-like syndrome of fever followed by defervescence and a rash

   E. positive IgG antibody titer for HHV-6

5. Diagnosis of *primary* HHV-6 infection in an immunocompetent infant or adult can be made by demonstration of

   A. a fourfold rise in IgG antibody to HHV-6

   B. seroconversion from negative to significant positive antibody response to HHV-6 in the absence of a cytomegalovirus infection

   C. PCR to detect HHV-6 DNA in peripheral blood leukocytes

D. characteristic pattern of lymphocytosis on an early white blood cell (WBC) profile

6. A 7-month-old child presents in late October with 3 days of fever to 103°F, a mildly injected pharynx, mild cervical adenopathy, and diarrhea. On the fourth day of the illness, the fever ceases and a measles-like rash appears. The most likely diagnosis is

   A. measles

   B. rubella

   C. drug reaction to antipyretics

   D. HHV-6 infection

   E. enteroviral infection

7. After diagnosis of pertussis in a toddler, erythromycin should be given to the patient and to which family members?

   A. Only those with a cough

   B. Only those younger than 7 years

   C. Only those who are incompletely immunized

   D. Only those with compromised immunity

   E. All regardless of age, symptoms, or immunization status

8. Acellular pertussis vaccines (DTaP) are currently licensed in the United States to be given in which one of the following situations instead of whole cell vaccines (DTP)?

   A. Second dose in a 4-month-old with inconsolable crying for more than 3 hours after the first dose of DTP

   B. Third dose in a 6-month-old with high fever after the second dose of DTP

   C. Fourth dose in a 12-month-old who had pain and swelling at the injection site after the third dose of DTP

   D. Fifth dose in a 4-year-old who has had no adverse effects after previous DTPs

   E. First dose in an 18-month-old toddler who has not received prior DTP

9. Complete series of whole cell pertussis vaccination can be expected to be at least 80% protective against

   A. infection with *Bordetella parapertussis*

   B. infection with *Bordetella pertussis*

   C. mild coughing illness due to *B. pertussis*

D. paroxysmal coughing illness of 14 or more days' duration due to *B. pertussis*

10. The majority of sporadic cases of pertussis-like illnesses in the United States currently are caused by

    A. *B. pertussis*

    B. *B. parapertussis*

    C. adenovirus

    D. *Chlamydia pneumoniae*

    E. respiratory syncytial virus

11. An 18-year-old sexually active female presents with her third episode in 4 months of painful shallow ulcers involving her right labia minora. A culture for herpes simplex virus (HSV) is positive. She is very upset about the episodes. Which statement is true?

    A. This illness can be generally prevented with prophylactic oral acyclovir.

    B. This illness can be permanently cured with high-dose intravenous acyclovir.

    C. This illness poses no threat to her future children.

    D. As long as lesions are absent, her sexual partner cannot be affected.

    E. Immunologic boosting with the varicella vaccine will decrease the risk of recurrences.

12. A 12-year-old child undergoing induction therapy for acute lymphocytic leukemia develops fever and an expanding, painful necrotic ulcer on his lower lip. ELISA is positive for HSV, as is a subsequent culture. Which of the following statements is true?

    A. This is probably colonization but not infection.

    B. This can be prevented by prophylactic acyclovir.

    C. Foscarnet is the drug of choice in initial HSV lesions in immunocompromised persons owing to the high incidence of acyclovir resistance.

    D. Therapy must include antiviral and antibacterial agents because of the synergistic nature of the infection.

    E. If treated with intravenous acyclovir, this type of infection responds dramatically and never develops recurrences.

13. A 3-year-old boy presents with a 7-day

history of fever, cervical adenopathy, foul breath, and painful oral lesions on his tongue, gums, and lips. For the past 3 days, he has had a red, painful swollen area about the nail of his right thumb with an area of fluid by the nail bed, unresponsive to warm soaks and a first-generation cephalosporin. The most likely useful diagnostic test would be

A. Gram stain of a finger aspirate

B. bacterial culture of the aspirated fluid

C. KOH preparation of the aspirated fluid

D. throat culture for group A streptococci

E. ELISA for HSV antigen of the aspirated fluid

14. A 13-month-old previously healthy child presents on New Year's Eve with a 1-day history of fever, lethargy, and left-side focal motor seizure activity. The cerebrospinal fluid (CSF) reveals 170 lymphocytes/mm^2, 400 red blood cells (RBCs)/mm^3, protein of 150 mg/dL, and normal glucose level. MRI scan reveals right temporal abnormalities. The single most appropriate therapy to begin empirically while awaiting definitive diagnosis would be

A. ceftriaxone

B. nafcillin, cefotaxime, and metronidazole

C. acyclovir

D. amphotericin B

E. isoniazid, rifampin, pyrazinamide, and streptomycin

15. A 7-year-old child presented to his pediatrician with a 1-week history of fever up to 39°C, joint pain involving the knees and elbows, and swelling of the right knee. He also had a rash consisting of papulopustular lesions over the extensor surfaces of the extremities including the dorsum of the hands. Which of the following statements is correct?

A. The patient clearly has juvenile rheumatoid arthritis and needs to be started on nonsteroidal anti-inflammatory agents.

B. The physician should inquire about the child's exposure to rodents (i.e., rats) and obtain blood, joint, and vesicular fluid to culture for the streptobacillary form of rat-bite fever.

C. This presentation is consistent with

erythema chronicum migrans and should be treated as such.

D. The patient should immediately be isolated for measles.

16. A full-term newborn male whose mother had reactive Venereal Disease Research Laboratory (VDRL) and microhemagglutination assay–*Treponema pallidum* (MHATP) results at the time of delivery was evaluated. He was anemic and had thrombocytopenia and mild hepatosplenomegaly. He also had a typical desquamative skin rash consistent with congenital syphilis. His CSF was clear, with 5 WBCs, 0 RBCs, protein of 80 mg/dL, and glucose of 49 mg/dL; the CSF VDRL result was nonreactive. Based on this examination, which of the following is true?

A. The patient has symptomatic congenital syphilis but not neurosyphilis and can therefore be treated with benzathine penicillin.

B. The patient may be treated with a combination of ampicillin and gentamicin for 7 to 10 days.

C. Neurosyphilis cannot be ruled out in this infant; therefore, he should be treated as though he has neurosyphilis.

D. All cases of neurosyphilis would have CSF pleocytosis and a reactive CSF VDRL result.

17. A full-term normal-appearing infant was born to a 26-year-old female with a history of syphilis during the first trimester of pregnancy, as evidenced by the seroconversion of her VDRL result (titer 1:4, previously nonreactive). The woman received one injection of 2.4 million units of benzathine penicillin. At delivery, her VDRL had a titer of 1:64. In evaluating this infant, the appropriate conclusion is that

A. the mother has been adequately treated, and the infant requires no further therapy

B. the infant has a high probability of having congenital syphilis and requires evaluation and treatment

C. if the infant's long bone radiographs show no abnormality, no treatment is indicated

D. this child may be given a shot of benzathine penicillin, and no further serologic evaluation is necessary

18. A 2.1 kg infant was born at term to a 20-year-old woman with no history of prenatal care. The maternal rapid plasma reagin test (RPR) result at delivery showed a titer of 1:32. The infant was completely normal on physical examination. In evaluating this infant, the most appropriate tests would be

   A. treponemal and nontreponemal serologic study of the infant's serum and CSF analysis including VDRL

   B. viral and bacterial cultures of CSF

   C. serologic tests for syphilis when the infant is 3 months of age

   D. complete blood count (CBC) and liver chemistry panel

19. *Nocardia* infection is an acute, subacute, or chronic suppurative infection that primarily causes pulmonary disease in immunocompromised patients. The hallmark of *Nocardia* infection is

   A. a tendency to remissions and exacerbations

   B. involvement of bone

   C. a self-limited disease with scar formation

   D. association in the pelvis with intrauterine device (IUD) placement

   E. an association with sickle cell disease

20. A 16-year-old female presents with signs and symptoms of appendicitis. Her past medical history is significant only for sexual activity and placement of an IUD 1 year previously. She undergoes an appendectomy, in which her appendix is found to be normal. One month postoperatively, she has local pain and has an irregular, hard mass in her ileocecal area. The most likely diagnosis is

   A. *Yersinia* pseudoappendicitis

   B. lymphoma

   C. inflammatory bowel disease

   D. pelvic actinomycosis

   E. amebiasis

21. A 2-year-old male with chronic granulomatous disease (CGD) presents with a history of multiple dental caries and a firm mandibular mass. He is experiencing localized pain and trismus. The mass is painless on palpation without erythema. The most likely diagnosis is

   A. staphylococcal preauricular lymphadenitis

   B. cervicofacial actinomycosis

   C. tuberculosis

   D. mandibular osteomyelitis

   E. nocardiosis

22. A 9-year-old male was diagnosed with a seizure disorder 1 year ago in El Paso, Texas. His seizures have been easily controlled, but he has since developed severe headaches. Computed tomography (CT) scan shows a punctate calcification and evidence of fourth ventricle enlargement. Serologic studies are positive for infection with *Taenia solium*. What is the most appropriate next step in treatment?

   A. Praziquantel, 50 mg/kg/day, then placement of a ventricular shunt

   B. Albendazole, 15 mg/kg/day plus prednisone

   C. Ventricular shunt

   D. Dexamethasone, 3 mg/kg

   E. Mebendazole, 100 mg b.i.d.

23. A 15-year-old female wishes to play soccer in school and needs medical clearance. On physical examination, her liver edge is palpable and seems minimally enlarged. Ultrasonography of the liver shows one cyst approximately 3 cm in diameter. Her menstruation is normal. Results of serologic tests for *Echinococcus* and hepatitis are negative, and liver enzyme values are normal. She has lived her whole life in Salt Lake City, Utah, and has never traveled abroad. Which factor is most important in allowing her to play this sport?

   A. Her travel history

   B. Negative echinococcal serology

   C. Negative hepatitis serology

   D. Normal liver enzymes

   E. Normal menstrual periods

24. ***Matching:*** Match the clinical syndrome or other information given with the appropriate classes of *Escherichia coli*

   1. Acute afebrile bloody diarrhea followed by development of hemolytic anemia, thrombocytopenia, and renal failure

   A. Enteropathogenic *E. coli* (EPEC)

   B. Enterotoxigenic *E. coli* (ETEC)

   C. Enteroinvasive *E. coli* (EIEC)

2. Large-volume watery stools without blood or mucus in an afebrile, acutely ill child who has recently returned from a trip to the developing world

3. Watery, nonbloody, afebrile diarrhea that persists for more than 2 weeks in a child recently returned from travel to the developing world

4. Acute diarrhea characterized by fever to 104°F, bloody mucous stool, painful defecation, abdominal pain, leukocytes identified in stool

5. *E. coli* 0157:H7, the only organisms detectable in routine hospital laboratories

6. The organisms that mimic shigellae in presentation

7. Produce a toxin closely related to the protein synthesis–inhibiting toxin of *Shigella dysenteriae* serotype 1; this toxin is thought to be responsible for the major manifestations of disease caused by this class of *E. coli*

8. Results of fecal leukocyte examination frequently positive

D. Entero-hemorrhagic *E. coli* (EHEC)

E. Entero-aggregative *E. coli* (EAggEC)

25. Many enteropathogens are not detected on stool culture by hospital laboratories unless the physician specifically requests testing for these pathogens. Which of the following are not commonly detected on standard culture media?

   A. Nontyphi salmonella, *Campylobacter jejuni*

   B. *Campylobacter coli*, *Shigella flexneri*

   C. *Aeromonas*, *Vibrio cholerae*

   D. *Shigella sonnei*, *Salmonella typhi*

   E. *E. coli* 0157:H7, *S. dysenteriae*

26. The prognosis in cholera is poor if

   A. illness is complicated by hypokalemia

   B. acidosis develops

   C. acute tubular necrosis develops

   D. tachycardia and tachypnea develop

   E. hypoglycemia and seizures occur

27. The differential diagnosis of diarrhea that persists for more than 2 weeks includes

   A. *S. dysenteriae* serotype 1, *V. cholerae*, *Pleisomonas shigelloides*

   B. enterotoxigenic *E. coli*, enterohemorrhagic *E. coli*

   C. enteropathogenic *E. coli*, enteroaggregative *E. coli*, nontyphi salmonella, *Aeromonas caviae*

   D. enteroinvasive *E. coli*, *Rotavirus*, Norwalk virus

   E. *C. jejuni*, *S. flexneri*, *Helicobacter pylori*

28. The best (most sensitive) culture specimen for diagnosing *S. typhi* (enteric fever) is

   A. blood

   B. stool

   C. cerebrospinal fluid

   D. gastric aspirate

   E. bone marrow aspirate

29. A 2-week illness characterized by gradually increasing fever that eventually reaches 104°F and is associated with headache, malaise, cough, and abdominal pain in a child who has recently returned from a visit to a developing country most likely is

   A. cholera

   B. diphtheria

   C. shigellosis

   D. typhoid fever

   E. tetanus

30. Antimotility agents have a role in therapy of acute diarrhea in infants and toddlers with gastroenteritis due to

    A. *Shigella*

    B. *Salmonella*

    C. enterohemorrhagic *E. coli*

    D. *Campylobacter*

    E. none of the above

31. Salmonella osteomyelitis is a common problem in children with

    A. sickle cell anemia

    B. animal contact

    C. a history of consuming unpasteurized milk

    D. prior antibiotic exposure

    E. sickle cell trait

32. Positive fecal leukocyte findings in a child with diarrhea allows the clinician to make a presumptive diagnosis of

    A. shigellosis

    B. *S. typhi*

    C. *Entamoeba histolytica*

    D. *Yersinia enterocolitica*

    E. colitis

33. Oral rehydration therapy is the treatment of choice for all children with gastroenteritis EXCEPT those with

    A. vomiting, high fever

    B. ileus, coma, or shock

    C. cholera

    D. shigellosis

    E. poor skin turgor, sunken fontanel, dry mouth, and decreased urine output

34. A 10-year-old child develops ascending paralysis with peripheral neuropathy (cranial nerves are normal); the CSF is normal except for an elevated protein level. The likely infectious agent precipitating this syndrome is

    A. *Corynebacterium diphtheriae*

    B. *Clostridium botulinum*

    C. *S. dysenteriae* serotype 1

    D. *Campylobacter jejuni*

    E. *Clostridium tetani*

35. **Part A.** A 10-year-old child presents with recurrent episodes of epigastric pain that occur at night and are relieved by antacids. He has also passed stools that look like road tar. Physical examination reveals positive stool guaiac results. The child has a hemoglobin of 8 g/dL. The most common infectious cause of this syndrome is

    A. *S. typhi*

    B. *C. jejuni*

    C. enteroaggregative *E. coli*

    D. *H. pylori*

    E. enterohemorrhagic *E. coli*

    Part B. Optimal therapy for this illness might include

    A. a third-generation cephalosporin such as cefotaxime given for 10 to 14 days

    B. erythromycin given orally for 5 days

    C. trimethoprim-sulfamethoxazole given orally for 5 days

    D. A bismuth compound, ampicillin, and metronidazole orally for 4 to 6 weeks

    E. antacids, H_2 blockers, diet manipulation, and psychotherapy

36. A 3-year-old male presents with a 12-hour history of severe watery diarrhea, sunken eyes, poor skin turgor, dry mouth, and anuria. He has no fever, polyuria, polydipsia, or polyphagia. Which of the following agents typically cause this syndrome?

    A. *S. dysenteriae*, enterohemorrhagic *E. coli*

    B. *S. typhi*, enteroinvasive *E. coli*

    C. Enterotoxigenic *E. coli*, *V. cholerae*

    D. *H. pylori*, *P. shigelloides*

37. A 20-month-old develops hemolytic anemia, anuria, azotemia, and thrombocytopenia after a bout of afebrile bloody diarrhea. What is the most likely cause of this illness?

    A. *C. jejuni*

    B. *S. typhi*

    C. Enterohemorrhagic *E. coli*

    D. *Aeromonas*

    E. Nontyphi *Salmonella*

38. A 10-month-old child presents with a temperature of 105°F, watery diarrhea, and a generalized seizure. The most likely cause of this syndrome is

A. *Salmonella* gastroenteritis

B. *Aeromonas* gastroenteritis

C. *Shigella* gastroenteritis

D. *Rotavirus* gastroenteritis

E. drug ingestion

39. Which one of the following statements is true about shigellosis?

   A. Neurologic complications occur in about 40% of patients.

   B. Animal reservoirs include poultry and shellfish.

   C. Neomycin, orally, is the antibiotic of choice.

   D. Bacteremia is common.

   E. The disease is rare in institutions for the retarded.

40. Hemorrhagic cystitis, conjunctivitis, pneumonia, and diarrhea all have been linked to which one of the following?

   A. Respiratory syncytial virus

   B. Adenovirus

   C. Rhinovirus

   D. Herpesvirus

   E. Parainfluenza virus

41. A 14-year-old farmer's son comes to the emergency room 26 hours after he tripped over a barbed wire fence and fell into a pile of cow manure, sustaining a puncture wound of his right hand. His parents tell you that he had "one, maybe two, baby shots" but none in recent memory. Appropriate treatment for this boy would include all of the following EXCEPT

   A. thorough washing and débridement of the wound

   B. administration of penicillin

   C. administration of tetanus immune globulin

   D. administration of tetanus toxoid and diphtheria toxoid (Td)

   E. hyperbaric oxygen

42. Congenital rubella syndrome is associated with which of the following?

   A. Patent ductus arteriosus (PDA) and branch pulmonary artery stenosis

   B. Ventricular septal defect (VSD) and PDA

C. Atrial septal defect (ASD) and PDA

D. VSD and ASD

E. VSD and pulmonary artery stenosis

43. Toxoplasmosis causes all of the following patterns of disease EXCEPT

   A. congenital infection in neonates manifested by chorioretinitis, cerebral calcifications, and hydrocephalus due to first-trimester infection

   B. congenital infection in neonates who appear normal at birth but become blind in adolescence because they have retinal (macular) lesions that recrudesce at that time. This infection was due to third-trimester infection

   C. brain abscess that results in confusion, seizures, and paralysis in a patient with acquired immunodeficiency syndrome (AIDS)

   D. asymptomatic acute infection in a pregnant woman that places her unborn child at significant risk for congenital toxoplasmosis

   E. myocarditis in a previously healthy young adult

   F. pectoral lymphadenopathy that is mistaken for breast cancer in a middle-aged woman

   G. congenital malformations, such as cleft palate

44. All of the following statements about cat-scratch disease are true EXCEPT that

   A. the majority of patients are younger than 21 years

   B. cat-scratch disease occurs worldwide

   C. cases are more prevalent in fall and winter in temperate zones

   D. it is observed more often in African-American children

45. Which procedure is most likely to yield *Pneumocystis carinii* from a patient with pneumonia caused by this organism?

   A. Bronchoalveolar lavage

   B. Induced sputum

   C. Hypopharyngeal swab

   D. Blood culture

   E. Gastric aspiration

46. Patients who should receive prophylaxis for *P. carinii* pneumonia are those afflicted with

    A. X-linked agammaglobulinemia

    B. severe combined immunodeficiency disorder

    C. chronic granulomatous disease

    D. sickle cell disease

    E. congenital neutropenia

47. The drug of choice for the treatment of *P. carinii* pneumonia is

    A. trimethoprim-sulfamethoxazole

    B. pentamidine isethionate

    C. amphotericin B

    D. acyclovir

    E. zidovudine

48. Which of the following is the most likely cause of bilateral diffuse pneumonitis in a patient with AIDS?

    A. *Mycobacterium avium-intracellulare*

    B. *Candida albicans*

    C. *Cryptococcus neoformans*

    D. *Pneumocystis carinii*

    E. *Streptococcus pneumoniae*

49. A 4-year-old male is brought to your office because of a circular reddish rash under his armpit. The child has been afebrile and has had no other systemic symptoms. The rash is not pruritic. The child's parents state that they have recently returned from a vacation in Massachusetts on Cape Cod and that a small tick had been removed from the same area where the rash is now. The only abnormality on the examination is the circular, flat, erythematous rash that is about 6 cm in diameter and is not tender. The appropriate next step in treating this patient is to

    A. order a test for serum antibodies against *Borrelia burgdorferi* to confirm that the child has Lyme disease

    B. begin treatment with doxycycline

    C. begin treatment with amoxicillin

    D. begin treatment with ceftriaxone

    E. perform a lumbar puncture to be certain that the child's central nervous system (CNS) is not involved

50. A 12-year-old male is brought to you by his mother, who is concerned that he has Lyme disease. The child has not been to an area where Lyme disease is endemic, but his parents have friends with similar symptoms who are being treated for Lyme disease. The major symptoms are chronic fatigue and intermittent headaches and arthralgias. He does well in school despite frequent absences. His parents were divorced 2 years ago, but he sees both parents regularly. He has received several courses of amoxicillin for sore throats and seems to feel better while he takes the antibiotic. He has had no arthritis or rashes. Findings on the physical examination are normal. The next appropriate step in the treatment of this patient is to

    A. order a test for serum antibodies against *B. burgdorferi*

    B. begin treatment with doxycycline

    C. begin treatment with amoxicillin

    D. begin treatment with ceftriaxone

    E. discuss further with his mother why she thinks this child has Lyme disease

51. A 6-year-old child is brought to your office because a tiny tick was found and removed from his forearm. The parents are unsure how long the tick had been attached, although they thought that it probably had not been there for more than 1 day. They live in an area where Lyme disease is common. The next step in the proper treatment of this patient should be to

    A. send the tick to be tested for infection with *B. burgdorferi*

    B. reassure the parents that the risk of infection is small and have them observe the area around the bite for the development of a rash

    C. begin prophylactic treatment with amoxicillin

    D. order a serologic test for antibodies against *B. burgdorferi* in the child

    E. wait 1 month and then order a serologic test for antibodies against *B. burgdorferi* in the child

52. Nodular lymphangitis in a child bitten by a cat is most likely caused by

    A. *Mycobacterium marinum*

    B. *Sporothrix schenckii*

    C. *Pasteurella multocida*

    D. *Nocardia brasiliensis*

    E. *Aeromonas hydrophilia*

53. Cryptococcosis occurs most often in

    A. infants

    B. children with diabetes

    C. HIV-infected children

    D. organ transplant recipients

    E. bone marrow transplant recipients

54. Primary pulmonary histoplasmosis in normal children is usually

    A. asymptomatic

    B. associated with severe flulike symptoms

    C. treated with assisted ventilation and steroid therapy

    D. associated with a sarcoid-like disease

    E. complicated by mediastinal fibrosis

55. All of the following are requirements for the diagnosis of allergic bronchopulmonary aspergillosis, EXCEPT

    A. asthma

    B. cutaneous reactivity to *Aspergillus fumigatus* antigens

    C. elevated serum IgE level

    D. peripheral eosinophilia

    E. hyperexpansion and hilar adenopathy

56. A small-for-gestational-age infant with congenital toxoplasmosis has obstruction of the aqueduct of Sylvius and consequent hydrocephalus. In addition to a ventricular peritoneal shunt, the most appropriate next step is to treat this patient with

    A. spiramycin

    B. spiramycin and leucovorin

    C. trimethoprim-sulfamethoxazole

    D. pyrimethamine, sulfadiazine, and leucovorin

    E. clindamycin and quinidine

57. All of the following are consistent with the diagnosis of congenital toxoplasmosis in an infant EXCEPT

    A. an infant with normal findings on newborn evaluation

    B. an infant who is small for gestational age

    C. a CSF protein level of 3 g/dL

    D. an infant whose mother has no serologic evidence of *Toxoplasma gondii* infection

    E. an infant whose mother has AIDS and is chronically infected with *T. gondii*

58. The most likely meningococcal serogroup to cause meningitis in a 5-month-old infant in the United States is serogroup

    A. A

    B. Y

    C. C

    D. B

    E. W-135

59. *T. gondii* is acquired by all of the following means EXCEPT

    A. ingestion of oocysts excreted by cats

    B. ingestion of oocysts excreted by dogs

    C. ingestion of cysts in undercooked meat

    D. transplacental transmission from an acutely infected mother to her fetus in utero

    E. organ transplantation of an infected heart to a previously uninfected recipient

60. Which of the following statements about *T. gondii* is FALSE?

    A. *T. gondii* transmitted in the first trimester causes the most severe disease in the infant.

    B. *T. gondii* transmitted in the third trimester very frequently causes chorioretinitis even if the infant appears normal at birth.

    C. *T. gondii* may cause lymphadenopathy in older children and adults.

    D. *T. gondii* may cause severe disseminated disease in immunocompromised children.

    E. *T. gondii* causes sinusitis and otitis media.

61. A 5-month-old previously healthy female is brought to her pediatrician because of fever, irritability, and poor feeding. She is the second child in her daycare center to be diagnosed with meningitis within a week. She has received all recommended immunizations. The most likely cause of her meningitis is

    A. *Haemophilus influenzae*

    B. *Neisseria meningitidis*

    C. group B streptococci

D. herpes simplex virus

E. *Listeria monocytogenes*

62. A 3-year-old male presents to the emergency department with a 1-day history of fever, headache, and myalgia. On examination, he is found to be lethargic and hypotensive. He has signs of meningeal irritation. A petechial and purpural rash is spreading rapidly on his trunk, face, and extremities. He has received all recommended immunizations. The most likely finding on Gram stain of the CSF is

A. large gram-negative rods

B. small pleomorphic gram-negative coccobacilli

C. gram-negative diplococci

D. gram-positive diplococci

E. gram-positive cocci in clusters

63. The Fitz-Hugh–Curtis syndrome is characterized by

A. right upper quadrant pain caused by gonococcal perihepatitis

B. polyarticular arthritis and rash of disseminated gonococcal infection

C. lower quadrant pain caused by gonococcal endometritis

D. gonococcal meningitis

E. monoarticular arthritis and urethral exudate caused by *N. gonorrhoeae*

64. Disseminated gonococcal infection in neonates usually occurs as

A. pneumonia

B. endocarditis

C. meningitis

D. septic arthritis

E. osteomyelitis

65. The drug that is recommended as initial therapy for disseminated gonococcal disease in children and adults is

A. penicillin

B. tetracycline

C. ceftriaxone

D. cefazolin

E. erythromycin

66. The drug that is recommended as initial therapy for nondisseminated gonococcal disease in children and adults is

A. penicillin

B. tetracycline

C. ceftriaxone

D. cefazolin

E. erythromycin

67. The source of the papillomavirus in most cases of juvenile-onset recurrent respiratory papillomatosis is

A. intrauterine exposure to infected amniotic fluid

B. sexual abuse in early childhood

C. close contact with other children with cutaneous warts and subsequent autoinoculation

D. intrapartum exposure to maternal genital lesions

68. Confirmation that an atypical-appearing lesion is caused by a human papillomavirus is best achieved by

A. a serologic test for papillomavirus antibodies

B. histologic examination of a lesion biopsy sample

C. culture of the lesion for papillomavirus

D. detection of papillomavirus antigens in a lesion scraping

69. The equine preparation of diphtheria antitoxin is indicated for which of the following individuals?

A. A patient in whom the clinical diagnosis of respiratory tract diphtheria is suspected but not proved

B. An asymptomatic household contact of a documented case, who is not immunized

C. An asymptomatic contact who is proved to be a carrier and who is not immunized

D. An asymptomatic nurse who is caring for a patient with respiratory tract diphtheria who has not received a booster of toxoid vaccine for more than 10 years

70. The largest subpopulation of individuals in the United States with nonprotective levels of diphtheria antitoxin is

A. infants younger than 2 months

B. children older than 2 years

C. children 2 to 5 years of age

D. individuals 5 to 14 years of age

E. individuals older than 60 years

71. Compared with respiratory tract diphtheria, cutaneous diphtheria is associated with

A. shorter duration of shedding of organisms

B. less contamination of the environment

C. greater transmission to close contacts

D. similar incidence of toxic complications

72. Diphtheria-producing strains of *C. diphtheriae* are distinguished from non–diphtheria-producing strains by

A. colony morphology

B. microscopic appearance

C. biochemical tests

D. biotype

E. immunoprecipitin test

73. Identification of an organism isolated from a patient as *Coccidioides immitis* can be accomplished by the following methods, but the most rapid is

A. inoculation of a mouse to produce endosporulating spherules

B. conversion of the hyphal to the spherule/endospore form in vitro

C. use of a DNA probe for coccidioidal RNA

D. exoantigen test for specific antigens

E. demonstration of germination of hyphae from a spherule

74. Systemic antifungal medication should be administered in all instances of coccidioidomycosis EXCEPT in

A. benign clinical pneumonitis

B. patients with AIDS

C. coccidioidomycosis meningitis

D. other extrapulmonary disease

75. Coccidioidomycosis is transmitted ("contagious") by which mechanism?

A. Exposure to contaminated soil

B. Human-to-human aerosols

C. Blood-borne transmission

D. Insect vectors

76. Because cerebral malaria can be fatal in as little as 24 hours, in any child having suggestive symptoms and/or history of recent tropical travel, what confirmatory procedure should immediately be invoked?

A. Serologic testing for specific antibodies

B. CT scan of the brain

C. Urinalysis for hematuria

D. Temperature readings at 6-hour intervals to ascertain fever intermittency

E. Microscopic examination of blood films

77. The first choice of treatment for a child admitted with a diagnosis of cerebral malaria should be

A. quinine or quinidine parenterally

B. chloroquine

C. tetracycline

D. pyrimethamine-sulfadoxine combination parenterally

E. primaquine for a 14-day course

78. Although malaria can be transmitted to a child through a blood transfusion or congenitally, the natural method of transmission is by

A. ingestion of contaminated food or water

B. inhalation of gas arising from a tropical swamp

C. the bite of a tsetse fly

D. the bite of an *Anopheles* mosquito

E. inhalation of airborne parasites

79. A child who returned 2 weeks ago from equatorial Africa is admitted in a coma, with high fever and a palpable spleen. The liver is not enlarged. Laboratory studies reveal hypoglycemia, but the CSF is essentially normal. An immediate working diagnosis would be

A. pancreatic neoplasm

B. pneumococcal meningitis

C. falciparum malaria

D. visceral leishmaniasis

E. dengue hemorrhagic fever

80. A 15-year-old male presents to your office with complaint of fever, malaise, headache, cough, and shortness of breath. A chest radiograph reveals left upper and lower lobe

infiltrates. His WBC count is elevated. He states he recently received a pet cockatiel that became ill and died. What is the most likely diagnosis?

A. *Mycoplasma* pneumonia

B. Pneumococcal pneumonia

C. Psittacosis

D. Q fever

E. Legionnaires' disease

81. What is the most appropriate step in the diagnosis of the case described in Question 80?

A. Blood culture

B. Routine throat culture

C. Sera sampling for chlamydial complement fixation (CF) test

D. Sputum or throat culture for *Chlamydia*

E. Viral cultures

82. A 5-year-old female with sickle cell disease is brought to the emergency room with a complaint of fever, cough, and difficulty breathing. A chest radiograph reveals a right middle lobe infiltrate. Her CBC is unremarkable. She has received Pneumovax and is currently on penicillin prophylaxis. Her pneumonia is most likely caused by

A. *Chlamydia pneumoniae*

B. *Mycoplasma pneumoniae*

C. a virus

D. all of the above

E. none of the above

83. What is the most appropriate presumptive treatment for the patient described in Question 82?

A. Penicillin

B. Amoxicillin

C. Cefaclor

D. Augmentin

E. Erythromycin

84. Which of the following tests can be used for the detection of *Chlamydia trachomatis* infection in the evaluation of suspected child sexual abuse?

A. Culture

B. DNA probe

C. Enzyme immunoassay (EIA)

D. Direct fluorescent antibody (DFA)

E. PCR

85. You are evaluating a 3-year-old female for suspected sexual abuse. She is asymptomatic. *C. trachomatis* is isolated from a vaginal culture. How could the child have acquired the infection?

A. From her mother at delivery

B. By sexual contact

C. Both of the above

D. None of the above

86. By what routes can infants acquire *C. trachomatis* infection?

A. Vertically from the mother at delivery

B. By respiratory droplets from other infants

C. Horizontally from the mother after birth

D. Horizontally from other family members after birth

E. From fomites

87. Which of the following statements about tests for antibodies against *B. burgdorferi* is true?

A. They are useful to determine whether an erythematous annular rash is erythema migrans, nummular eczema, or ringworm.

B. They should be routinely performed on children in endemic areas who present with fatigue and arthralgia.

C. They are useful to determine whether children with Lyme disease need additional antimicrobial treatment.

D. They commonly yield false-positive results, especially when performed on patients with nonspecific symptoms.

88. Which of the following statements correctly describes the proper treatment for children who are bitten by a deer tick?

A. They should routinely receive a course of antimicrobial prophylaxis.

B. They should be tested for antibodies against *B. burgdorferi* 4 to 6 weeks later and be treated if the test result is positive.

C. They should be observed for the development of erythema migrans at the site of the bite and be treated if this rash develops.

D. They should be treated if the tick that bit them tests positive for *B. burgdorferi*.

89. Which of the following statements about children who develop Lyme disease is true?

    A. A deer tick has usually been found on them in the preceding several weeks.

    B. They usually can be cured with a simple course of orally administered antimicrobials.

    C. They should have a determination of the concentration of antibodies against *B. burgdorferi* at follow-up.

    D. They should have regular slit-lamp examinations performed by an ophthalmologist to check for uveitis.

90. The most common clinical manifestation of *atypical* cat-scratch disease is

    A. seizures and coma

    B. systemic disease

    C. erythema nodosum

    D. oculoglandular syndrome of Parinaud

    E. neuroretinitis

91. The most common sites of adenopathy in cat-scratch disease are

    A. the head and neck in children

    B. multiple sites

    C. axillary in children

    D. the head and neck in adults

92. All of the following are true of cat-scratch disease EXCEPT that

    A. lymph nodes are tender in 80% of patients

    B. lymph nodes vary in size from 1 to 12 cm

    C. fever ($\geq$ 38.1°C) occurs in 90% of patients

    D. malaise and fatigue occur in 30% of patients

    E. splenomegaly occurs in 9% of patients

93. The incubation period for lymphadenopathy due to cat-scratch disease is variable. The average (and range) in days is

    A. 4 (1 to 7)

    B. 5 (2 to 9)

    C. 12 (5 to 60)

    D. 21 (10 to 80)

94. Cat contact/scratch occurs in what percent of patients with cat-scratch disease?

    A. 75% contact/25% scratches

    B. 90% contact/40% scratches

    C. 95% contact/75% scratches

    D. 100% contact/90% scratches

95. The cause of cat-scratch disease is

    A. a myxovirus

    B. a gram-positive pleomorphic bacillus

    C. unknown

    D. filamentous branching bacilli staining gram-negative and with silver stains (Warthin-Starry)

    E. mycobacteria

96. Which of the following statements correctly describes children with Lyme arthritis?

    A. They should be treated with orally administered amoxicillin or tetracycline.

    B. They should be hospitalized and treated with intravenously administered ceftriaxone or penicillin for 4 to 6 weeks.

    C. They frequently experience recurrent attacks of arthritis for years despite appropriate antimicrobial treatment.

    D. They require biopsy confirmation of erythema chronicum migrans.

97. Which of the following routes of transmission has been associated with several large outbreaks of human listeriosis?

    A. Aerosol transmission

    B. Person-to-person spread

    C. Zoonotic transmission

    D. Drinking contaminated water

    E. Food-borne transmission

98. All of the following are characteristic features of early-onset neonatal listeriosis EXCEPT

    A. premature labor in the mother

    B. isolation of *Listeria* from the mother

    C. maternal obstetric complication

    D. neonatal meningitis

    E. neonatal mortality exceeding 30%

99. All of the following are useful in establishing

a diagnosis of early-onset neonatal listeriosis EXCEPT

A. placental histology and culture

B. blood and CSF cultures from the newborn

C. maternal vaginal cultures

D. acute and convalescent blood for serologic study

E. alerting the laboratory to a suspected case

100. Which of the following antimicrobial regimens is NOT appropriate for treating brucellosis in a 10-year-old child?

A. Doxycycline plus streptomycin

B. Doxycycline plus gentamicin

C. Trimethoprim-sulfamethoxazole plus rifampin

D. Ceftriaxone

E. Tetracycline

101. Which of the following pairs of agglutination titers is most consistent with successful therapy for brucellosis?

A. IgM 1:8   IgG 1:256

B. IgM 1:128   IgG 1:8

C. IgM 1:256   IgG 1:512

D. IgM <1:2   IgG <1:2

E. IgM <1:2   IgG 1:128

102. All of the following statements about the isolation of *Brucella* species are true EXCEPT that

A. the lysis centrifugation method for blood cultures may improve the isolation rate

B. blood cultures should be held for as long as 4 weeks

C. culture diagnosis is improved by culturing bone marrow

D. common commercial media may be used for the isolation of *Brucella* species

E. anaerobic cultures improve the isolation of *Brucella* species

103. A 2-year-old child presents with signs and symptoms of brucellosis and a history of eating unpasteurized goat cheese. Which of the following species of *Brucella* is the most likely cause?

A. *Brucella abortus*

B. *Brucella suis*

C. *Brucella neotomae*

D. *Brucella melitensis*

E. *Brucella ovis*

104. Which of the following statements about plague is FALSE?

A. The etiologic agent is *Yersinia pestis*.

B. It is endemic in the southwestern United States.

C. It most often presents as bubonic plague.

D. Children in endemic areas should be routinely immunized.

E. The case-fatality rate is highest outside the endemic area.

105. Which of the following diagnostic tests is LEAST useful in establishing a diagnosis of mesenteric adenitis due to *Yersinia pseudotuberculosis*?

A. Stool culture

B. Mesenteric lymph node histology

C. Abdominal ultrasonography

D. Mesenteric lymph node culture

E. Endoscopy

106. Which of the following syndromes is most likely due to *Y. pseudotuberculosis?*

A. Solitary pulmonary calcification

B. Acute-onset watery diarrhea

C. Pseudoappendicitis without diarrhea

D. Plague

E. Acute gastritis

107. Enterocolitis due to *Y. enterocolitica* is most similar to diarrheal disease due to which of the following pathogens?

A. Enterotoxigenic *E. coli*

B. *S. sonnei*

C. *V. cholerae*

D. *Giardia lamblia*

E. *Rotavirus*

108. Which of the following blood products has been shown to be of greatest risk in transfusion-associated disease due to *Y. enterocolitica*?

A. Albumin

B. Fresh frozen plasma

C. Platelet concentrates

D. Intravenous immune globulin

E. Packed RBCs after 2-week storage

109. Which of the following diagnostic tests is most useful in the diagnosis and management of tularemia?

    A. Gram stain of involved lymph nodes

    B. Blood cultures

    C. Inoculation of guinea pig with ulcer material

    D. Serum agglutination test

    E. Skin test

110. Which of the following clinical syndromes is the most common clinical presentation of tularemia in children?

    A. Ulceroglandular disease

    B. Oropharyngeal disease

    C. Oculoglandular disease

    D. Glandular disease

    E. Typhoidal disease

111. All of the following have been shown to be routes of transmission for tularemia EXCEPT

    A. the bite of an infected tick

    B. the bite of a mosquito

    C. aerosol transmission from haying

    D. drinking contaminated water

    E. person-to-person transmission

112. On examining a full-term newborn, the physician noted mild hepatomegaly. The remainder of the physical findings were normal, including head circumference and retinas. A urine culture grew cytomegalovirus (CMV). Results of head ultrasonography were normal. Subsequent testing disclosed no metabolic disorders. What deficit is most likely to occur in the next year?

    A. Visual loss

    B. Hearing loss

    C. Cirrhosis

    D. Patent ductus arteriosus

    E. Immunoglobulin deficiency

113. Techniques for prenatal diagnosis include amniocentesis, cordocentesis, and chorionic villus sampling. These techniques have proved themselves very useful for early diagnosis of both genetic and infectious diseases. Unfortunately, each technique has some morbidity. Which one of the following is an unusual but serious complication of chorionic villus sampling?

    A. Hydrocephalus

    B. Limb anomalies

    C. Heart defects

    D. Hepatitis

    E. Bladder anomalies

114. Varicella-zoster virus is one of the human herpesviruses. When a pregnant woman contracts chickenpox during early gestation, her fetus can be infected. In turn, the infected fetus may be severely affected. If you were counseling a woman with gestational chickenpox, what percent value is a reasonable estimate of risk that her fetus will develop a major defect?

    A. Greater than 75%

    B. 50%

    C. 25%

    D. 10%

    E. Less than 5%

115. During one springtime, an infectious disease spread through a small community in the United States. The main signs and symptoms were fever, mild rash, and arthralgia. One pregnant woman in late gestation contracted the illness but recovered without difficulty. However, 1 month later she was delivered of a stillborn infant. The pathology report listed the diagnosis "hydrops fetalis." What is the most likely infectious disease?

    A. Congenital rubella virus

    B. Congenital CMV

    C. Congenital parvovirus

    D. Congenital HSV

    E. Congenital HIV

116. A baby is returned to the outpatient clinic at day 9 of life because of lethargy. On examination, a few vesicles are observed on the scalp. A rapid virology test confirms the diagnosis of HSV type 2. The baby should be admitted to the hospital and begun on which one of the following antiviral compounds?

    A. Ribavirin

B. Acyclovir

C. Ganciclovir

D. Amantadine

E. Zidovudine

117. HSV type 2 and varicella-zoster virus are human herpesviruses. Both viruses can cause congenital infections, especially when a pregnant woman has primary infection during the first trimester. The stigmata can be similar enough that the diagnosis is occasionally confusing. Which one of the following stigmata is strongly associated with congenital varicella infection only?

A. Encephalitis

B. Chorioretinitis

C. Microcephaly

D. Limb hypoplasia

E. Vesicular skin lesions

118. Rubella virus is one of the most teratogenic agents. Therefore, if an unimmunized pregnant female contracts a rubella infection, the risk of fetal damage is high. Because of lowered immunization rates, rubella has occurred more commonly in the 1990s, and a few new cases of congenital rubella are again being seen. CMV also can cause congenital infections with severe stigmata. Which one of the following problems in an infant is much more strongly associated with congenital rubella than congenital CMV infection?

A. Structural cardiac defects

B. Hearing loss

C. Hepatitis

D. Retinopathy

E. Encephalitis

119. An HIV-seropositive female comes to her physician for advice because she is pregnant. She has never been on any antiviral medication because she had remained healthy without symptoms of AIDS. However, she wonders whether antiviral treatment might diminish the likelihood of fetal HIV infection. Which one of the following statements is correct?

A. Treatment of the pregnant woman will produce maternal thrombocytopenia.

B. Treatment will result in viral resistance in all infected infants.

C. Treatment will decrease the likelihood of fetal infection but adversely affect the woman, so it should be avoided.

D. Treatment will decrease the likelihood of fetal infection by greater than 50%.

E. Treatment will adversely affect the fetus and should be avoided.

120. Which of the following descriptions concerning poliomyelitis is INCORRECT?

A. Sensory impairment is quite unusual but may rarely occur in paralytic poliomyelitis.

B. Difficulty in swallowing is the cardinal sign in bulbar poliomyelitis.

C. In the preparalytic stage of the major illness, the symptoms simulate those of aseptic meningitis.

D. CSF obtained during the meningitis stage of poliomyelitis often yields poliovirus in culture.

E. Poliovirus may be isolated from stools up to several months after acute illness.

121. A 5-year-old urban male was admitted to the hospital because of low-grade fever, flaccid paralysis of both legs, sensory changes, and absent ankle deep tendon reflexes. The child had received only two immunizations with TOPV at the age of 2 and 6 months. His diagnosis is most probably

A. acute paralytic poliomyelitis due to wild poliovirus

B. paralysis due to nonpolio enteroviruses

C. vaccine-associated poliomyelitis

D. Guillain-Barré syndrome

E. tick-bite paralysis

122. A 4-year-old child was seen by his physician because of fever, cervical lymphadenopathy, small ulcerative lesions on his buccal mucosa, and small vesicles on his fingers. Which of the following examinations would be most helpful in the diagnosis?

A. Serum IgG and IgM antirubella antibodies

B. IgM antibodies against measles virus in the serum

C. Throat and stool culture for enterovirus

D. Antistreptolysin-O titer in serum

E. Herpes simplex titers

123. All of the following statements are true of enteroviruses EXCEPT that

    A. enteroviruses are RNA viruses belonging to the Picornaviridae family

    B. enteroviruses lose activity within several hours at room temperature

    C. humans are the only natural host of human enteroviruses

    D. about 70 enteroviral types have been identified

    E. enteroviruses are spread from person to person by fecal-oral and possibly oral-oral (respiratory) routes

124. *Matching:* Match each syndrome with the appropriate parasite exposure history.

    1. Cercarial dermatitis

    2. Eosinophilic meningitis

    3. Jaundice, biliary stricture, and cholangiocarcinoma

    4. Iron deficiency anemia and protein malnutrition

    5. Fever, jaundice, eosinophilia, and multiple hypodense lesions on imaging of the liver

    A. Consumption of uncooked snails infested with *Angiostrongylus*

    B. Prolonged residence in Southeast Asia, consumption of raw fish

    C. Walking barefoot in hookworm-endemic areas

    D. Wading in freshwater streams infested with *Schistosoma mansoni*

    E. Consumption of wild watercress sandwiches in areas endemic for *Fasciola hepatica*

125. On a global basis, what are the odds of any child's having a hookworm infection?

    A. Less than 1%

    B. 5% to 10%

    C. 10% to 15%

    D. 20% to 25%

    E. Greater than 50%

126. A 10-year-old Korean female presents in stupor after a new-onset seizure. CNS imaging shows a distinct, contrast-enhancing, frontoparietal lesion. Careful CSF examination shows an eosinophilic pleocytosis. History from the parents reveals a past history of hemoptysis and a dietary history of ingesting food flavored with raw crab juice. The most likely cause of this girl's lesion is

    A. *Gnathostoma* species

    B. *Angiostrongylus cantonensis*

    C. *Paragonimus westermani*

    D. *Trichinella spiralis*

    E. tuberculous meningitis

127. The 12-year-old son of diplomat parents presents with crampy abdominal pain, fever, migratory arthralgias, and hepatosplenomegaly. During the past 5 years, his family has lived in the Philippines, Kampuchea, Senegal, and Mali. Ultrasound examination of his abdomen shows periportal fibrosis consistent with schistosomiasis. His kidneys and bladder are normal. Which of the following schistosome species is UNLIKELY to be the cause of his illness?

    A. *Schistosoma mansoni*

    B. *Schistosoma japonicum*

    C. *Schistosoma intercalatum*

    D. *Schistosoma haematobium*

    E. *Schistosoma mekongi*

128. Which of the following therapeutic options is the optimal method to manage symptomatic nontuberculous mycobacterial lymphadenitis?

    A. Complete surgical excision

    B. Isoniazid and rifampin for 6 months

    C. Await suppuration, then incise and drain

    D. Perform partial biopsy, begin antituberculous therapy

    E. Oral clarithromycin until the swelling resolves

129. A 3-year-old female with AIDS has developed fever, night sweats, anorexia, weight loss, and generalized lymphadenopathy. She has continued taking trimethoprim-sulfamethoxazole prophylaxis, and her CD4 cell count is 50/mm^3. The likely cause of her illness is

    A. *P. carinii* pneumonia

    B. Kaposi's sarcoma

    C. *Staphylococcus aureus* sepsis

    D. disseminated *M. avium* complex infection

    E. CMV retinitis

130. A 3-year-old male from Mississippi presents with a 1.8-cm left superior anterior cervical mass that is firm and nontender. The swelling has progressed for 2 weeks. He has no other symptoms and has had no exposure to tuberculosis. His chest roentgenogram findings are negative, and an intermediate-strength purified protein derivative (PPD) skin test results in 8 mm induration at 48 hours. The most likely diagnosis is

    A. rhabdomyosarcoma

    B. *Mycobacterium tuberculosis* lymphadenitis

    C. *M. avium* complex lymphadenitis

    D. *S. aureus* lymphadenitis

    E. cat-scratch disease lymphadenitis

131. A 14-year-old male with previously normal health presents in August with a 2-week history of progressive cough, low-grade fever, headache, and generalized malaise. His total WBC count is 11,000/mm^3 with a normal differential, and his chest roentgenogram reveals left and right perihilar infiltrates. The likely cause of this illness is

    A. *S. pneumoniae*

    B. *M. pneumoniae*

    C. *S. aureus*

    D. *M. avium*

    E. influenza virus

132. Which of the following problems is NOT a recognized complication of *M. pneumoniae* infection?

    A. Meningoencephalitis

    B. Stevens-Johnson syndrome

    C. Hepatitis

    D. Arthritis

    E. Osteomyelitis

133. An 8-year-old is brought to your office because of high fever, fatigue, and a peculiar discoloration of his skin. On examination, he is pale with yellowish skin. He has generalized adenopathy. His family just returned 2 weeks ago from a 3-week trek through the Peruvian Andes. Laboratory evaluation reveals severe anemia. Giemsa stain shows rodlike forms in the erythrocytes. The most likely diagnosis is

    A. leishmaniasis

    B. salmonellosis

    C. bartonellosis

    D. malaria

134. The most common systemic fungal infection in immunosuppressed patients with leukemia is

    A. aspergillosis

    B. candidiasis

    C. mucormycosis

    D. histoplasmosis

    E. coccidioidomycosis

135. A blood specimen was obtained for culture from a 6-year-old male with acute lymphocytic leukemia at the time of admission for a febrile episode. The absolute neutrophil count was 100 mm^3. Within 24 hours, microbial growth was obvious in the blood culture. The most likely organism and the drug to which it would be susceptible are

    A. *C. albicans*: amphotericin B

    B. *Staphylococcus epidermidis*: vancomycin

    C. *S. epidermidis*: ceftazidime

    D. *Pseudomonas aeruginosa*: cefuroxime

    E. *P. aeruginosa*: cefotaxime

136. When would the removal of central venous Broviac-Hickman catheters be indicated?

    A. Immediately on onset of fever

    B. In febrile episodes and tunnel track infection with *C. albicans* and candidemia

    C. In febrile episodes with *S. epidermidis* bacteremia

    D. In febrile episodes with *E. coli* bacteremia

    E. In colonization of the exit site with *Bacillus* species

137. Which of the following vaccines should NOT be given to children with severe combined immunodeficiency syndrome?

    A. DTP vaccine

    B. Measles virus vaccine

    C. Salk poliovirus vaccine

    D. Hepatitis B virus vaccine

    E. Pneumococcal vaccine

138. A 6-month-old breast-fed infant presents with a 24-hour history of diarrhea but no

emesis. On examination, the child is afebrile, has normal vital signs, but has slightly sunken eyes and fontanel. She continues to nurse fairly well. The most appropriate therapy is

A. slow intravenous rehydration and nothing by mouth

B. clear liquid diet for 24 hours, followed by dilute formula or breast milk for several days until stools reduce in frequency

C. rapid infusion of intravenous saline

D. oral electrolyte solution given by mouth to make up a 5% to 10% volume deficit over 6 hours and continuation of breast-feeding

E. begin tincture of opium or Imodium

139. For which person is a 6-mm tuberculin skin test reaction considered positive, likely indicating tuberculous infection?

A. A 3-year-old who received bacillus Calmette-Guérin (BCG) vaccine as a newborn

B. An 8-year-old whose skin test reaction last year was 0 mm

C. A 2-year-old whose asymptomatic father is a prison guard

D. A 3-year-old whose mother has acid-fast bacilli in her sputum smear

E. A 10-year-old who was born in Vietnam

140. The best management for a child born to a mother with a positive tuberculin skin test result, normal findings on a chest radiograph, and no symptoms is to

A. immediately isolate the infant from the mother

B. give the child BCG vaccination

C. permit contact between the mother and child; do not treat the child, but try to evaluate other family members for tuberculosis

D. start the baby on isoniazid and rifampin

E. give the baby isoniazid until the mother finishes treatment

141. All of the following are risk factors for tuberculous infection in a small child EXCEPT

A. birth in a country with high rates of tuberculosis

B. having a father who just left a state prison

C. exposure to a child with primary pulmonary tuberculosis

D. HIV infection in the mother and father

E. having an uncle with hemoptysis and pneumonia

142. Which statement applies to a 2-year-old female whose father has been diagnosed with pulmonary tuberculosis in the past 2 weeks?

A. A tuberculin skin test reaction less than 15 mm indicates that she is at no risk for tuberculous disease.

B. Contact with her father should be stopped immediately.

C. She should receive a tuberculin skin test and chest radiograph and begin treatment only if results of one or both are positive.

D. She should be started on isoniazid therapy even if her skin test result is nonreactive and her findings on a chest radiograph are normal.

143. Examination of nail fold capillaries using an ophthalmoscope can be helpful in making a diagnosis of

A. visceral larva migrans

B. connective tissue diseases

C. Kawasaki syndrome

D. rheumatic fever

E. shock

144. A severe systemic response to any kind of microorganism is called sepsis. The systemic immune responses syndrome (SIRS) can be triggered by bacteria, viruses, fungi, or parasites. Which of the following systems are activated in SIRS?

A. Coagulation

B. Complement

C. Cytokines

D. Polymorphonuclear cells

E. All of the above

145. The most common cause of fever of unknown origin (FUO) in children after infection is

A. malignancies

B. connective tissue disease

C. inflammatory bowel disease

D. teething

E. allergies

146. The most useful information in diagnosing the cause of FUO comes from

    A. history and physical examination

    B. laboratory test results

    C. diagnostic scanning

    D. provocative tests

    E. radiographs

147. In regions where penicillin-resistant pneumococci are prevalent, patients strongly suspected of having bacterial meningitis should receive which of the following antimicrobial agents in addition to age-appropriate empirical (ceftriaxone or cefotaxime) antimicrobial therapy?

    A. Clindamycin

    B. Azithromycin

    C. Vancomycin

    D. Streptomycin

    E. Any of the above

148. Which of the following vaccines has resulted in the greatest changes in the evaluation and management of febrile infants and children suspected of having serious bacterial infections?

    A. Typhoid fever

    B. *H. influenzae* type b

    C. Pneumococcal

    D. Meningococcal

    E. BCG

149. Febrile children with sickle cell anemia are at an increased risk for having overwhelming sepsis. Some of these children can be given intramuscular ceftriaxone and treated as outpatients. Which of the following should lead to hospitalization?

    A. Temperature greater than 40°C

    B. WBC count less than 5000 cells/μL

    C. WBC count greater than 30,000 cells/μL

    D. Apparent respiratory distress

    E. All of the above

150. Children should be evaluated for suspected sepsis, hospitalized, and receive empirical antimicrobial therapy if they have signs of

    A. lethargy

    B. poor perfusion

    C. hypoventilation or hyperventilation

    D. cyanosis

    E. any of the above

151. Evaluation of a febrile infant who is younger than 60 days and who appears generally well and has no specific symptoms should include all of the following EXCEPT

    A. past medical history

    B. physical examination

    C. CBC count with differential

    D. urinalysis

    E. stool culture

152. Pyelonephritis is a frequent cause of fever in young infants. All of the following infants have an increased risk for urinary tract infections EXCEPT

    A. uncircumcised male infants

    B. those with urinary tract anomalies

    C. young girls

    D. those with Mediterranean ancestors

    E. those with vesiculoureteral reflux

153. Which of the following bacterial pathogens is UNLIKELY to cause sepsis in an infant less than 60 days old, born at term, discharged from the hospital with the mother, and now febrile?

    A. Group B streptococci

    B. *S. pneumoniae*

    C. *E. coli*

    D. *P. aeruginosa*

    E. *L. monocytogenes*

154. Serious bacterial infection should always be considered when evaluating a febrile infant younger than 3 months. What percentage of febrile infants in this age group will be found to have serious bacterial infections when evaluated?

    A. 0% to 5%

    B. 5% to 10%

    C. 10% to 15%

    D. 15% to 20%

    E. 20% to 25%

155. A 5-year-old Hispanic female presents with fever and myalgias, nausea, vomiting, diarrhea, anorexia, and abdominal pain for the previous several days. She has not traveled recently and lives in a suburban area of Corpus Christi in southern Texas. She has had no recent tick bites, the family does not own a dog, and she has not been in any rural areas recently. The family cat has had a problem with fleas, and all family members have had flea bites in the past 2 weeks. Currently her temperature is 102.2°F, her heart rate is 140, and respirations are 28 per minute. A 1.5-cm nontender, motile lymph node is found in the left inguinal region, but no other physical abnormalities are present. She has no rash. Her WBC count is 4500/mm^3, with 25% segmented neutrophils, 30% band neutrophils, and 35% lymphocytes. Her platelet count is 195,000/mm^3. The serum sodium concentration is 131 mEq/L, and a urinalysis is unremarkable. What is the most likely diagnosis?

    A. Plague

    B. Hantavirus infection

    C. Tularemia

    D. Rocky Mountain spotted fever

    E. Murine typhus

156. A 5-year-old black male has had fever, headache, abdominal pain, and muscle aches for the preceding 3 to 4 days. His temperature is 103.4°C, heart rate is 130, and respirations are 40 per minute. He appears acutely ill and dehydrated. He has no rash. No history of tick bite is obtained, but the child had recently been camping in rural Wisconsin. Laboratory findings include WBC count of 2300/mm^3, 24% segmented neutrophils, 65% bands, 8% lymphocytes, and platelet count 57,000/mm^3. Elevations in serum AST (465 IU/L; normal 0 to 40 IU/L) were also present. A peripheral blood smear reveals small blue clusters of bacteria-like bodies in an aggregate within the cytoplasm of 1% of circulating mononuclear WBCs. What is the most appropriate diagnosis?

    A. Staphylococcal septicemia

    B. Ehrlichiosis

    C. Meningococcemia

    D. Hemolytic uremic syndrome

    E. Rocky Mountain spotted fever

157. A 14-year-old white female presents in good

health, complaining of a recent tick bite between the great toe and second toe on her left foot. The tick-bite wound is not infected and is healing well. The patient is afebrile, all vital signs are normal, and she feels well. She lives in an area not endemic for Lyme disease. What is the most appropriate next step in patient management?

    A. Reassure the patient that she is well and discharge her.

    B. Counsel the patient on diseases transmitted by ticks and how to avoid tick bites in the future.

    C. Start doxycycline prophylactic therapy for Rocky Mountain spotted fever and Lyme disease.

    D. Reassure the patient that she is well and tell her that if she should experience fever or other symptoms within 2 weeks, she should return.

    E. Perform biopsy of the tick-bite lesion and request immunofluorescent or immunohistologic evaluation to rule out rickettsia.

158. A 3-year-old, previously healthy white male presents with fever and a generalized macular rash, including rash on the palms and soles. He has slight tender posterior auricular adenopathy but no conjunctivitis, pharyngitis, or evidence of otitis media. His mother states that she removed a tick from the patient approximately 1 to 2 weeks previously. His temperature is 101.4°F, and laboratory findings include a WBC count of 7,700/mm^3 with 62% bands, 15% segmented neutrophils, and a platelet count of 25,000/mm^3. What is the most appropriate next step in patient management?

    A. Immediately perform a Weil-Felix test to confirm the diagnosis of Rocky Mountain spotted fever before starting therapy.

    B. Start doxycycline or chloramphenicol therapy simultaneously with other diagnostic evaluation.

    C. Examine a peripheral blood smear for evidence of intraleukocytic rickettsiae.

    D. Start broad-spectrum antimicrobial therapy with a cephalosporin and an aminoglycoside.

    E. Obtain a skin biopsy specimen for immunofluorescent or immunohistologic examination to preclude Rocky Mountain spotted fever and delay therapy until a positive result is returned.

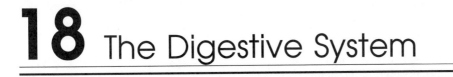

18 The Digestive System

We are now moving to organ system–based *parts* of the *Nelson Textbook* and this accompanying review book. Gastrointestinal diseases are quite common if we consider all the children whom we see with vomiting, abdominal pain, diarrhea, or constipation. Parents and society are quite preoccupied with what goes into and out of the mouth and what exits the bottom. Fortunately, we now have other diagnostic approaches that enable us to test, image, or visualize the gastrointestinal system.

The questions should help build on the educational foundation of the *Nelson Textbook*. In addition, we are reminded of the quote from Dr. Krugman's previous introduction to this section, "Have fun and don't get trapped in a blind loop."

1. The recommended procedure for a physician to follow for an avulsed central incisor in an 8-year-old child is to

   A. call the dentist for an appointment

   B. keep the tooth moist until dental care is available

   C. replant the tooth to resemble the one on the other side

   D. place the tooth in apple juice

2. The most common cause of facial swelling without facial tenderness or erythema in the maxillary area of a 12-year-old is

   A. localized trauma

   B. an abscessed tooth

   C. a bee sting

   D. *Haemophilus influenzae* type b

   E. angioedema

3. Although the toxic dose of fluoride is many times greater than the dose needed to cause mild fluorosis (mottling), the dose associated with mottling in young infants is how many times the dose from fluoridated water?

   A. 2 to 5 times

   B. 10 to 20 times

   C. 100 to 200 times

   D. 1000 times

4. Natal teeth are most often part of the natural primary dentition rather than supernumerary teeth. They are frequently loose on eruption, necessitating extraction. The occurrence of natal teeth is approximately one in

   A. 20 live births

   B. 200 live births

   C. 2000 live births

   D. 20,000 live births

5. Complications of appendicitis include

   A. wound infection

   B. intraabdominal abscess

   C. infertility

   D. liver abscess

   E. all of the above

6. The most reliable physical finding in appendicitis is

   A. the psoas sign

   B. abdominal distension

   C. direct tenderness

   D. abnormal bowel sounds

   E. rebound tenderness

7. Abdominal pain, weight loss, anemia, and chronic or recurrent symptoms in an adolescent female suggest

   A. Henoch-Schönlein purpura

   B. inflammatory bowel disease

   C. pregnancy

   D. pelvic inflammatory disease

   E. irritable bowel disease

8. Appendicitis can effectively be eliminated as a cause of abdominal pain that

   A. is crampy in nature

   B. began after vomiting

   C. is localized to the right flank

   D. is characterized by none of the above

9. An 18-month-old is discovered with his mouth over a storage bottle containing a strong alkali. The parents remove the bottle, and the boy seems well. Some fluid is missing from the bottle, but no external signs are found on the child's clothing and the child has no burns on his face or lips. The most appropriate advice to give the parents, who are on their way to the hospital, is to

    A. administer ipecac

    B. administer milk

    C. administer toast

    D. administer acetaminophen

10. After the child described in Question 9 arrives in the emergency room, results of his physical examination, including an examination of his posterior pharynx, are found to be unremarkable. The most appropriate approach now is to

    A. administer prednisone to decrease stricture formation

    B. administer penicillin to prevent infection

    C. administer an acidic fluid to neutralize the alkali

    D. perform endoscopy to assess the severity of the ingestion

    E. place a nasogastric tube to feed the child

11. *Matching:* Gastrointestinal tumors

    1. Familial polyposis
    2. Gardner syndrome
    3. Lip and gum pigmentation
    4. Diarrhea, achlorhydria
    5. Facial flushing
    6. Hypertension

    A. VIPoma
    B. Carcinoid
    C. Pheochromocytoma
    D. Osteomas
    E. Annual colonoscopy
    F. Peutz-Jeghers syndrome

12. A full-term infant becomes cyanotic in the delivery room. After intubation and attempts at stabilization, it is noticed that the infant has a scaffold abdomen and decreased breath sounds over the left hemithorax. The most likely diagnosis is

    A. pneumothorax

    B. cardiomegaly

    C. diaphragmatic hernia

    D. neuroblastoma

    E. atelectasis

13. A 16-year-old female with a past history of hypothyroidism, which developed at age 10, now manifests fever, anorexia, amenorrhea, and jaundice of 4 months' duration. Her direct bilirubin level is 6 mg/dL, and her total bilirubin value is 11 mg/dL. Results of tests for hepatitis A and B are negative, and her serum IgG level is 16.5 g/L. The most likely diagnosis is

    A. mononucleosis

    B. chronic active hepatitis

    C. α_1-antitrypsin deficiency

    D. cystic fibrosis

    E. Wilson disease

14. A 13-year-old female developed a viral respiratory tract illness that lasted 7 days. She had a temperature of 39.7°C, which was treated with an unknown antipyretic given every 4 to 6 hours for 3 days. After an initial recovery period, she then began to manifest protracted emesis, confusion, combativeness, and lethargy. Blood glucose and serum electrolyte values were normal. The most important laboratory test to perform is

    A. a complete blood count

    B. blood culture

    C. blood ammonia level

    D. blood urea nitrogen

    E. serum carnitine level

15. An 18-year-old male complains of right upper quadrant pain and fever for 2 weeks. Physical examination reveals hepatomegaly, no icterus, and right lower quadrant fullness. Four weeks before admission, he returned from Mexico, where he received an over-the-counter medication for an illness characterized by abdominal pain, nausea, and emesis. The most likely diagnosis is

    A. giardiasis

    B. hepatitis

    C. hepatic abscess

    D. cholangitis

    E. Crohn disease

16. A 12-year-old male develops increasing difficulty in school performance and chronic jaundice of 6 months' duration. Laboratory data are consistent with active hepatitis and

reveal hemolytic anemia. The urinalysis reveals glycosuria. The most likely diagnosis is

A. chronic hepatitis E virus infection

B. hepatic encephalopathy

C. Reye syndrome

D. Wilson disease

E. galactosemia

F. glycogen storage disease

17. A 10-year-old female who had biliary atresia treated with the Kasai procedure in infancy now manifests increasing clumsiness, reduced deep tendon reflexes, and ataxia. The most likely diagnosis is

A. hepatic encephalopathy

B. vitamin A deficiency

C. encephalitis

D. vitamin E deficiency

E. kernicterus

18. *Matching:* Neonatal cholestasis

1. Small for gestational age
2. Other malformations
3. May be familial
4. Polysplenia
5. Giant cells on biopsy

A. Neonatal hepatitis

B. Biliary atresia

C. Both

19. *Matching:* Jaundice

1. Hemolysis
2. Breast milk jaundice
3. Viral hepatitis
4. Sepsis
5. Hypothyroidism
6. Pyloric stenosis
7. Cystic fibrosis
8. Biliary atresia
9. Crigler-Najjar syndrome
10. Zellweger syndrome
11. Galactosemia
12. Gilbert disease

A. Indirect hyperbilirubinemia

B. Mixed (cholestatic) jaundice

C. Either

20. Metabolic diseases associated with recurrent pancreatitis include all of the following EXCEPT

A. diabetes mellitus

B. glycogen storage disease

C. hypercalcemia

D. hypoglycemia

E. hypertriglyceridemia

21. A previously healthy 10-year-old male develops excruciating abdominal pain and protracted emesis of 3 days' duration. The emesis is originally clear fluid, but the day of admission the emesis becomes blood colored. The most likely diagnosis is

A. peptic ulcer disease

B. hepatitis

C. gastroenteritis

D. pancreatitis

E. pyelonephritis

22. A 15-year-old female is placed in a total body cast after repair of scoliosis. The cast is to be in place for 2 months. Two weeks after cast placement, she develops abdominal pain, emesis, and nausea. The most likely diagnosis is

A. peptic ulcer disease

B. pancreatitis

C. pyelonephritis

D. appendicitis

E. sepsis

23. A 2.9-kg term male infant is born to a mother who developed polyhydramnios at 34 weeks' gestation. At birth, the Apgar scores were 9 and 9 at 1 and 5 minutes. At 2 hours of life, the infant is noted by the nurses to be continuously drooling saliva. In addition, they are unable to place a nasogastric tube. The most likely diagnosis is

A. choanal atresia

B. laryngomalacia

C. tracheal atresia

D. tracheoesophageal atresia

E. vascular ring

24. Associated anomalies in children with the

condition described in Question 23 include all of the following EXCEPT

A. congenital heart disease

B. vertebral anomalies

C. rectal agenesis

D. hydrocephalus

E. limb anomalies

25. *Matching:* Malabsorption

1. Acanthocytes
2. Pellagra-like rash
3. IgA-endomysial antibody
4. Attends daycare
5. Chronic sinopulmonary disease
6. Responds to oral zinc sulfate
7. Neutropenia

A. Cystic fibrosis

B. *Giardia*

C. Celiac disease

D. Hartnup disease

E. Abetalipoproteinemia

F. Acrodermatitis enteropathica

G. Shwachman-Diamond syndrome

26. A previously healthy, well-developed 6-month-old infant develops diarrhea that proves to be due to rotavirus infection that lasts 3 weeks and requires treatment with intravenous and oral rehydration fluids. Thereafter, the infant is again fed with the regular infant formula that was used before this illness. Each time the infant receives this formula, the infant develops watery diarrhea, which is now rotavirus negative. The most likely diagnosis is

A. stagnant bowel syndrome

B. primary disaccharidase deficiency

C. pancreatic insufficiency

D. dumping syndrome

E. secondary lactase deficiency

F. milk protein allergy

27. An 11-year-old Tanner stage 2 female develops intermittent periumbilical abdominal pain 2 days before visiting her pediatrician. Six hours later, she is nauseated and has one or two episodes of emesis. She also has had two soft bowel movements without blood or relief of symptoms. She walks cautiously into your office and lies still on your examining table. When you begin your examination, she is apprehensive and watches every move of your examining hand. You note guarding and

tenderness throughout her abdomen; the most tender area is the right lower quadrant. The most likely diagnosis is

A. pelvic inflammatory disease

B. ruptured ectopic pregnancy

C. Crohn disease

D. appendicitis

E. mesenteric adenitis

28. *Matching:* Inflammatory bowel disease

1. Fever, weight loss, no diarrhea
2. Ileal involvement
3. Transmural involvement
4. Risk of cancer
5. Colonic involvement
6. Fistula
7. Cured by colectomy

A. Crohn disease

B. Ulcerative colitis

C. Both of the above

29. A 12-year-old male develops epigastric abdominal pain relieved by food. The pain becomes more intense at night. He has an endoscopically demonstrated ulcer and receives cimetidine for 3 months. Once he discontinues cimetidine, his symptoms return. The most beneficial next therapy is to

A. switch to ranitidine

B. start omeprazole

C. start bismuth, amoxicillin, and metronidazole

D. start anticholinergic agents

E. add antacids to the cimetidine

30. A 2-year-old female was well until 12 hours ago, when she developed lethargy, vomiting, and intermittent crying episodes during which she appears to be in pain. During these painful episodes, she draws her legs up to her abdomen. In the office, she passes a maroon-colored stool and has a slightly tender but full abdomen. The most likely diagnosis is

A. pyloric stenosis

B. appendicitis

C. urinary tract infection

D. intussusception

E. peptic ulcer disease

31. **Matching:** Constipation

    1. Onset at birth   A. Hirschsprung disease
    2. Enterocolitis   B. Functional constipation
    3. Stool in ampulla
    4. Encopresis
    5. Poor weight gain

32. A 6-week-old male born to a para 1 gravida 1, 44-year-old woman presents with a week of recurrent nonbilious emesis and dehydration. The serum levels of sodium are 138, potassium 2.9, and bicarbonate 34. The most likely diagnosis is

    A. duodenal stenosis
    B. annular pancreas
    C. adrenogenital syndrome
    D. galactosemia
    E. pyloric stenosis

33. The proper instructions to the family of a child with an avulsed permanent tooth includes all of the following EXCEPT

    A. rinse the tooth
    B. insert the clean tooth in the tooth socket
    C. scrub the root of the tooth
    D. place the tooth in cold cow's milk
    E. avoid having the child swallow the tooth

34. A 2.7-kg full-term infant is noted to have respiratory distress when placed in a supine position. Physical examination reveals micrognathia and a cleft palate. The most likely diagnosis is

    A. CHARGE syndrome
    B. hemifacial microsomia syndrome
    C. Down syndrome
    D. Pierre Robin syndrome
    E. hypothyroidism

35. **Matching:** Tooth development

    1. Anodontia   A. Porphyria
    2. Partial anodontia   B. Hypothyroidism
    3. Mottled enamel   C. Ectodermal dysplasia
    4. Enamel hypoplasia   D. Cleidocranial dysostosis
    5. Red-brown discoloration   E. High-fluoride water source

36. The metabolic alteration found in infants with pyloric stenosis is

    A. hypochloremic acidosis
    B. hypochloremic alkalosis
    C. hyperchloremic acidosis
    D. hyperchloremic alkalosis

37. Persistent jaundice with hypergammaglobulinemia, positive results of a lupus erythematosus cell preparation, anti-DNA antibodies, and an elevated transaminase value are compatible with which disease?

    A. Hepatitis A
    B. Hepatitis B
    C. Chronic persistent hepatitis
    D. Chronic active hepatitis
    E. Amebic abscess

38. Which of the following statements about pyloric stenosis is FALSE?

    A. The incidence is higher in males than females.
    B. Onset is generally in the first month of life.
    C. The vomitus is bile stained.
    D. Vomiting usually becomes projectile.
    E. Jaundice occurs in association.

39. A telephone call comes from the mother of a 19-month-old infant who was fine (except for an upper respiratory tract infection last week) until 6 hours ago, when he suddenly began screaming every 10 minutes. He is afebrile; he vomited twice but has no diarrhea, although he clearly has cramping abdominal pain. Which one of the following would you do?

    A. See the child immediately.
    B. Recommend clear fluids and see the child in the morning.
    C. Prescribe an antispasmodic, anticholinergic drug and see the child if he does not improve.
    D. Suggest a tap water enema.
    E. Refer the mother to a surgeon.

40. On physical examination of the child described in Question 39, you feel a mass in the right upper quadrant. You find bloody stool in the rectum. The most likely diagnosis is

A. appendicitis

B. gastroenteritis *(Shigella)*

C. gastroenteritis (viral)

D. intussusception

E. Meckel diverticulum

41. Appropriate therapy for the disorder described in Question 40 in most cases is

    A. surgical resection

    B. antibiotics and intravenous fluids

    C. clear fluids by mouth

    D. anticholinergic drugs

    E. barium enema

42. Metabolic alkalosis occurs in which one of the following?

    A. Pyloric stenosis

    B. Methyl alcohol poisoning

    C. Ketogenic diet

    D. Hyperalimentation

    E. Excessive intake of ethyl alcohol

43. A 4-year-old child with failure to thrive has bulky stools that leave oil in the toilet bowl. The most likely diagnosis is

    A. gluten-sensitive enteropathy

    B. giardiasis

    C. cystic fibrosis

    D. sucrase-isomaltase deficiency

    E. hypothyroidism

44. Which of the following tests is most likely to be helpful as an index of activity of Crohn disease in a child with chronic right lower quadrant abdominal pain?

    A. Erythrocyte sedimentation rate

    B. White blood cell count

    C. Antineutrophil cytoplasmic antibodies (ANCA)

    D. Platelet count

    E. Serum albumin level

45. Which of the following findings is most helpful in distinguishing Crohn disease from ulcerative colitis?

    A. Joint tenderness

    B. Perianal skin tags

    C. Episcleritis

D. Erythema nodosum

E. Fever

46. A 2-year-old child has persistent diarrhea. Stool electrolyte values include $[Na^+] = 25$ mEq/L and $[K^+] = 10$ mEq/L. Which of the following diagnoses is most likely?

    A. Lactose intolerance

    B. Bile acid malabsorption

    C. Neuroblastoma

    D. Ulcerative colitis

    E. Pseudomembranous enterocolitis

47. A 10-year-old child is seen for a routine school physical examination. While taking the family history, you learn that the father died of colon cancer at age 29. Further information about the father's illness should be obtained in order to determine whether the child will require endoscopic screening of the colon for

    A. Peutz-Jeghers syndrome

    B. familial polyposis coli

    C. juvenile polyposis coli

    D. neurofibromatosis

    E. ulcerative colitis

48. The most common immunosuppressive regimen used after liver transplantation is

    A. cyclosporine and steroids

    B. azathioprine and steroids

    C. cyclosporine and azathioprine

    D. cyclophosphamide and steroids

    E. cyclosporine and FK506

49. Lymphoproliferative disease may be an ominous late complication of liver transplantation and immunosuppression. Which of the following viruses is most closely related to the development of lymphoproliferative disease?

    A. Cytomegalovirus

    B. Adenovirus

    C. Rubeola (measles) virus

    D. Epstein-Barr virus (EBV)

    E. Parvovirus B19

50. A 2-year-old child is evaluated 18 months after an unsuccessful portoenterostomy (Kasai) procedure to treat extrahepatic biliary atresia. He is jaundiced and has signs of cirrhosis and

portal hypertension. In addition, he is not walking well, has an ataxic gait, and shows no deep tendon reflexes. He has received inadequate medical care and no nutritional supplementation. The most likely explanation of his neuromuscular disorder is

A. vitamin A deficiency

B. vitamin B_{12} deficiency

C. vitamin D deficiency

D. biotin deficiency   .

E. vitamin E deficiency

51. The most common indication for liver transplantation in pediatric patients is

A. chronic hepatitis

B. α_1-antitrypsin deficiency

C. biliary atresia

D. fulminant hepatic failure

E. familial cholestasis

52. False-positive elevations of serum amylase levels may be found in all of the following EXCEPT

A. viral pneumonia

B. renal failure

C. mumps

D. appendicitis

E. anorexia nervosa

53. A 10-year-old male is admitted to the hospital for his third episode of pancreatitis. The test most likely to lead to a diagnosis of the cause of these episodes is

A. serum amylase determination

B. abdominal CT scan with intravenous contrast

C. abdominal ultrasonography

D. endoscopic retrograde cholangiopancreatography (ERCP)

E. a sweat test

54. Malabsorption is usually present in all of the following EXCEPT

A. cystic fibrosis

B. pancreas divisum

C. Shwachman-Diamond syndrome

D. chronic pancreatitis

55. The bentiromide test is useful in making the diagnosis of

A. acute pancreatitis

B. disaccharidase deficiency

C. pancreatic insufficiency

D. nesidioblastosis

E. pancreatic pseudocyst

56. All of the following conditions are associated with a higher incidence of inguinal hernia EXCEPT

A. cystic fibrosis

B. a family history of inguinal hernia

C. adrenogenital syndrome

D. testicular feminization syndrome

57. The differential diagnosis of an inguinal hernia in an infant includes

A. inguinal adenitis

B. retractile testis

C. hydrocele of the cord

D. isolated hydrocele

E. all of the above

58. Inguinal hernias should be repaired

A. when a child weighs 10 pounds

B. when a child is 6 months of age

C. on an elective basis

D. as an emergency at the time of diagnosis

59. Hernias in infants result from

A. failure of gonadal development

B. hormonal insufficiency

C. failure of the processus vaginalis to obliterate

D. weakness of the inguinal canal

60. The hernia most commonly encountered in infants and children is

A. a direct hernia

B. an indirect hernia

C. a femoral hernia

D. a Richter hernia

61. Which one of the following has the most value in establishing the functional prognosis in a child with an imperforate anus?

A. Electromyographic evaluation of the perineum

B. The presence of lumbar hemivertebrae

C. The characteristics of the sacrum

D. The sex of the patient

E. Association with esophageal atresia

62. The anorectal defect most frequently encountered in male patients is

A. perineal fistula

B. rectourethral fistula

C. rectum–bladder neck fistula

D. rectal atresia

E. imperforate anus without a fistula

63. The anorectal malformation most frequently encountered in females is

A. perineal fistula

B. vestibular fistula

C. persistent cloaca

D. rectal atresia

E. imperforate anus without a fistula

64. The second most important question to be answered during *the first 24 hours of life* in a newborn with an anorectal malformation is whether

A. the baby has spinal abnormalities

B. the baby has a tethered cord

C. the baby has obstructive uropathy

D. the baby's sacrum is normal

E. the baby has patent ductus arteriosus

65. Which one of the following conditions is associated with rectal prolapse?

A. Tuberculosis

B. Cystic fibrosis

C. Crohn disease

D. Perianal fistula

E. Hemorrhoids

66. Which one of the following conditions is most likely to be a factor predisposing to a perianal fistula?

A. Tuberculosis

B. Crohn disease

C. Imperforate anus

D. Ulcerative colitis

E. Myelomeningocele

67. At what age is idiopathic perianal abscess or fistula most frequently encountered?

A. In the first 2 years of life

B. From 2 to 6 years of age

C. From 6 to 12 years of age

D. From 12 to 15 years of age

E. Between 15 and 18 years of age

68. Which one of the following is most likely to be effective in the treatment of an anal fissure in a baby?

A. Antibiotic treatment for the local flora

B. Fissurotomy

C. Treatment for associated constipation

D. Local steroids

E. Sphincterotomy

69. Which statement about *Helicobacter pylori* and peptic ulcer disease is true?

A. Patients with *H. pylori* and active ulcers improve promptly on treatment with antacids or H_2-blocking drugs.

B. Treatment of ulcers with bismuth heals the ulcers and eradicates *H. pylori*.

C. The presence of antibodies to *H. pylori* identifies patients with recurrent ulcer disease.

D. Treatment with amoxicillin routinely eradicates *H. pylori* from the stomach.

E. Patients with peptic ulcer disease and *H. pylori* respond poorly to antacid therapy.

70. A 12-hour-old, 2100-g male was frequently suctioned for excessive mucus since birth and immediately vomited the first feeding. Which associated problem would he be LEAST likely to have?

A. Hemivertebrae

B. Cardiac malformation

C. Malformation of the forearm

D. Schizencephaly

E. Imperforate anus

71. An asymptomatic 2-year-old swallowed a hearing aid battery 4 hours previously. A radiograph at 11:00 p.m. located it in the upper third of the esophagus. The most appropriate next step is to

A. observe the patient to see if it will pass

through the esophagus during the next 24 hours

B. schedule esophagoscopy the next morning to remove the battery

C. observe the patient in expectation that it will pass into the stomach during the next 6 hours

D. attempt to retrieve the battery using a Foley catheter and fluoroscopy

E. schedule immediate esophagoscopy to retrieve the battery

72. A 12-year-old lost 2.5 kg during a 1-year period and developed a night cough and dysphagia. An esophageal fluid level was noted on a chest radiograph, and barium swallow showed a dilated esophagus that narrowed sharply at the gastroesophageal junction. Barium slowly entered the stomach. The most appropriate treatment is

A. metoclopramide

B. colonic interposition

C. resection of the distal esophagus

D. an H_2 blocker (cimetidine)

E. myotomy of the gastroesophageal junction

73. Which statement about peptic ulcer disease in pediatric patients is FALSE?

A. Intestinal perforation and hemorrhage are the major presenting symptoms in infancy.

B. Vomiting, slow growth, and hemorrhage are the major symptoms in children younger than 2 years.

C. A history of epigastric pain relieved by antacids can be elicited in fewer than one third of children.

D. It has not been demonstrated that *H. pylori* causes ulcer disease.

E. The majority of stress ulcers in severely ill children occur in the duodenal bulb.

74. A 5-year-old female with cirrhosis and portal hypertension develops increasing abdominal distension. Shifting dullness and a puddle sign are noted on physical examination. Paracentesis reveals cloudy fluid. Culture of the ascitic fluid is most likely to reveal

A. *Pseudomonas*

B. *Candida albicans*

C. pneumococci

D. *Serratia*

E. *H. influenzae*

75. A 4-year-old male with a history of poorly controlled nephrotic syndrome develops abdominal pain, vomiting, diarrhea, and a temperature of 39°C. Abdominal tenderness and diminished bowel sounds are noted. Paracentesis is performed. Which of the following ascitic fluid analyses would be most consistent with primary peritonitis?

A. 300 white blood cells/mm³, pH 7.35, high lactate

B. 500 white blood cells/mm³, pH 7.25, high lactate

C. 500 white blood cells/mm³, pH 7.29, low lactate

D. 500 white blood cells/mm³, pH 7.35, low lactate

E. 200 white blood cells/mm³, pH 7.29, high lactate

76. Which of the following dietary compositions is most appropriate for the treatment of an infant with postsurgical chylous ascites?

A. High calorie, low protein, low fat

B. High calorie, high protein, low fat

C. Normal calorie, high protein, high fat

D. High calorie, low protein, high fat

E. Normal calorie, normal protein, normal fat

77. A 3-day-old 34-week-gestation infant is noted to have abdominal distension. Ultrasound examination reveals the presence of ascitic fluid. Paracentesis is performed 2 hours after the infant has received a feeding of breast milk. Which of the following laboratory characteristics is most consistent with a diagnosis of chylous ascites?

A. Ascitic fluid glucose level of 250 mg/dL

B. Ascitic fluid protein level of 3.6 g/dL

C. Ascitic fluid lymphocyte count of 250 cells/mm³

D. Ascitic fluid with milky appearance

E. Ascitic fluid of pH 7.44

19 The Respiratory System

Respiratory problems are leading causes of death among children throughout the world. Respiratory physiology has been a challenging topic for most medical students. This *part* of the *Nelson Textbook* does an excellent job of integrating the physiology, anatomy, and pathology with the clinical disease entities. This *part* moves through an initial section on pulmonary development and function to more specific anatomically based sections on the upper and lower respiratory tracts, diseases of the pleura, and neuromuscular or skeletal diseases that affect pulmonary function.

Questions in this area should help readers review their knowledge in clinical pulmonology and otorhinolaryngology. In addition, readers will be in a better position to recognize respiratory illnesses.

1. A 3.5-kg full-term infant is born after an uncomplicated delivery with Apgar scores of 9 and 9 at 1 and 5 minutes. The infant cries vigorously after birth but then goes into a quiet state. Within 10 minutes, the infant develops cyanosis and respiratory arrest. During resuscitation, the nurse is unable to pass a nasogastric tube. The most likely diagnosis is

   A. tracheoesophageal fistula

   B. pneumothorax

   C. persistent fetal circulation

   D. choanal atresia

   E. laryngotrachomalacia

2. Associated malformations that may be present in the infant described in Question 1 include all of the following EXCEPT

   A. coloboma

   B. congenital heart disease

   C. asplenia

   D. ear anomalies

   E. central nervous system (CNS) anomalies

3. A 3-month-old develops respiratory distress with fever, tachypnea, stridor, and retractions during an upper respiratory tract infection. The parents report that the child is a noisy breather; these sounds become worse when the child is positioned supine. The most likely diagnosis is

   A. asthma

   B. laryngotracheomalacia

   C. group A streptococcal pharyngitis

   D. epiglottitis

   E. tuberculosis

4. An 8-year-old presents with fever, cough, and tachypnea. Physical examination reveals rales in the left posterior lung base, and a chest radiograph confirms pneumonia. Past history is positive for two other episodes of pneumonia at the left base at ages 4 and 6 years. The most likely diagnosis is

   A. eventration of the diaphragm

   B. pulmonary sequestration

   C. pulmonary embolism

   D. diaphragmatic hernia

   E. resistant pneumococcal pneumonia

5. *Matching:* Upper airway infection

   1. Parainfluenza virus
   2. *Staphylococcus aureus*
   3. Steeple sign
   4. Thumb sign
   5. Ragged tracheal air column
   6. *Haemophilus influenzae* type B
   7. Requires urgent endotracheal intubation
   8. Corticosteroids of some benefit
   9. Barking cough
   10. Drooling

   A. Croup
   B. Epiglottitis
   C. Bacterial tracheitis

6. A 1-year-old presents with an acute onset of cough, choking, and respiratory distress. Physical examination reveals a respiratory rate of 45 and wheezing. There is no family history of asthma, and no one at home is ill.

The older sister states that they were both playing house and that they both had eaten granola. The most likely diagnosis is

A. anaphylaxis

B. bronchiolitis

C. cystic fibrosis

D. foreign body aspiration

E. angioedema

7. A 2-year-old is noted to ingest kerosene from a container in the garage. The child vomits and then develops a respiratory rate of 45. In the emergency room, the child is tachypneic and has rales at both lung bases. The child is alert but anxious and cyanotic. The best approach to this patient is to

A. administer ipecac to induce vomiting

B. administer activated charcoal

C. place a nasogastric tube for gastric lavage

D. administer oxygen

E. administer penicillin

8. A 12-year-old with recurrent wheezing has required 10 separate courses of prednisone this year. Each time the prednisone dose is tapered off, the child develops an exacerbation of severe wheezing, cough, and low-grade fever. Laboratory studies reveal marked eosinophilia. The most likely diagnosis is

A. cystic fibrosis

B. bronchiolitis

C. congestive heart failure

D. allergic bronchopulmonary aspergillosis

E. adrenal insufficiency

9. A 16-year-old female presents with cough, dyspnea, and blood-streaked sputum. On physical examination, her respiratory rate is 25, pulse is 120, and blood pressure is 150/100 mm Hg, and she is afebrile. A chest radiograph reveals multiple bilateral pulmonary densities. A urinalysis reveals proteinuria and hematuria. The most likely diagnosis is

A. rheumatic fever

B. nephrotic syndrome

C. hemolytic-uremic syndrome

D. Goodpasture syndrome

E. aspiration pneumonia

10. An 18-year-old female presents with an acute onset of chest pain, tachypnea, and cyanosis 1 week after the birth of her first child. Her chest radiograph is nondiagnostic, but her PaO_2 is 60 on 40% oxygen. The most likely diagnosis is

A. preeclampsia

B. *Legionella* pneumonia

C. a fractured rib

D. a pulmonary embolism

E. hysterical hyperventilation

11. All of the following are associated with hemoptysis EXCEPT

A. foreign body aspiration

B. tuberculosis

C. Henoch-Schönlein purpura

D. milk allergy

E. pulmonary alveolar proteinosis

12. All of the following are gastrointestinal manifestations of cystic fibrosis EXCEPT

A. intussusception

B. appendicitis

C. colonic mucosal thickening

D. gastric outlet obstruction

E. inguinal hernias

13. All of the following are noted in patients with cystic fibrosis EXCEPT

A. hyponatremia dehydration

B. male infertility

C. nasal polyps

D. rectal prolapse

E. *Pseudomonas aeruginosa* bacteremia

14. The approach to hemoptysis in patients with cystic fibrosis includes all of the following EXCEPT

A. vitamin K

B. blood transfusion

C. chest physiotherapy

D. bronchial artery embolization

E. antimicrobial agents

15. An 8-year-old white male is noted to be underweight and not growing well. Past medical history reveals three episodes of "pneumonia" and wheezing thought to be

asthma. His appetite is good, but he has had intermittent diarrhea since weaning from breast milk. The most appropriate laboratory test is

A. antiendomysial antibody

B. breath hydrogen test

C. stool α_1-antitrypsin measurement

D. sweat chloride measurement

E. endoscopy and small bowel biopsy

16. A 13-year-old male presents with fever, sore throat, difficulty swallowing, and a garbled "hot potato" voice. He was well until 7 days before admission, when he had a mild sore throat that did not remit and then rapidly worsened 1 day before admission. The most likely diagnosis is

A. foreign body

B. rheumatic fever

C. retropharyngeal abscess

D. peritonsillar abscess

E. diphtheria

17. A 12-year-old male presents with a 12-hour history of facial swelling, pain, and fever. Physical examination reveals a nonerythematous but edematous swelling over his lower left cheek. The area is minimally tender, and no trismus is noted. Examination of his mouth and throat reveals multiple caries and minimally enlarged nonerythematous tonsils. The most appropriate immediate therapy is

A. penicillin

B. dental extraction

C. dental fillings

D. gentamicin

E. diphenhydramine

18. Which of the following is the most likely diagnosis in an otherwise normal adolescent with the sudden onset of respiratory distress, cyanosis, retractions, and markedly decreased breath sounds over his left lung?

A. Empyema

B. Chylothorax

C. Left pneumothorax

D. Staphylococcal pneumonia

E. Aspiration of a foreign body

19. A 3-year-old has had a cough for 2 months. It is a loose cough, but he does not seem to produce sputum. The cough is getting worse, especially at night. It keeps his parents awake, although the child sleeps through the cough. Family history revealed that the mother has eczema and the father has had "hay fever." Additional historical facts that should be elicited to determine whether this represents a serious illness include all of the following EXCEPT

A. reduced exercise tolerance

B. failure to gain weight

C. chronic diarrhea

D. persistent fevers

E. serous otitis media

20. None of the additional symptoms listed in Question 19 is present. On physical examination, you hear an occasional wheeze in both lung fields. Other physical findings that would be indicative of *chronic* lung disease include which of the following? (Choose one or more.)

A. Posterior pharyngeal drainage

B. Hyperexpansion of the chest with an increased anteroposterior diameter

C. Clubbing

D. Tachypnea

E. Cyanosis

21. The patient described in Questions 19 and 20 has none of the findings indicative of chronic lung disease. What would be the most likely diagnosis at this time?

A. Bronchiectasis

B. Pertussis

C. Foreign body aspiration

D. Asthma

E. Interstitial pneumonia

22. A 2-year-old previously well male is brought to you with cough and fever. His history is unremarkable. Physical examination reveals a toxic, ill child with fever, dyspnea, and decreased breath sounds in the right middle lung fields. Posteroanterior and lateral chest radiographs reveal an infiltrate in the right middle lobe. His right lung is clear. Leukocyte count is 19,000/mm³ with 54% polymorphonuclear neutrophils, 18% band

forms, and 28% lymphocytes. The child is admitted to the hospital. Which of the following would you do first?

A. Repeat the leukocyte count.

B. Obtain a blood culture.

C. Obtain a throat culture.

D. Obtain a radiograph of his sinuses.

E. Schedule bronchoscopy.

23. Which antibiotic would you choose for the patient described in Question 22?

A. Methicillin

B. Ceftriaxone

C. Gentamicin

D. Penicillin

E. Tetracycline

24. Within 24 hours, the patient described in Questions 22 and 23 improves, and he is discharged after 3 days on oral antibiotics. He fares well until 2 weeks later, when 4 days after stopping antibiotics he gets another fever and his cough becomes worse. You should now

A. begin steroids

B. order a sweat chloride test

C. perform bronchoscopy

D. order a lung biopsy

E. order a leukocyte count and blood culture

25. Which of the following is the most likely diagnosis for the patient described in Questions 22 to 24?

A. α_1-Antitrypsin deficiency

B. Tuberculosis

C. Foreign body in the left mainstem bronchus

D. *Pneumocystis carinii* pneumonia

E. Congenital lung cyst

26. A male born at term after an uncomplicated pregnancy, labor, and delivery within a few hours develops severe cyanosis requiring supplemental oxygen and supported ventilation. Results of routine cultures are negative. The chest roentgenogram reveals a normal heart shadow and a fine reticulonodular pulmonary infiltrate radiating from the hilum. Family history reveals that a

male and a female sibling with a similar clinical course died at 2 and 4 months of age, respectively. What is the most likely diagnosis?

A. Neonatal alveolar proteinosis

B. Neonatal herpes simplex infection

C. Type II glycogenosis

D. Meconium aspiration syndrome

E. Carnitine palmityltransferase deficiency

27. Which of the following is most likely to occur in the patient described in Question 26?

A. An excellent response to bronchoalveolar lavage

B. An excellent response to exogenous surfactant

C. Progressive renal failure

D. The need for extracorporeal membrane oxygenation

28. What is the most appropriate next step in the treatment of the patient described in Questions 26 and 27?

A. Provide parenteral heparin.

B. List the patient for a lung transplant.

C. Administer acyclovir.

D. Perform bronchoalveolar lavage.

29. What is the most likely cause of the condition affecting the patient described in Questions 26 to 28?

A. Surfactant protein SP-B deficiency

B. Acid maltase deficiency

C. α_1-Antitrypsin deficiency

D. Congenital lobar emphysema

E. Congenital infection

30. Which of the following is appropriate in the treatment of bronchial foreign body?

A. Flexible fiberoptic bronchoscopy

B. Rigid open tube bronchoscopy

C. Bronchodilators and postural drainage

D. Fogarty catheter

E. Foley catheter

31. Etiologic factors in spasmodic croup are thought to include

A. allergy

B. viral infection

C. psychologic factors

D. gastroesophageal reflux

E. all of the above

32. Which of the following has NOT been associated with gastroesophageal reflux?

A. Hoarseness

B. Cystic fibrosis

C. Stridor

D. Apnea

E. α-Antitrypsin deficiency

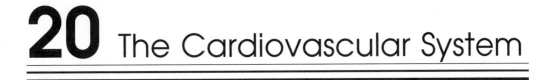

20 The Cardiovascular System

What clinician hasn't been perplexed by a heart murmur in a newborn infant or an athlete during a preparticipation sports examination? The ability to differentiate pathologic lesions from benign murmurs is occasionally difficult and may require consultation or ancillary testing. This extensively updated *part* is usefully divided into eight sections: evaluation, the transitional circulation, congenital heart disease (left-to-right shunts, obstructive lesions, cyanotic congenital heart disease), cardiac arrhythmias, acquired heart disease, myocardial diseases, therapy, and diseases of the peripheral vascular system including hypertension. The chapters on heart and heart-lung transplantation are quite exciting and state of the art.

In developing questions, we could not provide you with auscultatory findings. Nonetheless the questions in this *part* of the *Nelson Review* will help add to your foundation of knowledge in pediatric cardiology.

1. A 1-day-old is noted to be cyanotic. Physical examination reveals a grade 2-3/6 systolic murmur and a single loud second heart sound. The chest radiograph reveals a normal-sized heart and decreased pulmonary vascular markings. The electrocardiogram (ECG) reveals left ventricular dominance. The next step in the management of this neonate is to administer

    A. sodium bicarbonate

    B. morphine

    C. prostaglandin E_1

    D. digoxin

    E. positive-pressure ventilation

2. The most likely diagnosis in the patient described in Question 1 is

    A. persistent pulmonary hypertension

    B. transposition of the great arteries

    C. truncus arteriosus

    D. pulmonary atresia

    E. total anomalous venous return

3. An 18-month-old is noted to assume a squatting position frequently during play time at the daycare center. The mother also notices occasional episodes of perioral cyanosis during some of these squatting periods. The day of admission, the child becomes restless, hyperpneic, and deeply cyanotic. Within 10 minutes, the child becomes unresponsive. The most likely underlying lesion is

    A. cardiomyopathy

    B. anomalous coronary artery

    C. tetralogy of Fallot

    D. cystic fibrosis

    E. aspiration pneumonia

4. Therapy of a "blue" or "tet" spell could include all of the following EXCEPT

    A. epinephrine

    B. knee-chest position

    C. oxygen

    D. morphine

    E. sodium bicarbonate

    F. phenylephrine

5. Tricuspid atresia is associated with all of the following EXCEPT

    A. ventricular septal defect (VSD)

    B. cyanosis

    C. left-axis deviation

    D. left ventricular hypertrophy

    E. "tet" spells

    F. heart failure

    G. total surgical correction

6. Ebstein anomaly is associated with all of the following EXCEPT

    A. dysrhythmias

    B. patent ductus arteriosus (PDA) dependence in neonates

    C. massive heart size on radiographs

    D. VSD

    E. tall, broad P waves

7. A 1-day-old has manifested severe cyanosis (Pao$_2$ 22 mm Hg) since birth. The infant has marked tachypnea and tachycardia but no cardiac murmur. The chest radiograph reveals a small heart with a diffuse white-out pattern of pulmonary venous congestion. The response to PGE$_1$ is poor. The most likely diagnosis is

   A. total anomalous venous return

   B. partial anomalous venous return

   C. pulmonary atresia

   D. transposition of the great arteries

   E. truncus arteriosus

8. A 2-day-old develops cyanosis, hypotension, and metabolic acidosis. On examination, the infant is lethargic, tachycardic, and gray-blue, with hepatomegaly, a grade 2-3/6 systolic murmur, and poor radial and femoral pulses. A chest radiograph reveals cardiomegaly, and an ECG demonstrates right ventricular dominance with markedly reduced R waves in V$_5$ and V$_6$. The most likely diagnosis is

   A. myocarditis

   B. hypoplastic left heart syndrome

   C. anomalous coronary arteries

   D. total anomalous venous return

   E. tetralogy of Fallot

9. *Matching:* Cardiosplenic heterotaxias

1. Severe cyanosis	A. Asplenia
2. Dextrocardia	B. Polysplenia
3. Decreased pulmonary blood flow	C. Both
4. Males	D. Neither
5. Malrotation (intestinal)	
6. Absent inferior vena cava	
7. Howell-Jolly bodies	
8. Biliary atresia	
9. Trisomy 21	

10. A 3-day-old presents with fussiness and poor feeding. On examination, the heart rate is noted to be 250. The ECG reveals a rate of 250, a QRS of 0.07 second, and no visible P waves. The most likely diagnosis is

    A. ventricular tachycardia

    B. supraventricular tachycardia with aberrant conduction

    C. supraventricular tachycardia

    D. heart block

    E. none of the above

11. The first approach to the therapy of the dysrhythmia described in Question 10 is

    A. fluid challenge

    B. iced saline bag placed over the face

    C. carotid massage

    D. propranolol

    E. verapamil

12. If vagal maneuvers do not correct the situation described in Questions 10 and 11, the treatment of choice in a hemodynamically stable neonate is

    A. verapamil

    B. synchronized DC cardioversion

    C. adenosine

    D. quinidine

    E. propranolol

13. High-risk lesions for bacterial endocarditis include all of the following EXCEPT

    A. PDA

    B. VSD

    C. ASD

    D. Blalock-Taussig shunt

    E. left-sided valvular lesions

14. *Matching:* Congenital heart disease—syndromes

1. Endocardial Cushing defect	A. DiGeorge syndrome
2. Bicuspid aortic valve	B. Congenital rubella
3. Conotruncal anomalies	C. Trisomy 21
4. Complex multiple cyanotic lesions	D. Turner syndrome
5. PDA	E. Asplenia syndrome
6. Dextrocardia	F. Williams syndrome
7. Supravalvular aortic stenosis	G. Kartagener syndrome

15. Risks for spontaneous cerebrovascular accidents in children with congenital heart disease include all of the following EXCEPT

A. left-to-right shunts

B. tetralogy of Fallot

C. polycythemia

D. hypoxia

E. iron deficiency

F. dehydration

16. *Matching:* Systemic illnesses and heart disease

1. Pericarditis	A. Lyme disease
2. Heart block (acquired)	B. Homocystinuria
3. Coronary thrombosis	C. Juvenile rheumatoid arthritis
4. Aortic insufficiency	D. Hypothyroidism
5. Cardiac rhabdomyoma	E. Marfan syndrome
6. Bradycardia	F. Tuberous sclerosis
7. Short PR interval	G. Carnitine deficiency
8. Cardiomyopathy	H. Pompe disease
9. Congenital heart block	I. Maternal systemic lupus erythematosus

17. A 4-month-old infant is noted to have a grade 4 holosystolic murmur that is harsh over the left parasternal border. Results of both the chest radiograph and ECG are normal, and the child is otherwise asymptomatic. The most likely cause of this murmur is

A. large VSD with 3:1 shunt

B. an ASD secundum defect

C. a small VSD

D. pulmonic stenosis

E. pink tetralogy of Fallot

18. A previously well 3 1/2-month-old presents with poor feeding, diaphoresis during feeding, and poor growth. Vital signs reveal respirations of 70, pulse of 175, and blood pressure of 90/65 mm Hg in the upper and lower extremities. The cardiac examination reveals a palpable parasternal lift and a systolic thrill. A grade 4 holosystolic murmur and a middiastolic rumble are noted. The chest radiograph reveals cardiomegaly. The most likely diagnosis is

A. cardiomyopathy

B. myocarditis

C. VSD

D. coarctation of the aorta

E. transposition of the great arteries

19. All of the following conditions may require antimicrobial prophylaxis against endocarditis EXCEPT

A. PDA 1 year after surgical ligation

B. ASD primum

C. VSD

D. prior endocarditis

E. prosthetic mitral valve

F. tetralogy of Fallot

20. The initial treatment of choice for a symptomatic patient with isolated pulmonic stenosis is

A. closed surgical blade valvotomy

B. open surgical valvotomy

C. balloon catheter valvuloplasty

D. Blalock-Taussig shunt

E. valve replacement

21. A 12-year-old female is noted to have a blood pressure of 170/110 mm Hg during a routine grade physical examination for school sports participation. She is asymptomatic but has been noted to have a grade 1-2/6 short systolic murmur at the left sternal border. The next important step in her evaluation should include

A. chest radiograph

B. ECG

C. funduscopic examination

D. lower extremity blood pressure

E. a tilt test

22. Complications after repair of a coarctation of the aorta include all of the following EXCEPT

A. immediate rebound postoperative hypertension

B. recoarctation

C. essential hypertension

D. migraines

E. mesenteric arteritis syndrome

23. A 3-month-old has recurrent episodes of crying, painful facial expressions, and

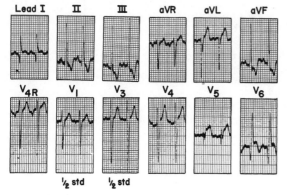

Figure 20-1

discomfort. The infant has dyspnea, a gallop rhythm, and cardiomegaly on chest radiography. The accompanying ECG was obtained (Fig. 20–1). The most likely diagnosis is

A. anomalous origin of the left coronary artery

B. aortic sling

C. pulmonary ring

D. myocarditis

E. endocardial fibroelastosis

24. Complications of cyanotic heart disease or Eisenmenger syndrome include all of the following EXCEPT

A. gout

B. obesity

C. hemoptysis

D. clubbing

E. polycythemia

25. Pulsus paradoxus is associated with

A. pericarditis

B. endocarditis

C. rheumatic fever

D. myocarditis

E. postperfusion syndrome

26. The finding of substernal thrust on palpation of the precordium is most likely to be associated with

A. left ventricular hypertrophy

B. right ventricular hypertrophy

C. an ejection click

D. systemic hypertension

E. pericardial effusion

27. A Still murmur is

A. an early diastolic murmur signifying mitral stenosis

B. an innocent murmur that disappears on jugular pressure

C. an innocent, musical, vibratory ejection murmur heard best in a recumbent patient

D. an innocent, blowing, early systolic murmur that increases in intensity on expiration

E. a blowing diastolic murmur most frequently heard in the newborn period

28. Which of the following is the most common congenital heart defect in infants and children (excluding the neonatal period)?

A. ASD

B. VSD

C. PDA

D. Coarctation of the aorta

E. Tetralogy of Fallot

29. The syndrome of idiopathic hypercalcemia, hypertelorism, and mental retardation is associated with

A. supravalvular aortic stenosis

B. valvular aortic stenosis

C. subvalvular aortic stenosis

D. aortic insufficiency

E. patent ductus arteriosus

30. Which of the following is the most common immediate valvular lesion resulting from acute rheumatic fever?

A. Mitral insufficiency

B. Mitral stenosis

C. Aortic insufficiency

D. Aortic stenosis

E. Tricuspid insufficiency

31. The roentgenographic finding of notching of the ribs is associated with

A. pulmonary hypertension

B. anomalous pulmonary venous return above the diaphragm

C. coarctation of the aorta

D. systemic hypertension

E. aortic insufficiency

32. Which of the following is the most important procedure in the diagnosis of subacute bacterial endocarditis?

    A. Complete blood count

    B. Urinalysis (microscopic)

    C. Erythrocyte sedimentation rate

    D. Blood culture

    E. Electrocardiogram

33. Which of the following statements about primary hypertension diagnosed in a moderately overweight 15-year-old is true?

    A. It should be treated with a combination of antihypertensive agents for 2 years.

    B. It may be effectively managed initially with a weight-loss program.

    C. It must be treated with a diuretic along with a weight-loss program.

    D. It means that the patient will remain hypertensive throughout adulthood.

    E. It will prevent participation in physical exercise until the resting blood pressure is less than 132/82 mm Hg.

34. Hypertension associated with increased activation of the renin-angiotensin-aldosterone system is most appropriately treated with

    A. an angiotensin-converting enzyme (ACE) inhibitor

    B. a calcium channel blocking drug

    C. an α-adrenergic blocking drug

    D. a thiazide diuretic

    E. a β-adrenergic receptor agonist

35. If a 5-year-old female is consistently found to have blood pressure greater than the 95th percentile for her age, which of the following should be investigated early?

    A. Thyroid function

    B. Urinary excretion of vanillylmandelic acid

    C. Parathyroid function

    D. Urinary excretion of aldosterone

    E. Kidneys and urinary tract

36. A 16-year-old adolescent is examined before participating in high-school football. His resting blood pressure is 142/85 mm Hg. There is no known family history of hypertension. The next step in evaluation of the adolescent should be to

    A. refer him for an intravenous pyelogram

    B. prohibit his participation in the fall season

    C. arrange a return visit for blood pressure measurement in 1 week

    D. obtain blood for serum electrolytes and creatinine

    E. tell him that additional assessment is not needed

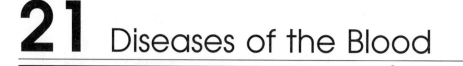

21 Diseases of the Blood

This *part* covers all aspects of hematology—from the many common and uncommon anemias, to polycythemia, pancytopenias, transfusion therapy, coagulopathies and thrombosis, the spleen, and the lymphatics. The individual chapters are well written and can help reinforce for readers the multiple genetic and structural relationships of hemoglobin in the different thalassemias. A clinical approach to all of these disorders is emphasized; the history and physical examination and some simple inexpensive laboratory studies become paramount tools for hematologists.

The questions help confirm your understanding of the coagulation pathways, microcytic and macrocytic and normocytic anemias, and other general pediatric hematology topics.

1. A 5-year-old white female has multiple bruises on her lower extremities and oral-mucosal bleeding of 3 days' duration. Two weeks before these signs, she had a mild respiratory tract infection. Physical examination reveals multiple ecchymoses and petechiae; no lymphadenopathy or hepatosplenomegaly is noted. The next diagnostic step is

   A. a complete blood count

   B. a prothrombin time

   C. a bleeding time

   D. a partial thromboplastin time

   E. an antinuclear antibody titer

2. The most likely diagnosis for the patient described in Question 1 is

   A. leukemia

   B. neuroblastoma

   C. aplastic anemia

   D. idiopathic thrombocytopenia

   E. systemic lupus erythematosus

3. A 10-month-old white male presents with a 1-day history of persistent bleeding after cutting his lip slightly. The family history is unremarkable, and the patient is receiving no medications. Laboratory data reveal a hemoglobin value of 11 g/dL, platelets of 350,000, a prothrombin time of 11.8 seconds, and a partial thromboplastin time (PTT) of 100 seconds, which is corrected by mixing of normal plasma. The most likely diagnosis is

   A. von Willebrand disease

   B. hemophilia A

   C. Hageman factor deficiency

   D. scurvy

   E. anticardiolipin antibody syndrome

4. Appropriate long-term management of the disease described in Question 3 includes all of the following EXCEPT

   A. avoiding aspirin

   B. hepatitis B vaccination

   C. home replacement factor VIII therapy

   D. splenectomy

   E. desmopressin for mild hemorrhage

5. Ten years later, the patient described in Questions 3 and 4 develops recurrent hemarthroses that become refractory to standard doses of factor VIII. The most likely cause of this is

   A. worsening hemophilia

   B. factor VIII antibodies

   C. development of AIDS

   D. development of hepatitis

   E. aspirin therapy

6. Possible solutions to treat patients with acquired anti-factor VIII antibodies include all of the following EXCEPT

   A. porcine factor VIII

   B. factor IX concentrates

   C. immunosuppression

   D. immune tolerance

   E. plasmapheresis with factor VIII replacement

7. *Matching:* Bone marrow failure

   1. Diagnosis after age 10 years

   2. Pancreatic insufficiency

   3. Chromosomal breaks

   4. Iron deficiency possible

   5. Hepatitis viruses

   6. Bone marrow replacement

   A. Fanconi anemia

   B. Dyskeratosis congenita

   C. Shwachman-Diamond

   D. Paroxysmal nocturnal hemoglobinuria

   E. Leukemia

   F. Aplastic anemia

8. A 5-day-old full-term male presents with intense cyanosis, tachypnea, and tachycardia. Physical examination reveals cyanosis of the skin and mucous membranes; the lungs, heart, pulses, and general examination show no abnormalities. Arterial blood gas determination reveals a PaO_2 of 95 while breathing room air. The most likely diagnosis is

   A. transposition of the arteries

   B. pulmonary atresia

   C. pulmonary hypoplasia

   D. methemoglobinemia

   E. Heinz body anemia

9. An 8-month-old black male presents with pallor of 1 month's duration and fever with lethargy of 2 days' duration. Physical examination reveals a poorly responsive infant with a bulging anterior fontanel, nuchal rigidity, splenomegaly, and a temperature of 40.1°C. Laboratory studies reveal a WBC count of 21,000 and a hemoglobin level of 6.3 g/dL; the cerebrospinal fluid is cloudy, and the Gram stain demonstrates gram-positive diplococci. The disease that predisposed this patient to meningitis is most likely

   A. AIDS

   B. sickle cell anemia

   C. DiGeorge syndrome

   D. leukocyte adhesion defect

   E. thalassemia

10. Sequelae of the foregoing patient's meningitis include all of the following EXCEPT

   A. deafness

   B. seizures

   C. cortical blindness

   D. pseudotumor cerebri

   E. mental retardation

11. After the diagnosis of pneumococcal meningitis, you place the patient described in Questions 9 and 10 on intravenous ceftriaxone. Three days later, he is still obtunded and febrile. A repeat lumbar puncture is performed, and no change is found in the cell count, glucose, or protein levels. The Gram stain reveals occasional gram-positive diplococci. The most appropriate treatment strategy would be to begin

   A. steroids

   B. intrathecal antibiotics

   C. intraventricular antibiotics

   D. intravenous vancomycin

   E. intravenous chloramphenicol

12. All of the following are examples of vaso-occlusive crisis in patients with sickle cell anemia EXCEPT

   A. acute chest crisis

   B. stroke

   C. dactylitis

   D. priapism

   E. aplastic crisis

13. A 1-year-old presents with pallor of 3 months' duration. Past medical history reveals neonatal hyperbilirubinemia that was treated with phototherapy for 1 week and a father who had a splenectomy at the age of 2 years for unknown reasons. On physical examination, the child is pale and has splenomegaly (4 cm below the left costal margin). The most likely diagnosis is

   A. sickle cell anemia

   B. thalassemia

   C. paroxysmal nocturnal hemoglobinuria

   D. spherocytosis

   E. Diamond-Blackfan syndrome

14. *Matching:* Hemolytic anemia

   1. Dactylitis

   2. Decay-accelerating factor deficiency

   3. Oxidant stressors

   A. Hereditary spherocytosis

   B. Autoimmune hemolytic anemia

   C. Hereditary pyropoikilocytosis

4. Spectrin deficiency

5. Microcytosis

6. Coombs positive

7. Thermal sensitivity

D. Sickle cell anemia

E. Paroxysmal nocturnal hemoglobinuria

F. Glucose-6-phosphate dehydrogenase (G6PD) deficiency

G. Hemoglobin E

15. A former 28-week premature infant presents with pallor and reduced activity at the age of 14 months. The diet includes cow's milk and juices. The mother had a history of anemia during pregnancy. The child's CBC reveals a hemoglobin value of 5.2 g/dL and a mean corpuscular volume (MCV) of 50. The platelet and WBC counts are normal. The reticulocyte count is 3.2%. The most likely cause of this child's anemia is

A. thalassemia

B. hemoglobin E

C. iron deficiency

D. sickle-thalassemia

E. lead poisoning

16. A 6-month-old from rural Wisconsin has had intermittent diarrhea for 1 month. After multiple formula changes, the local general practitioner changed the formula to goat's milk. At 12 months of age, the child presents with pallor and decreased activity. The most likely diagnosis is

A. Crohn disease

B. giardiasis

C. iron deficiency anemia

D. folate deficiency

E. copper deficiency

17. A 13-year-old female with chronic juvenile rheumatoid arthritis receiving steroids and nonsteroidal anti-inflammatory drugs has progressive pallor and becomes dyspneic with exercise. A CBC reveals a hemoglobin value of 6.5 g/dL. You begin therapy with recombinant erythropoietin and repeat the CBC 1 month later to discover that the hemoglobin level is still 6.5 g/dL. The most likely cause is

A. antierythropoietin antibodies

B. iron deficiency

C. parvovirus infection

D. vitamin E deficiency

E. folate deficiency

18. A 3-month-old white female presents with pallor and poor feeding of 1 month's duration. Past medical and neonatal history are unremarkable, as is the review of systems. She has no history of hematemesis or melena. Physical examination reveals a heart rate of 170, a grade 2/6 systolic ejection murmur, and triphalangeal thumbs. She has no hepatosplenomegaly or lymphadenopathy. The most important test to perform as part of the initial assessment is

A. iron and iron-binding capacity

B. ferritin

C. complete blood count

D. electrocardiogram

E. chest radiography

19. The most likely diagnosis for the patient described in Question 18 is

A. congenital hypoplastic anemia

B. transient erythroblastopenia of childhood

C. iron deficiency

D. sideroblastic anemia

E. ABO incompatibility

20. *Matching:* Anemia

1. Thalassemia

2. Aplastic anemia

3. Copper deficiency

4. Enzymopathy

5. Orotic aciduria

6. Iron deficiency

7. Hypothyroidism

8. Leukemia

A. Microcytic

B. Normocytic

C. Macrocytic

21. *Matching:*

1. Onset before age 4 months

2. X-linked recessive

3. Rarely needs transfusions

4. Elevated hemoglobin F

5. Normal MCV

A. Diamond-Blackfan syndrome

B. Transient erythroblastopenia of childhood

C. Both

D. Neither

6. Elevated expression of i antigen

7. Congenital anomalies

8. Parvovirus B19

9. Both sexes affected

22. The hematocrit is normally at its lowest level at which age in childhood?

    A. 1 hour

    B. 1 week

    C. 1 month

    D. 3 months

    E. 3 years

23. An 18-month-old Caucasian male is brought to your office for a routine health maintenance visit. The mother reveals that the child always appears hungry; in fact, he drinks a quart of whole milk a day and also eats dirt. Intake of solid foods is sporadic, but the mother states that she thought all 18-month-olds were "picky eaters." Physical examination reveals mild pallor of the conjunctivae. He has no hepatosplenomegaly, and the rest of the examination findings are normal. Based on the information, which of the following would be the most likely to determine the diagnosis?

    A. Complete blood count, including blood smear

    B. Reticulocyte count

    C. Lead screen

    D. Ophthalmologic consultation

    E. Testing stools for occult blood

24. A blood smear taken from the patient described in Question 23 shows a microcytic hypochromic anemia. Iron supplementation therapy is started. When will the reticulocyte response be maximum?

    A. 1 to 2 days

    B. 5 to 7 days

    C. 14 to 21 days

    D. 3 to 4 weeks

    E. About 6 weeks

25. In the patient described in Questions 23 and 24, when the hemoglobin and hematocrit return to normal, which should be done?

    A. Stop iron supplementation

    B. Continue iron for 1 to 2 weeks

    C. Continue iron for 4 to 8 weeks

    D. Continue iron for 4 to 6 weeks

26. If the patient described in Questions 23 to 25 does not have improvement in his anemia, which of the following should be explored? (Choose as many as are appropriate.)

    A. Gastrointestinal blood loss

    B. Thalassemia

    C. Sickle cell anemia

    D. Urinary tract infection

    E. Parasitic infection

27. *Matching:* For each of the following disorders, select the appropriate platelet presentation.

    1. Anaphylactoid purpura

    2. Aspirin toxicity

    3. ITP

    4. Wiscott-Aldrich syndrome

    5. Kawasaki disease

    6. Disseminated intravascular coagulation (DIC)

    7. TTP

    8. Kasabach-Merritt syndrome

    A. Platelets decreased in number

    B. Platelet count normal

    C. Platelets increased

28. What is the approximate risk of posttransfusion hepatitis per one-donor exposure?

    A. 1 in 100

    B. 1 in 1500

    C. 1 in 4000

    D. 1 in 10,000

29. The child most likely to benefit from a fresh frozen plasma transfusion is

    A. a child with chronic liver disease with no bleeding but prothrombin time 20 seconds (normal 12 seconds) and PTT 60 seconds (normal 30 seconds)

    B. a 1-week-old neonate with purpura fulminans and family history of warfarin-induced skin necrosis

    C. a 2-week-old neonate with heart failure

and a plasma albumin concentration of 18 g/dL

D. a 15-year-old who has von Willebrand disease and is scheduled to undergo a liver biopsy

30. The 3-day-old neonate who is most likely to benefit from a platelet transfusion is one who

A. has an intracranial hemorrhage with a platelet count 155 × 10⁹/L

B. is clinically stable with a platelet count 30 × 10⁹/L

C. is on a ventilator for severe respiratory disease with a platelet count 40 × 10⁹/L

D. has suspected sepsis with a platelet count 65 × 10⁹/L

31. Which of the following children is most likely to benefit from an RBC transfusion?

A. A neonate with severe respiratory disease and a hemoglobin level of 100 g/L

B. A stable and growing neonate with a hemoglobin level of 80 g/L

C. An 18-month-old infant with iron deficiency anemia (hemoglobin level 60 g/L) noted on routine examination

D. A 3-year-old child with Wilms tumor and hemoglobin level of 90 g/L

32. A 5-year-old has a temperature of 39.6°C. Physical examination reveals a tender, nonfluctuant 3×4-cm left cervical node. The child has no pharyngitis. The best approach to the problem would be

A. treatment with penicillin

B. treatment with amoxicillin

C. treatment with dicloxacillin

D. observation

E. incisional biopsy

33. A 5-year-old has a 3×4-cm left anterior cervical lymph node. What additional finding would lead you to consider a biopsy?

A. Temperature greater than 40°C

B. Erythema of the overlying skin

C. A firm, rubbery consistency

D. Tenderness on palpation

E. Carious teeth

34. A 14-year-old has had fevers for 3 weeks. Physical examination is normal except for a

firm, nontender 3×4-cm right supraclavicular node. The most appropriate radiographic study would be

A. chest computed tomography

B. posteroanterior and lateral chest films

C. flat and upright abdominal films

D. abdominal ultrasonography

E. abdominal computed tomography

35. A 1250-g, 32-week-gestation newborn is transferred to your care. Physical findings at 24 hours are normal except for mild icterus. Laboratory values include hemoglobin 18.5 g/dL, reticulocytes 7%, platelets 200 × 10⁹/L, and bilirubin 5.4 mg/dL (all indirect). The peripheral smear shows Howell-Jolly bodies in the RBCs. The most likely explanation for the latter finding is

A. physiologic hyposplenism of the premature

B. hemoglobin SS disease

C. hypersplenism

D. Ivemark syndrome

E. portal vein obstruction

36. A 10-year-old black female presents with hematemesis. Her birth weight was 1250g. The neonatal course was complicated by hyperbilirubinemia requiring three exchange transfusions. Physical findings are normal except for a firm spleen edge palpable 10 cm below the left costal margin. The CBC includes hemoglobin 8.3 g/dL, WBCs 3.4 × 10⁹/L (30% polymorphonuclear neutrophils), platelets 43 × 10⁹/L. The most likely diagnosis is

A. aplastic anemia

B. acute nonlymphocytic leukemia

C. Wilson disease

D. portal vein thrombosis

E. sickle cell anemia

37. A 10-year-old has a total splenectomy because of trauma. The best statement about the risk of postsplenectomy infection is that

A. the risk is increased in older children

B. the most common organisms are staphylococci

C. posttraumatic splenosis reliably protects patients

D. postsplenectomy vaccinations reliably protect patients

E. the risk is increased and may be lifelong

38. A 10-year-old has been monitored for a diagnosis of hereditary spherocytosis. Laboratory data include hemoglobin 8.3 g/dL, reticulocytes 14%, bilirubin 5.3 mg/dL—total/ 0.3 mg/dL direct. The best procedure to improve the patient's hematologic status would be

    A. cholecystectomy

    B. partial splenectomy

    C. splenic artery embolization

    D. portacaval shunt

    E. total splenectomy

39. An asymptomatic 10-year-old has a spleen edge palpable 3 cm below the left costal margin. She has no other abnormal physical findings. Results of a CBC are normal. The best next test to evaluate the spleen would be

    A. ^{99}Tc sulfur colloid spleen scan

    B. abdominal computed tomography

    C. abdominal ultrasonography

    D. RBC pit test

    E. Monospot or Epstein-Barr virus titers

40. **Matching:** Anemia may be classified by the RBC size. For each of the following anemias, select the appropriate RBC size category.

    1. Folate deficiency   A. Microcytic
    2. G6PD deficiency   B. Normocytic
    3. Hereditary spherocytosis   C. Macrocytic
    4. Thalassemia trait
    5. Iron deficiency
    6. Vitamin B$_{12}$ deficiency
    7. Sickle cell anemia
    8. Lead poisoning

41. A 2-year-old is referred for microcytosis that has not responded to iron therapy. Findings on physical examination are normal. Laboratory values include hemoglobin 11.5 g/dL, MCV 72 fL, and reticulocytes 1.0%. RBC morphology is normal. The most likely explanation for the microcytosis is

    A. iron deficiency

    B. lead exposure

    C. thalassemia trait

    D. chronic disease

    E. normal values for age

42. A term newborn is jittery and has acral cyanosis. Physical examination reveals normal vital signs, clear lungs, no murmur, and no organomegaly. The hemoglobin value is 26 g/ dL. The most likely cause of the high hemoglobin level is

    A. placental insufficiency

    B. Wilms tumor

    C. pulmonary disease

    D. methemoglobinemia

    E. congenital heart disease

43. A 15-year-old is referred for evaluation of a hemoglobin value of 19.5 g/dL. Results of a physical examination are normal. The remainder of the CBC values are normal. The next step in your evaluation should be

    A. chest radiography

    B. hemoglobin determinations in parents and siblings

    C. cardiac catheterization

    D. pulmonary function tests

    E. leukocyte alkaline phosphatase determination

44. Hemolysis may be characterized by

    A. shortened RBC life span

    B. accelerated RBC destruction

    C. increased reticulocyte count if the marrow is not suppressed

    D. hemoglobinemia ± hemoglobinuria

    E. all of the above

45. Large numbers of spherocytes on the blood film are found in all of the following disorders EXCEPT

    A. immune hemolytic anemia

    B. Wilson disease

    C. hereditary spherocytosis

    D. sickle cell anemia

    E. clostridial sepsis

46. A previously normal African-American army recruit was assigned to Southeast Asia and given malarial prophylaxis. He developed pallor, fatigue, and dark urine. His hemoglobin level decreased from 14.8 to 9 g/dL. The most likely diagnosis is

    A. hereditary spherocytosis

    B. sickle cell disease

C. hepatitis

D. G6PD deficiency

E. immune hemolytic anemia

47. The diagnosis of the condition described in Question 46 can be confirmed by

    A. hemoglobin electrophoresis

    B. enzyme assay

    C. sucrose hemolysis test

    D. osmotic fragility

    E. Coombs test

48. The best treatment for the patient described in Questions 46 and 47 includes

    A. immediate transfusion

    B. discontinuing malarial prophylaxis

    C. iron therapy

    D. oxygen

    E. prednisone

49. A previously normal 10-year-old male develops pallor, fatigue, and a fall in hemoglobin level from 13 to 8 g/dL without evidence of bleeding. His spleen is slightly enlarged. The reticulocyte count is 10%, and his WBC and platelet counts are normal. Many spherocytes are observed on the blood film. The most likely diagnosis is

    A. hereditary spherocytosis

    B. G6PD deficiency

    C. pyruvate kinase (PK) deficiency

    D. occult bleeding

    E. acquired immune hemolytic anemia

50. The definitive diagnostic test for the condition described in Question 49 is

    A. an enzyme assay

    B. a stool Hemoccult test

    C. chest radiography

    D. direct and indirect Coombs tests

    E. an osmotic fragility test

51. For the patient described in Questions 49 and 50, initial treatment at the time of diagnosis may include (may choose more than one)

    A. splenectomy

    B. intravenous gammaglobulin

    C. ferrous sulfate

D. glucocorticoids

E. transfusion

52. Aplastic crises are correctly characterized as

    A. never life threatening

    B. always associated with high reticulocyte counts

    C. often the result of parvovirus infection in children

    D. never occurring in hereditary spherocytosis

    E. always resulting in profound anemia

53. In the absence of bleeding, hemolysis may be present with

    A. falling hemoglobin and hematocrit values

    B. normal hemoglobin and hematocrit values

    C. an elevated reticulocyte count

    D. a reticulocyte count near 0

    E. all of the above

54. A 12-year-old female of Pakistani parents is found to have mild microcytic anemia (hemoglobin 10.2 g/dL; MCV 60 fL). Which of the following laboratory values would support a diagnosis of β-thalassemia trait in this patient?

    A. Hemoglobin A2 value of 4.5% (normal = 1.8% to 3.5%)

    B. The presence of an abnormal hemoglobin band in a hemoglobin electrophoresis determination

    C. Fetal hemoglobin (hemoglobin F) value of 3% (normal <1.5%)

    D. Choices A and C above

    E. A reticulocyte count of 2.5%

55. A 2-year-old female is observed to have generalized cyanosis, but she appears otherwise clinically well. Which of the following would be expected to produce this clinical picture?

    A. Congenital methemoglobinemia due to heterozygous hemoglobin M

    B. Hemoglobin Kansas, an abnormal hemoglobin that has very low oxygen affinity

    C. A deficiency of NADH cytochrome b5 reductase (methemoglobin reductase)

    D. Tetralogy of Fallot

    E. Choices A, B, and C above

56. An 8-year-old African-American male is admitted to the emergency department after an automobile accident. He is found to have positive results on a screening test for sickle hemoglobin. His blood count shows hemoglobin 14 g/dL, MCV 85 fL, and normal RBC morphology in a stained blood smear. The differential diagnosis for this patient should include which of the following?

    A. Hemoglobin SC disease

    B. Sickle cell anemia (Hb SS)

    C. Sickle cell trait (Hb AS)

    D. G6PD deficiency

    E. Sickle-thalassemia

57. A 2-month-old child is found to have sickle cell anemia (hemoglobin SS) from a cord blood screening study. Appropriate measures for the treatment of this infant should include which of the following?

    A. Prophylactic oral penicillin G to be given twice daily

    B. Prophylactic transfusions of packed RBCs to be given at 4- to 6-week intervals

    C. Monthly deferoxamine injections to prevent iron overload

    D. Splenectomy

    E. None of the above

58. A 4-year-old child of Thai parents exhibits pallor and hepatosplenomegaly. His blood count shows a hemoglobin value of 5.0 g/dL and MCV of 55 fL. His blood smear shows severe anisopoikilocytosis, and his serum ferritin level is within the range of normal for his age. Which of the following are likely possible causes of this child's anemia?

    A. α-Thalassemia

    B. Hemoglobin E

    C. β-Thalassemia

    D. Sickle cell anemia

    E. Choices A, B, and C above

59. Coagulation of factor VIII has all of the following characteristics EXCEPT

    A. reduced activity in hemophilia A

    B. reduced activity in classic von Willebrand disease

    C. needed for normal platelet adhesion

    D. reduced levels in disseminated intravascular coagulation

    E. normal level in liver disease

60. The prothrombin time, which is a test of the extrinsic or tissue coagulation pathway, is abnormally prolonged in

    A. hemophilia A

    B. von Willebrand disease

    C. congenital factor XIII deficiency

    D. congenital factor VII deficiency

    E. congenital factor XI deficiency

61. A patient with fat malabsorption bruises easily. Laboratory studies show a PTT of 190 seconds (normal 25 to 35 seconds); prothrombin time of 100 seconds (normal 12 to 14 seconds); fibrinogen of 400 mg/dL (normal 174 to 450 mg/l); and platelet count of 175×10^9/L (normal 150 to 400 $\times$ 10^9/L). The most likely cause of the hemostatic defect is

    A. cirrhosis

    B. disseminated intravascular coagulation

    C. vitamin K deficiency

    D. vitamin A deficiency

    E. vitamin E deficiency

62. Coagulation studies on a patient with a bleeding disorder show factor VIII coagulant activity of 10 units/dL, factor IX coagulant activity of 60 units/dL, and von Willebrand factor activity of 100 units/dL. (Normal range for all three tests is 70 to 150 units/dL.) The bleeding time was 6 minutes (normal <10 minutes). These findings are diagnostic of

    A. liver disease

    B. von Willebrand disease

    C. hemophilia A

    D. hemophilia B

    E. thrombasthenia

63. Primary hemostatic mechanism defects are characterized by (may choose more than one)

    A. immediate onset of bleeding with trauma

    B. delayed onset of bleeding with trauma

    C. petechiae in the skin and mucous membranes

    D. abnormal bleeding time

    E. abnormal PTT or prothrombin time

64. When plasma is converted to serum, certain coagulation factors are consumed during the clotting process. This occurs in patients with

the entity DIC. Of the coagulation factors listed below, which ones are consumed? (Choose one or more.)

A. Fibrinogen

B. Prothrombin (factor II)

C. Factor V

D. Factor VIII

E. Factor X

65. In differentiating hemophilia from vitamin K deficiency, the most useful laboratory test is

A. PTT

B. prothrombin time

C. platelet count

D. fibrinogen concentration

E. bleeding time

66. *Matching:*

1. Prolonged PTT   A. Hemophilia A

2. Prolonged   B. von Willebrand
   prothrombin time   disease

3. Prolonged   C. Both
   bleeding time   D. Neither

4. Reduced factor
   VIII coagulant
   activity

67. The bleeding time is a test for

A. fibrinolysis

B. antithrombin III activity

C. platelet function

D. factor VIII coagulant activity

E. Lupus-type anticoagulant

68. The PTT is a useful screening test for detecting abnormally low plasma levels of

A. factor VII

B. factor VIII

C. factor XIII

D. platelets

E. protein C

22 Neoplastic Diseases and Tumors

The good news is that many childhood cancers are curable. The bad news is that cancer is still a leading cause of disease-based childhood mortality. In addition, survivors of childhood malignancies now face the long-term complications of their therapy, including secondary new malignancies. This *part* has been extensively updated, and chapters on epidemiology, molecular pathogenesis, principles of diagnosis, and principles of treatment have added to our general understanding of childhood malignancies.

Questions in this *part* do not expect you to be up to date on the latest Pediatric Oncology Group (POG) or Childhood Cancer Study Group (CCSG) protocols. Rather, they are directed at general pediatricians who usually diagnose the malignancy, work with the child and family, and monitor the ever-increasing number of survivors of childhood cancer.

1. Sites of leukemic recurrence usually include all of the following EXCEPT

   A. bone marrow

   B. central nervous system (CNS)

   C. testis

   D. kidneys

2. A 15-year-old white female reports that she has had fever, weight loss, and night sweats for 3 months. On physical examination, she has painless swelling of the left cervical and supraclavicular lymph nodes. Her liver and spleen are not enlarged. The initial evaluation of the patient should include

   A. bone marrow aspiration

   B. abdominal CT

   C. chest radiograph

   D. head CT

   E. erythrocyte sedimentation rate

3. The chest radiograph of the patient described in Question 2 reveals mediastinal lymphadenopathy. The next appropriate diagnostic test is

   A. abdominal CT

   B. head CT

   C. bone marrow biopsy

   D. lymph node biopsy

   E. thoracic CT

4. A 19-year-old female presents with pallor and ecchymosis of 2 weeks' duration. A complete blood count (CBC) reveals a hemoglobin value of 7.5, a platelet count of 25,000, and a white blood cell (WBC) count of 45,000. Ten years earlier, she was successfully treated for Hodgkin disease. The most likely diagnosis is

   A. secondary leukemia

   B. recurrent Hodgkin disease

   C. breast cancer

   D. mononucleosis

   E. aplastic anemia

5. *Matching:*

   1. Hypertension
   2. Congenital
   3. Aniridia
   4. Opsoclonus
   5. Diarrhea
   6. Ataxia
   7. Leukemic transformation
   8. Favorable prognosis
   9. Denys-Drash syndrome
   10. Pancytopenia
   11. Bilateral disease

   A. Neuroblastoma
   B. Wilms' tumor
   C. Both A and B
   D. Neither A nor B

6. A 5-year-old previously healthy white female manifests progressive painless proptosis and decreased visual acuity of the left eye during a 2-month period. The most likely diagnosis is

   A. pseudotumor of the orbit

B. trichinosis

C. retinoblastoma

D. rhabdomyosarcoma

E. orbital cellulitis

7. *Matching:*

   1. All races
   2. Limp
   3. Fever of unknown origin
   4. Differential diagnosis of osteomyelitis
   5. May be secondary malignancy
   6. Radiosensitive
   7. Metastasis to orbit
   8. Sunburst radiographic pattern
   9. Bone pain
   10. Small round cell tumor

   A. Osteogenic sarcoma
   B. Ewing sarcoma
   C. Both A and B
   D. Neither A nor B

8. A mother states that her 14-month-old infant's eye has a "cat's eye" appearance. On routine office ophthalmoscopic examination, you have a hard time seeing the fundus but observe no gross abnormalities. The extraocular muscles and remaining head and neck and general physical findings are normal. You should

   A. reassure the mother that nothing is wrong

   B. obtain toxoplasmosis titers

   C. culture for rubella

   D. refer the patient to an infectious disease specialist

   E. refer the patient to an ophthalmologist for examination under general anesthesia

9. *Matching:*

   1. Seminoma
   2. Hepatoblastoma
   3. Neuroblastoma
   4. Ovarian dysgerminoma
   5. Yolk sac carcinoma
   6. Choriocarcinoma

   A. Elevated α-fetoprotein
   B. Elevated β-human chorionic gonadotropin
   C. Neither A nor B
   D. Both A and B

10. A 16-year-old survivor of childhood leukemia presents with short stature and failure to develop puberty. Treatment for leukemia at the age of 8 years included vincristine, prednisone, 6-mercaptopurine, L-asparaginase, and craniospinal radiation for suspected CNS leukemia. The most likely diagnosis is

    A. recurrent leukemia

    B. secondary cerebral astrocytoma

    C. panhypopituitarism

    D. pseudotumor cerebri

11. A 19-year-old patient presents with tachycardia and a temperature of 39.7°C with disorientation. Ten years earlier, he was successfully treated for Hodgkin disease. The most likely diagnosis is

    A. recurrent Hodgkin disease

    B. tuberculosis

    C. secondary acute myeloblastic leukemia

    D. pneumococcemia

    E. mononucleosis

12. A 4-year-old presents with weight loss, anorexia, and weakness for 2 months. Left-sided ptosis and an ipsilateral miotic pupil are noted on physical examination. The most likely diagnosis is

    A. leukemia

    B. neuroblastoma

    C. Wilms' tumor

    D. cerebral astrocytoma

    E. cerebellar astrocytoma

13. A patient with newly diagnosed acute lymphocytic leukemia has a CBC that reveals a hemoglobin value of 9.0, a WBC count of 75,000, and a platelet count of 5000. During the initial high-intensity chemotherapy, the patient becomes obtunded and has bradycardia with hypertension. The most likely diagnosis is

    A. cerebral thrombosis

    B. cerebral leukemia

    C. anaphylaxis

    D. cerebral hemorrhage

    E. meningitis

14. A patient with newly diagnosed acute lymphocytic leukemia has a WBC count of 100,000. During induction high-dose chemotherapy, the patient develops oliguria. Laboratory data reveal blood urea nitrogen

(BUN) level of 65 and a serum creatinine value of 5.2. The most likely diagnosis is

A. leukemic renal infiltrates

B. hypotension

C. anaphylaxis

D. tumor lysis syndrome

E. sepsis

15. *Matching:* Cancer chemotherapy

1. Peripheral neuropathy	A. Cytoxan
2. Coagulopathy	B. Vincristine
3. Myelosuppression	C. Bleomycin
4. Pneumonitis	D. L-Asparaginase
5. Cardiomyopathy	E. Adriamycin

16. *Matching:* Presentation of malignancy

1. Diarrhea	A. Rhabdomyo-sarcoma
2. Vaginal bleeding	
3. Headache	B. Cerebellar astrocytoma
4. Night sweats	C. Lymphoma
5. Leukocoria	D. Neuroblastoma
6. Periorbital ecchymosis	E. Leukemia
7. Pancytopenia	F. Retinoblastoma

17. *Matching:* Familial-genetic factors and malignancy

1. Melanoma	A. Monosomy 5
2. Leukemia	B. Gardner syndrome
3. Myelodysplasia	C. Li-Fraumeni syndrome
4. Adenocarcinoma of the colon	D. Dysplastic nevus syndrome
5. Wilms' tumor	E. Fanconi anemia
6. Hemangioblastoma of the cerebellum	F. Hemihypertrophy
7. Sarcomas	G. von Hippel–Lindau disease

18. *Matching:* Neoplastic diseases

1. Li-Fraumeni syndrome	A. Diethylstilbestrol
2. Vaginal clear cell carcinoma	B. Radiation for a large thymus
3. Thyroid carcinoma	C. Anabolic androgenic steroids
4. Hepatoma	

5. Nasopharyngeal carcinoma

6. Cervical cancer

7. Melanoma

D. Papovavirus

E. Ultraviolet irradiation

F. Familial malignancies

G. Epstein-Barr virus

19. A 16-year-old white male presents with a history of 3 months of pain and swelling in the midportion of his tibia. A plain radiograph of the tibia reveals bone destruction in the midportion of his tibia, with an adjacent soft tissue mass. The lesion is sampled, and a small round cell tumor that stains positively for glycogen is described. Tumor cell karyotype reveals a t(11;22). The diagnosis is

A. osteosarcoma

B. Ewing sarcoma

C. acute lymphoblastic leukemia

D. benign bone cyst

E. neuroblastoma

20. A 14-month-old presents with a right-sided Horner syndrome and has a mass noted on chest film in the superior mediastinal region. The most likely diagnosis is

A. Wilms' tumor

B. neuroblastoma

C. acute leukemia

D. salivary gland tumor

E. rhabdomyosarcoma

21. A 5-year-old presents with a 1-month history of bone pain, increased bruising, swollen lymph glands, and recurrent fever. Laboratory studies reveal a hemoglobin value of 6.8 g/dL, platelet count 60,000/mm^3, and leukocyte count 3500/mm^3 with 2% neutrophils and atypical cells described. The most likely diagnosis is

A. acute myelocytic leukemia

B. Wilms' tumor

C. Hodgkin disease

D. aplastic anemia

E. acute lymphoblastic leukemia

22. The most common pediatric cancers include

A. colon cancer

B. breast cancer

C. acute lymphoblastic leukemia

D. lung cancer

E. adrenocortical carcinoma

23. Treatment of Wilms' tumor typically includes

A. actinomycin D

B. 6-mercaptopurine

C. cytosine arabinoside

D. methotrexate

E. allopurinol

24. A factor that is consistently related to prognosis in childhood lymphoblastic leukemia is

A. race

B. leukocyte level at diagnosis

C. uric acid level

D. bilirubin level

E. sex

23 Nephrology

This *part* is particularly valuable in bringing together the functional anatomy with the disease process. Renal physiology, another area in need of curriculum enhancement and better understanding by many house staff, is well integrated into the clinical chapters in this *part*. Causes of hematuria, proteinuria, tubular dysfunction, and toxic nephropathies are main sections in this *part* of the *Nelson Textbook*.

Questions for review relate to the parallel chapters in the *Nelson Textbook*. It is hoped that the knowledge gained by answering these questions will contribute to your comfort in managing renal diseases in children.

1. The predominant immunoglobulin deposited in the glomeruli of patients with Berger nephropathy is

   A. IgA

   B. IgD

   C. IgE

   D. IgG

   E. IgM

2. The triad of microangiopathic hemolytic anemia, renal failure, and thrombocytopenia is characteristic of which one of the following?

   A. Membranous lupus nephritis

   B. Focal glomerulonephritis secondary to septicemia

   C. Hemolytic-uremic syndrome

   D. Acute poststreptococcal glomerulonephritis

   E. Berger disease

3. An infant is admitted to the hospital because of vomiting and lethargy. The child shows evidence of failure to thrive, and physical examination reveals an abdominal mass. Blood and urinary cultures grow *Escherichia coli*. The most likely cause of this disorder is

   A. mesenteric cyst

   B. Wilms' tumor

   C. adrenal hemorrhage

   D. obstruction at the ureteropelvic junction

   E. retrocaval ureter

4. The best treatment for pediatric patients showing evidence of end-stage renal disease (ESRD) is

   A. long-term peritoneal dialysis and a low-protein diet

   B. long-term hemodialysis and a low-protein diet

   C. a low-protein diet and dihydroxycholecalciferol (vitamin D₃)

   D. living related donor renal transplantation

   E. renal transplantation with a cadaveric kidney

5. The most frequent cause of graft loss in pediatric renal transplant recipients is

   A. trauma to the graft

   B. recurrence of the original renal disease in the graft

   C. technical difficulties

   D. infection

   E. rejection reaction

6. Which of the following statements is correct?

   A. Renal metabolic diseases are the most frequent causes of ESRD in children.

   B. The congenital nephrotic syndrome (minimal change nephropathy) is the most frequent cause of ESRD in young children.

   C. Causes of ESRD in children vary with age.

   D. Congenital and obstructive processes are the most frequent causes of ESRD in 13- to 17-year-old children.

   E. The glomerulonephritides produce ESRD most frequently in children younger than 5 years.

7. A 10-year-old child with a serum creatinine level of 2.1 mg/dL 4 weeks after renal transplant (2 weeks before this, the creatinine level was 0.9 mg/dL) has a persistent temperature of 39° to 40°C, a tender graft, and blood pressure of 130/80. He has been on

cyclosporine-azathioprine-prednisone therapy. He most likely is experiencing

A. recurrence of his original renal disease in the graft

B. cyclosporine A toxicity

C. acute rejection reaction

D. thrombosis of the graft

E. graft artery stenosis

8. *Matching:*

1. Membranous glomerulonephritis	A. Immune complex deposition
2. Goodpasture disease	
3. Rapidly progressive glomerulonephritis	B. Antiglomerular basement membrane antibody deposition
4. Membranoproliferative glomerulonephritis	
5. Idiopathic nephrotic syndrome	C. Both immunologic mechanisms
	D. Neither immunologic mechanism

9. *Matching:* For the following items, choose the associated form of nephrotic syndrome.

1. Hypocomplementemia	A. Membranoproliferative glomerulonephritis
2. Most common in children	B. Membranous glomerulonephritis
3. Most common in adults	C. Minimal change disease
4. Gross hematuria	D. Focal sclerosis
5. Renal vein thrombosis	E. Congenital nephrotic syndrome
6. Juxtamedullary glomeruli	

10. A 10-month-old male presents with a 3-day history of vomiting, diarrhea, fever, lethargy, and declining urine output. Examination shows dry mucous membranes, poor skin turgor, and a blood pressure of 60/40 mm Hg. Laboratory studies include a serum sodium level of 137 mEq/L, potassium 3.1 mEq/L, chloride 91 mEq/L, bicarbonate 18 mEq/L, blood urea nitrogen (BUN) 62 mg/dL, creatinine 2.6 mg/dL, calcium 7.9 mg/dL, phosphorus 7.0 mg/dL, and uric acid 9.7 mg/dL. Urinalysis reveals a specific gravity of 1.006, 5 to 10 red blood cells and 5 to 10 white blood cells per high-power field, and + + protein. The urine sodium concentration is 42 mEq/L, and the fractional excretion of sodium is 3.2%. Findings on renal ultrasound examination are normal. The most likely diagnosis would be

A. acute tubular necrosis

B. urethral valves

C. uric acid nephropathy

D. dehydration-associated prerenal azotemia

E. renal venous thrombosis

11. A 4-year-old male developed an upper respiratory tract infection that was followed in 2 weeks by general edema. His blood pressure is normal. Urinalysis reveals 2 to 5 red blood cells per high-power field and 4+ protein. His BUN is 19 mg/dL, creatinine 0.6 mg/dL, cholesterol 402 mg/dL, serum albumin 0.9 g/dL, antistreptolysin O titer 1:16, and C3 92 mg/dL. The most likely diagnosis would be

A. poststreptococcal glomerulonephritis

B. membranous glomerulonephritis

C. minimal lesion nephrotic syndrome

D. membranoproliferative glomerulonephritis

E. focal sclerosis

12. A 4-year-old with a serum creatinine level of 5.1 mg/dL has a serum calcium level of 10.1 mg/dL and phosphorus level of 8.2 mg/dL. For this patient, it would be most appropriate to begin therapy with

A. dialysis

B. aluminum hydroxide

C. calcitriol

D. calcium carbonate

E. dihydrotachysterol

13. A 6-month-old male is evaluated for growth failure. The following laboratory results are obtained: serum sodium 136 mEq/L, potassium 6.5 mEq/L, chloride 108 mEq/L, carbon dioxide 15 mEq/L, BUN 8 mg/dL, and creatinine 0.2 mg/dL. The most appropriate next step in evaluating this patient would be

A. renal ultrasonography

B. blood gas determination

C. measurement of urine electrolytes

D. measurement of urine amino acids

E. determination of creatinine clearance

24 Urologic Disorders in Infants and Children

Urinary anomalies, infection, and reflux greatly contribute to end-stage renal disease. This *part* of the *Nelson Textbook* emphasizes early recognition, intensive evaluation, and compulsive management and follow-up.

Questions for this *part* are clinically based and reemphasize the principles outlined in the previous paragraph.

1. A woman at 24 weeks of gestation has poor uterine growth and decreased fetal movement. Screening fetal ultrasonography reveals oligohydramnios. The next step should include

   A. taking a careful drug history

   B. higher-level ultrasonography to examine the fetal kidneys and bladder

   C. an α-fetoprotein level

   D. an abortion

   E. amniocentesis

2. Potter syndrome is due to

   A. renal agenesis

   B. renal dysplasia

   C. obstructive uropathy

   D. severe amniotic fluid leak

   E. none of the above

   F. all of the above

3. Risk factors for urinary tract infections include all of the following EXCEPT

   A. uncircumcised male infants

   B. sexual activity

   C. reflux nephropathy

   D. double-ureteral systems

   E. chronic use of antibiotics

   F. spina bifida

4. In infants with urinary tract infection, the most common manifestation is

   A. fever

   B. dysuria

   C. frequency

   D. costovertebral angle tenderness

   E. incontinence

5. The imaging study of choice for the first urinary tract infection in an 18-month-old during the hospitalization is

   A. renal ultrasonography

   B. DMSA scan

   C. computed tomography

   D. voiding cystourethrogram (VCUG)

   E. none of the above

6. The presence of renal parenchymal scarring due to vesicoureteral reflux is best determined by

   A. DMSA scan

   B. renal ultrasonography

   C. VCUG

   D. CT scan

   E. intravenous pyelography

7. Risk factors for vesicoureteral reflux include all of the following EXCEPT

   A. spina bifida

   B. ureteral duplication

   C. ureteral diverticula

   D. ureterocele

   E. bladder outlet obstruction

   F. sexual intercourse

   G. positive family history of reflux

8. A fetus at 30 weeks' gestation is noted by fetal ultrasonography to have unilateral hydronephrosis. After birth, the child appears normal, and on the first day of life the renal ultrasonographic findings of the neonate are now normal. The next step is to

   A. begin prophylactic antibiotics

B. assure the parents that the fetal ultrasound findings were false positive

C. perform a VCUG

D. repeat the ultrasound examination in 1 to 3 months

E. do none of the above

9. The most common abdominal mass in a neonate is

A. renal dysplasia—hydronephrosis

B. Wilms' tumor

C. neuroblastoma

D. Meckel diverticulum

E. ovarian teratoma

10. Prune belly syndrome is usually associated with all of the following EXCEPT

A. oligohydramnios

B. deficient abdominal muscles

C. undescended testes

D. urethral atresia

E. bowel malrotation

11. A 6-month-old male presents with failure to thrive. His blood urea nitrogen (BUN) level is 60 mg/dL, and his creatinine value is 5.3 mg/dL. Past history reveals an episode of *Escherichia coli* sepsis and urinary tract infection at 1 month of age. The mother also comments that compared with his older brother, his urinary stream isn't as strong. His most likely diagnosis is

A. chronic pyelonephritis

B. meningomyelocele

C. atonic bladder

D. AIDS

E. posterior urethral valves

12. A 7-year-old male presents with episodes of abdominal pain, nausea, and vomiting that last several hours and subside spontaneously. The past medical history, review of systems, family history, and physical examination are unremarkable. What imaging study would be most appropriate to begin his evaluation?

A. Gastroscopy

B. Abdominal ultrasonography

C. Barium enema

D. Diuresis renography

E. None of the above

13. An adolescent boy notices a painless, ropelike mass in the left side of his scrotum. The most likely diagnosis is

A. epididymitis

B. torsion of an appendage

C. torsion of the testis

D. hydrocele

E. varicocele

14. The recommended age to perform corrective surgery in a child with a unilateral undescended testis is

A. the first month of life

B. between 12 and 18 months of age

C. between 5 and 7 years of age

D. before puberty

E. after puberty

15. Which of the factors listed below is most likely to contribute to renal deterioration in an infant with myelomeningocele?

A. The level of the lesion

B. The child's gender

C. High intravesical pressure

D. The presence of hydrocephalus

E. All of the above

16. An infant with treated posterior urethral valves is at risk for which of the following complications?

A. Urinary incontinence

B. Renal failure

C. Urinary tract infections

D. Arterial hypertension

E. All of the above

17. An otherwise normal newborn known to have had left hydronephrosis on prenatal ultrasonograms at 28 and 36 weeks of gestation has a renal ultrasonogram on the day of birth that shows no dilatation of the renal collecting systems. The most appropriate course of action is

A. no further evaluation

B. immediate diuresis renography and voiding cystourethrography

C. repeat renal ultrasonography within the first 4 weeks of life

D. antibacterial prophylaxis

E. intravenous urography

18. A 3-year-old female presents with vomiting, diarrhea, and fever. A urinalysis shows pyuria and hematuria, and a culture grows greater than 10^5 colonies of *E. coli*. She responds well to hydration and intravenous antibiotics. What imaging studies, if any, are appropriate during the acute phase of the infection?

   A. Renal and bladder ultrasonography

   B. Intravenous urogram

   C. VCUG

   D. CT scan of the abdomen

   E. None

25 Gynecologic Problems of Childhood

Traditional gynecologic problems are relatively uncommon before puberty. In the large population of adolescents, many of whom are also sexually active, gynecologic problems become similar to those in young adult women. Pediatricians initially see many young women with gynecologic problems and should carefully study this *part* of the *Nelson Textbook.*

Questions in this *part* do not make you an expert in the art of bimanual palpation but help reinforce your understanding of the signs, symptoms, and management of pediatric gynecologic problems.

1. A 17-year-old Tanner stage 2 female presents with a history of bilateral spontaneous milky discharge from her breasts for 2 months. Menarche was at age 12 years, and her periods had been regular until 4 months before this visit to your office. In addition, she complains of headache on awakening for the past 2 weeks. The most useful screening test is a

   A. urine pregnancy test

   B. serum pregnancy test

   C. serum prolactin level

   D. serum estrogen level

   E. serum luteinizing hormone level

2. The prolactin level of the young woman described in Question 1 is 1000 times higher than normal. The next test in her evaluation should be

   A. cranial MRI

   B. abdominal CT

   C. pelvic ultrasonography

   D. uterine biopsy

   E. mammography

3. Vaginal bleeding in prepubertal females may be due to all of the following EXCEPT

   A. von Willebrand disease

   B. foreign body

   C. urethral prolapse

   D. sexual abuse/trauma

   E. endodermal carcinoma

   F. mesonephric carcinoma

4. A 10-year-old white female is found to have pink-white flat-topped papules over her labia majora and perianal area. The atrophic-appearing lesions have coalesced to form a figure-of-eight lesion around the labia and anus. The most likely diagnosis is

   A. excessive masturbation

   B. lichen planus

   C. lichen sclerosus

   D. child abuse

   E. contact dermatitis

5. *Matching:* Vulvovaginitis

1. Umbilicated pink-white small nodule	A. Enterobiasis (pinworm)
2. Nits on hair shaft	B. Molluscum contagiosum
3. Associated bloody mucous stools	C. Pediculosis pubis
4. Purulent vaginal discharge	D. *Shigella*
5. Nocturnal perineal pruritus	E. Group A streptococcus

6. A 7-year-old female complains of a brown-green vaginal discharge on her underwear. She has no fever or labial tenderness and denies sexual contact. Her mother states that for the past 4 months, her daughter has been taking ballet classes and frequently sleeps in her leotards. The most likely diagnosis is

   A. nonspecific vaginitis

   B. *Gardnerella vaginalis* vaginitis

   C. gonorrhea

   D. chlamydial vaginitis

   E. *Candida* vaginitis

7. Initial therapy for the girl described in Question 6 should include all of the following EXCEPT

   A. instruction in perineal hygiene

   B. sitz baths

   C. use of mild soaps

   D. avoiding tight clothing

   E. metronidazole

8. After the onset of menarche at 13 years of age, a patient is noted to have irregular menses (i.e., occurring every 12 to 14 weeks). She is now 16 years old and is noted to have onset of acne, oily hair, and associated hirsutism, which began soon after menarche. She shows no evidence of deepening of the voice or clitoromegaly (virilization). With respect to polycystic ovary syndrome, which of the following statements is correct?

   A. It is associated with altered luteinizing hormone release.

   B. It is associated with a luteinizing hormone to follicle-stimulating hormone ratio of 4:1 or greater.

   C. It is clearly of central nervous system origin.

   D. It is associated with a heterozygous form of 21-hydroxylase deficiency.

9. A sexually active adolescent who has had multiple partners is currently being evaluated. As part of her routine gynecologic examination, a Papanicolaou smear is obtained, the result of which identifies human papillomavirus. In addition, a review of systems notes evidence of vaginal discharge without associated pruritus. With respect to human papillomavirus and vulvovaginitis, which types are particularly associated with premalignant lesions of the vulva?

   A. 1 and 6

   B. 6 and 11

   C. 16 and 18

   D. 18 and 22

   E. None of the above

10. When cervical intraepithelial neoplasia is identified on a Papanicolaou smear, which of the following procedures would be performed first?

    A. Cold conization of the cervix

    B. Colposcopic examination

    C. Repeat the Papanicolaou smear

    D. Cryotherapy

    E. Laser therapy

11. You are asked to evaluate a vulvar lesion in a 6-year-old. She has pruritus and a lesion characterized by scaly macules over her vulvar area. The history does not include evidence of vaginal discharge, and this appears to be an overall recent (2 weeks) problem that has been identified by the parents. Which of the following statements is NOT associated with pityriasis versicolor?

    A. It is caused by *Pityrosporum orbiculare.*

    B. It is manifested by scaly macules on the trunk as well as lesions in the genital area in postpubertal patients.

    C. Diagnosis requires visualization on wet preparation of hyphae and spores with 10% potassium hydroxide solution.

    D. Treatment requires application of topical imidazoles.

    E. Its presence implies sexual abuse.

12. A $5^{7}/_{12}$-year-old female is brought to you for evaluation. She has a history of approximately 3 weeks of labial agglutination. There is no evidence of recurrent urinary tract infection or of sexual abuse. Her external genitalia were noted to be normal at birth. The parents express concern about the diagnosis and underlying cause of the gynecologic problem. Overall nonspecific vulvovaginitis accounts for what percentage of all pediatric vulvovaginitis cases?

    A. 25%

    B. 40%

    C. 50%

    D. 70%

    E. 90%

13. The most common bacterial organism associated with nonspecific vulvovaginitis is

    A. β-hemolytic streptococcus

    B. coagulase-positive *Staphylococcus*

    C. *Escherichia coli*

    D. *Pseudomonas aeruginosa*

    E. *Neisseria gonorrhoeae*

26 The Endocrine System

Disorders of the hypothalamus-pituitary gland, thyroid gland, parathyroid glands, adrenal glands, and gonads in addition to diabetes mellitus are well described in this *part* of the *Nelson Textbook*. These problems, taken together as endocrine-related diseases, are relatively common and are rarely encountered in an inpatient setting but occupy a significant amount of outpatient pediatrics.

In addition to clinical recognition and management, the diagnostic utility of hormone assays or provocative testing is highlighted.

The questions in this *part* should reinforce your reading of the *Nelson Textbook* chapters and the 1-month rotation in outpatient endocrinology that you probably had as an elective during residency.

1. ***Matching:*** Adrenocortical insufficiency

   1. Holoprosencephaly
   2. Male predominance
   3. Familial glucocorticoid deficiency
   4. Allgrove syndrome
   5. Most common cause of adrenocortical insufficiency

   A. ACTH receptor mutations
   B. ACTH resistance
   C. Corticotropin deficiency
   D. Adrenal hypoplasia congenita
   E. Congenital adrenal hyperplasia

2. A 12-year-old female has a hypoglycemic seizure, weakness, and increased cutaneous pigmentation. She is also noted to have a chronic history of mucocutaneous candidiasis, which is especially severe on her nails. In addition, she has been on thyroid replacement medication since the age of 9 years. The most likely diagnosis is

   A. insulinoma
   B. growth hormone deficiency
   C. AIDS
   D. autoimmune polyendocrinopathy
   E. DiGeorge syndrome

3. A 1-day-old full-term neonate manifests ambiguous genitalia. The infant has complete labial fusion and a phallus that resembles a small penis with hypospadias. No gonads are palpable. The vital signs including the blood pressure are normal, and the serum electrolytes reveal no abnormalities. The laboratory evaluation of this patient should include

   A. karyotype
   B. pelvic ultrasonography
   C. serum 17-hydroxyprogesterone
   D. daily electrolyte determinations
   E. all of the above

4. Cushing syndrome in children is associated with all of the following EXCEPT

   A. functioning adrenocortical tumor
   B. age less than 3 years
   C. McCune-Albright syndrome
   D. basophilic adenoma of the pituitary
   E. mucocutaneous candidiasis

5. ***Matching:***

   1. Hypokalemia
   2. Alkalosis
   3. Hyponatremia
   4. Hypochloremia
   5. Hypertension
   6. High renin level
   7. High urinary prostaglandin levels
   8. Growth failure

   A. Primary hyperaldosteronism
   B. Bartter syndrome
   C. Neither
   D. Both

6. The appropriate approach to removal of a pheochromocytoma is best accomplished with

   A. α-adrenergic receptor blockade
   B. β-adrenergic receptor blockade
   C. saline fluid loading
   D. identification of bilateral tumors
   E. all of the above
   F. none of the above

7. Adrenal calcification may be a sequela of all of the following EXCEPT

    A. meningococcal sepsis

    B. neonatal adrenal hemorrhage

    C. meconium peritonitis

    D. Wolman syndrome

    E. tuberculosis

    F. neuroblastoma

8. A 16-year-old male has a tall stature but no facial, axillary, or pubic hair. His penis and scrotum are obscured by pubic adipose tissue, but they appear infantile. Chromosome analysis reveals an XY karyotype. His serum follicle-stimulating hormone (FSH) and luteinizing hormone (LH) levels are elevated. The most likely diagnosis is

    A. galactosemia

    B. primary hypogonadism

    C. adrenal hyperplasia

    D. Noonan syndrome

    E. none of the above

9. All of the following are associated with Klinefelter syndrome EXCEPT

    A. 47 XXY karyotype

    B. mental retardation

    C. small testes and penis

    D. precocious puberty

    E. gynecomastia

    F. azoospermia

10. A 14-year-old male has unilateral gynecomastia and is Tanner stage 3 in pubertal development. He complains of occasional episodes of breast tenderness, which last less than 30 minutes and occur once a month. His serum estradiol and prolactin levels are normal. The most likely next step in the treatment of this patient is

    A. reassurance and explaining the transient nature

    B. mammography

    C. abdominal CT including the pelvis

    D. head CT focusing on the pituitary

    E. karyotype

11. Causes of hypergonadotropic hypogonadism in females include all of the following EXCEPT

    A. gonadal dysgenesis

    B. galactosemia

    C. cytotoxic drugs

    D. polycystic ovaries

    E. type I autoimmune polyendocrinopathy

    F. ataxia-telangiectasia

12. Male pseudohermaphroditism in neonates is associated with all of the following syndromes EXCEPT

    A. camptomelic

    B. WAGR

    C. Denys-Drash

    D. Swyer

    E. 11-hydroxylase deficiency

13. *Matching:* Diabetes

    1. Autoimmune
    2. Obesity
    3. Insulin resistance
    4. Honeymoon period
    5. Glucokinase mutation
    6. Antibody to glutamic acid decarboxylase
    7. Familial
    8. Hypothyroidism
    9. Blindness
    10. Cure available

    A. Insulin-dependent diabetes

    B. Non–insulin-dependent diabetes

    C. Both A and B

    D. Neither A nor B

14. All of the following are associated with type I diabetes EXCEPT

    A. high incidence in Finland

    B. male predominance

    C. onset in autumn and winter

    D. congenital rubella

    E. specific HLA susceptibility

15. A 12-year-old Tanner stage 2 female has weight loss, polyuria, and polydipsia. Her blood glucose level is 1000 mg/dL, and her blood urea nitrogen (BUN) value is 75 mg/dL. She is tachypneic and has a serum bicarbonate level of 5. It is estimated that she is 15% dehydrated. Therapy is begun with insulin and aggressive fluid management. Five hours later,

she complains of a headache, has double vision, and quickly becomes unresponsive. The most likely new problem is

A. hypoglycemia

B. hyponatremia

C. uremia

D. cerebral edema

E. cerebral hemorrhage

16. Long-term complications of type I diabetes include all of the following EXCEPT

A. hypoglycemia

B. retinopathy

C. neuropathy

D. nephropathy

E. arthropathy

F. hypocalcemia

17. Causes of hypercalcemia include all of the following EXCEPT

A. multiple endocrine neoplasia type I

B. parathyroid adenoma

C. DiGeorge syndrome

D. vitamin D intoxication

E. sarcoidosis

18. A patient with hypocalcemia demonstrates short stature and brachydactyly with a short middle finger. The serum parathyroid hormone level is elevated. The most likely diagnosis is

A. rickets

B. hypoparathyroidism

C. hypomagnesemia

D. DiGeorge syndrome

E. pseudohypoparathyroidism

19. A 12-year-old female has muscle cramps and tingling of her hands and feet unrelated to exertion. When she grabs a door handle to open the door, she is unable to release her grasp because her hand is in spasm. The most important laboratory test is

A. serum glucose determination

B. serum calcium determination

C. electromyography (EMG)

D. nerve conduction velocity testing

E. arterial blood gas determination

20. The most likely diagnosis for the patient described in Question 19 is

A. rickets

B. hysterical hyperventilation

C. hypoparathyroidism

D. renal failure

E. furosemide (Lasix) abuse

21. Acquired hypothyroidism is associated with all of the following EXCEPT

A. diabetes mellitus

B. cystinosis

C. hyperparathyroidism

D. lymphocytic thyroiditis

E. Langerhans cell histiocytosis

22. Complications of drug therapy (propylthiouracil or Tapazole) for hyperthyroidism include all of the following EXCEPT

A. hypotension

B. urticaria

C. leukopenia

D. hepatitis

E. lupus-like syndrome

23. Physical findings in Graves disease include all of the following EXCEPT

A. motor hyperactivity

B. cold intolerance

C. tremor

D. weight loss

E. tachycardia

F. smooth, flushed, warm skin

24. Ocular manifestations of Graves disease include all of the following EXCEPT

A. lid lag

B. exophthalmos

C. impaired convergence

D. infrequent blinking

E. detached retina

25. A 10-year-old white female is noted not to have grown in the past year. Physical findings are otherwise normal except for fullness over the area of her thyroid gland. Her T_4 level is normal. The next important test to perform is

A. antithyroglobulin and antithyroid peroxidase antibodies

B. thyroid scan

C. thyroid ultrasonography

D. glucose tolerance test

E. TSH level

26. Laboratory evidence of classic congenital hypothyroidism in a sample of blood taken on the third day of life includes

    A. elevated TSH, low T_4

    B. elevated TSH, high T_3

    C. low TSH, low T_4

    D. low T_4, high T_3

    E. low TBG, low T_4

27. All of the following are commonly associated with congenital hypothyroidism EXCEPT

    A. a lower incidence in African-Americans

    B. absence of symptoms at birth

    C. frequent prolongation of physiologic jaundice

    D. temperature instability

    E. a palpable goiter

28. McCune-Albright syndrome is associated with all of the following EXCEPT

    A. precocious puberty in females

    B. hyperthyroidism

    C. diabetes mellitus

    D. Cushing syndrome

    E. phosphaturic osteomalacia

    F. neonatal cholestasis

    G. bony fibrous dysplasia

29. Treatment of true precocious puberty is best achieved with

    A. gonadotrophin-releasing hormone (GnRH)

    B. hypothalamic surgery to remove the hamartoma

    C. dexamethasone suppression

    D. prolactin

    E. thyroid hormone

30. Gonadotropin-independent precocious puberty in females (precocious pseudopuberty) is associated with all of the following EXCEPT

    A. pulsatile secretion of LH and FSH

B. McCune-Albright syndrome

C. ovarian cysts

D. exogenous estrogens

E. granulosa-theca cell tumor

31. Gonadotropin-dependent precocious puberty (true precocious puberty) is associated with all of the following EXCEPT

    A. female predominance

    B. hypothalamic hamartoma

    C. hypothyroidism

    D. menstruation as the first sign

    E. shorter than expected stature

32. An 18-month-old female with sickle cell anemia develops pneumococcal meningitis. Her initial vital signs on presentation are pulse 160, respirations 45, blood pressure 65/35 mm Hg, and temperature 40°C. Her initial electrolyte values were normal. After fluid resuscitation and antibiotic therapy, she begins to improve. On the second day of the illness, the electrolyte results reveal Na^+ 115 mEq/dL, K^+ 2.9 mEq/dL, Cl^- 95 mEq/dL, and BUN 5. Her urine sodium level is 86. The most likely electrolyte disturbance at this time is

    A. acute tubular necrosis

    B. dilutional hyponatremia (iatrogenic)

    C. cardiogenic shock

    D. inappropriate ADH secretion

    E. hyponatremic dehydration

33. The syndrome of inappropriate ADH secretion is associated with all of the following EXCEPT

    A. meningitis

    B. head trauma

    C. pneumonia

    D. Guillain-Barré syndrome

    E. Ewing sarcoma

    F. hypernatremic dehydration

34. A 2-month-old has a temperature of 39.9°C, severe dehydration, but no history of vomiting or diarrhea. He also has constipation and is constantly crying for his bottle. His serum sodium level is 167 mEq/dL and urine specific gravity is 1.001. The most likely diagnosis is

    A. acute tubular necrosis

    B. diabetes insipidus

C. diabetes mellitus

D. hydronephrosis

E. adrenal insufficiency

35. Diabetes insipidus is associated with all of the following EXCEPT

A. optic glioma

B. craniopharyngioma

C. diabetes mellitus

D. Langerhans cell histiocytosis

E. encephalitis

F. atypical mycobacteria

36. Russell-Silver syndrome is characterized by all of the following EXCEPT

A. hemihypertrophy

B. short stature

C. pituitary adenoma

D. frontal bossing

E. a small triangular face

37. Constitutional growth delay is characterized by all of the following EXCEPT

A. normal length at birth

B. growth below the third percentile after 1 year of age

C. delayed bone age

D. positive family history

E. insulin resistance

38. Risk factors with current treatment protocols with growth hormone include all of the following EXCEPT

A. pseudotumor cerebri

B. slipped capital femoral epiphysis

C. worsening of scoliosis

D. development of antibodies

E. Creutzfeldt-Jakob disease

39. All of the following are associated with hypopituitarism EXCEPT

A. histiocytosis X

B. CNS irradiation

C. septo-optic dysplasia

D. child abuse

E. nesidioblastosis

F. optic glioma

40. Neonatal clues to the diagnosis of hypopituitarism include all of the following EXCEPT

A. microphallus

B. hypoglycemia

C. bifid epiglottis

D. hydrocephalus

E. optic nerve hypoplasia

F. postaxial polydactyly

41. A 12-year-old manifests poor growth for the past 2 years. At the age of 7 years, she developed acute lymphocytic leukemia and received cranial irradiation of 45 Gy. The most likely diagnosis is

A. isolated GH deficiency

B. TSH deficiency

C. recurrent leukemia

D. psychosocial dwarfism

E. spinal stenosis

42. All of the following are true about the genetic forms of isolated growth hormone (IGH) deficiency EXCEPT that

A. IGF-1 levels are elevated

B. inheritance is autosomal recessive

C. inheritance is autosomal dominant

D. inheritance is X linked

E. some have complete deletions of the GH gene

43. Laron syndrome is associated with all of the following EXCEPT

A. low IGF-1 levels

B. high GH levels

C. short stature

D. absent GH binding

E. correction with exogenous recombinant GH

44. Definitive and confirmatory laboratory evidence of growth hormone deficiency is documented by

A. CT scan

B. low IGF-1 levels

C. low IGF-binding protein 3

D. absent or low GH levels after provocative tests

E. growth less than 3 SD below the mean

F. bone age

45. A mother and her 14½-year-old daughter come to you because the girl has not begun to menstruate. Findings on her medical history and complete physical examination are normal. Breast development and pubic hair have been present for 18 months and are normal. Which would be most appropriate?

   A. Reassurance that she likely will begin menstruating within the year

   B. Laboratory evaluation for systemic disease

   C. Urinary estriol determination

   D. Buccal smear

   E. Referral for psychologic counseling

46. A child is below the third percentile for height. Growth velocity is normal, but chronologic age is greater than skeletal age. This condition is called

   A. primary hypopituitarism

   B. secondary hypopituitarism

   C. constitutional delay in growth

   D. genetic short stature

   E. primordial dwarfism

47. The growth hormone levels in the child described in Question 46 are most likely

   A. elevated

   B. normal

   C. depressed

   D. variable

48. A 10-year-old female is noted to have lagging of the upper eyelid when she looks down. Her eyes cannot converge, and she has retraction of her upper eyelid. This constellation of signs is diagnostic for

   A. lymphocytic thyroiditis

   B. congenital hypothyroidism

   C. simple goiter

   D. Graves disease

   E. solitary thyroid nodule

49. An infant is brought to the emergency room with vomiting, lethargy, dehydration, and failure to thrive. Intravenous administration of fluids is begun. Serum electrolyte values are sodium 124 mEq/L, chloride 88 mEq/L, and potassium 6.8 mEq/L. Serum glucose level is 35 mg/dL. The child is hypotensive and has areas of depigmentation. The most likely diagnosis is

   A. Addison disease

   B. Waterhouse-Friderichsen syndrome

   C. 17-hydroxylase deficiency

   D. Cushing syndrome

   E. adrenoleukodystrophy

50. Treatment for the infant described in Question 49 should include which of the following? (Choose as many as are appropriate.)

   A. Desoxycorticosterone acetate (DOCA)

   B. Hydrocortisone hemisuccinate

   C. Adrenalectomy

   D. Insulin

   E. Glucagon

51. The most common form of congenital adrenal hyperplasia is deficiency of

   A. 3β-hydroxysteroid dehydrogenase

   B. 11β-hydroxylase

   C. 17-hydroxylase

   D. 21β-hydroxylase

   E. aldosterone

27 The Nervous System

This *part* of the *Nelson Textbook* is an important reminder of the complexities of neurologic disorders. This *part* has chapters that discuss examination and evaluation, congenital anomalies, seizures, headaches, neurocutaneous syndromes, movement disorders, encephalopathies, coma, brain death, injuries, neurodegenerative disorders, stroke, abscesses, tumors, pseudotumor cerebri, and spinal cord disorders.

Questions for the nervous system *part* emphasize the recognition and differential diagnosis of neurologic disorders.

1. A 4-year-old female has experienced progressive loss of ambulation for a 2-year period. On examination, the child is apathetic and disinterested in her surroundings. She has horizontal nystagmus and optic atrophy. Her voice is dysarthric. She is hypotonic, and her deep tendon reflexes are absent. A sibling died at the age of 6 years with a similar history. The motor nerve conduction velocities show marked slowing, and computed tomography (CT) of the head shows diffuse symmetric attenuation of the cerebral and cerebellar white matter. The most likely diagnosis is

   A. multiple sclerosis

   B. metachromatic leukodystrophy

   C. GM$_2$ gangliosidosis (Tay-Sachs disease)

   D. neuronal ceroid lipofuscinosis

   E. Pelizaeus-Merzbacher disease

2. A 12-year-old female notes repetitive jerks of her upper extremities on awakening, which make hair combing and teeth brushing difficult. The myoclonus disappears by midmorning. At the age of 14 years, while at school, she had a 5-minute generalized tonic-clonic seizure. Results of her neurologic examination are normal, and the electroencephalogram (EEG) shows irregular spikes and waves, four to six per second, particularly with photic stimulation. Which anticonvulsant is the drug of choice?

   A. Ethosuximide

   B. Felbamate

   C. Valproic acid

   D. Phenobarbital

   E. Carbamazepine

3. A 4-year-old female has a 2-week history of fever associated with bifrontal headache,
lethargy, and vomiting. She has a history of perioral cyanosis and dyspnea with exertion beginning in infancy. She suddenly has a 10-minute focal tonic-clonic seizure. The child is obtunded and has a temperature of 100.8°F (38.2°C), pulse of 118, and blood pressure of 96/70 mm Hg in her right arm, supine. Perioral cyanosis is noted at rest. A harsh pansystolic murmur is heard best along the left sternal border. Examination of her eye grounds reveals bilateral papilledema. She has right-sided weakness associated with hyperreflexia and an extensor plantar reflex. The most likely cause of the hemiparesis is

   A. moyamoya disease

   B. a brain tumor

   C. an intracranial hemorrhage

   D. methemoglobinemia

   E. a brain abscess

4. A 14-year-old female is suspected of having pseudoseizures. The most precise procedure for confirming the diagnosis is

   A. response to intravenous phenytoin

   B. simultaneous video/EEG recording during seizure

   C. absence of Babinski sign and normally reactive pupils during seizure

   D. measurement of baseline and postseizure serum prolactin levels

   E. psychiatric evaluation

5. An active 6-year-old male has complained of an intermittent right frontal pounding headache for 2 months. The headache is often associated with nausea and is relieved by acetaminophen. On the day of admission, he had a throbbing frontal headache followed by a left hemiparesis associated with stupor.

Physical examination showed a temperature of 101°F (38.4°C), nuchal rigidity, a high-pitched bruit over the right side of his forehead, a Glasgow coma scale score of 8, and a left hemiparesis. What is the most likely diagnosis?

A. Encephalitis

B. Migraine

C. Subdural hematoma

D. Ruptured arteriovenous malformation

E. Brain tumor

6. A 15-month-old patient with a repaired low lumbar meningomyelocele was well until 5 days ago. At this time, the patient developed stridor, poor feeding, and stiffness of the arms. Physical examination revealed inspiratory stridor with intermittent apnea. Direct laryngoscopy demonstrated vocal cord paralysis. The most likely diagnosis is

A. laryngotracheobronchitis

B. tethered spinal cord

C. Chiari crisis

D. syringomyelia

E. spinal cord lipoma

7. *Matching:*

1. Prevented by folic acid	A. Hydrocephalus
2. Detected by antenatal ultrasonography	B. Spina bifida
	C. Both A and B
	D. Neither A nor B
3. Elevated maternal serum α-fetoprotein	
4. May be X linked	
5. Valproic acid as teratogen	
6. Radiation exposure	

8. *Matching:*

1. Optic nerve hypoplasia	A. Lissencephaly
2. Sequela of cerebral infarction	B. Schizencephaly
	C. Porencephaly
	D. All of the above
3. Seizures	
4. Absent cerebral convolutions	
5. Clefts in cerebral hemispheres	

9. A 15-year-old presents with recurrent headache, progressive neck pain, and bladder dysfunction for the past 7 months. Physical examination reveals nuchal rigidity and lower extremity spasticity. The most appropriate diagnostic test is

A. skull radiographs

B. lumbar puncture

C. myelogram

D. head MRI

E. lateral neck radiographs

10. Causes of megalocephaly include all of the following EXCEPT

A. thalassemia

B. chronic subdural effusions

C. hydrocephalus

D. Canavan disease

E. congenital CMV

F. familial

11. A 4½-year-old undergoes a shunt revision for congenital hydrocephalus. Ten weeks later, the patient suffers a headache, abdominal pain, and low-grade fever for 5 days. Physical examination reveals a temperature of 38.7°C and a shunt tract without erythema or tenderness and is otherwise unremarkable. The most likely diagnosis is

A. shunt thrombosis

B. shunt infection

C. shunt dislodgement

D. migraine

E. malingering

12. A full-term neonate born to a healthy mother with an unremarkable pregnancy, labor, and delivery develops a left-sided focal seizure lasting 15 minutes. Two hours later, the physical examination is unremarkable other than for a left-sided hemiparesis. The infant is afebrile and alert. Blood glucose and serum calcium and electrolyte values are normal, as are the complete blood count (CBC) and platelet count. The next diagnostic step is to perform

A. a lumbar puncture

B. a TORCH titer

C. angiography

D. MRI

E. electroencephalography

13. Additional potential causes of neonatal stroke include all of the following EXCEPT

    A. protein S deficiency

    B. protein C deficiency

    C. homocystinuria

    D. paroxysmal nocturnal hemoglobinuria

    E. cyanotic congenital heart disease

14. A 5-year-old female presents with a sensation of "feeling funny" followed by clonic movements of the left side of her face with head turning. These have recurred four to five times a day for the past week and last 10 seconds. She cannot suppress the episodes. The most likely diagnosis is

    A. tics

    B. Bell palsy

    C. simple partial seizures

    D. complex partial seizures

    E. Rasmussen syndrome

15. A 3-month-old presents with a temperature of 39.5°C and a generalized seizure that lasts 35 minutes. After the seizure, the infant remains lethargic. The family history is unremarkable. After 5 hours of observation, the patient develops another generalized seizure. A consultant suggests that the patient has had febrile seizures. This diagnosis is questioned. All of the following suggest another diagnosis EXCEPT the

    A. patient's age

    B. duration of the seizures

    C. recurrence of the seizure

    D. family history

    E. persistence of lethargy

16. All of the following cause neonatal seizures EXCEPT

    A. pyridoxine deficiency

    B. lissencephaly

    C. hypoglycemia

    D. hypoxia-ischemia

    E. spina bifida

    F. incontinentia pigmentosa

17. An 18-month-old female develops sudden episodes of falling, ataxia, and refusal to walk or sit. The episodes last 10 minutes and have occurred occasionally during the past 2

months. Physical findings are normal except for horizontal nystagmus. The most likely diagnosis is

    A. epilepsy

    B. acoustic neuroma

    C. cerebellar astrocytoma

    D. benign paroxysmal vertigo

    E. diskitis

18. A 16-year-old white female complains of headaches of 2 years' duration. The headaches occur once every few months. She often feels that the headache is coming and occasionally has blurred vision before the peak of the headache. The headache is usually on one side but not necessarily the same side and is relieved by rest. The physical findings are nondiagnostic. The most appropriate approach to the patient is to

    A. perform a head CT

    B. perform a lumbar puncture

    C. reassure her that her headaches are psychosomatic

    D. administer ergotamine daily

    E. reassure her that migraines are usually benign

19. *Matching:* Neurocutaneous lesions

    1. Seizures   A. Neurofibromatosis

    2. Facial nevi   B. Tuberous sclerosis

    3. Café au lait spots   C. Sturge-Weber

    4. Ash leaf spot   D. None of the above

    5. Lisch nodules

    6. Shagreen patch   E. All of the above

    7. Glaucoma

    8. Melanoma

    9. Axillary freckling

    10. Kyphoscoliosis

20. *Matching:* Encephalomyopathies

    1. Ragged red muscle fibers   A. MELAS

    2. Heart block   B. MERRF

    3. Mitochondrial inheritance   C. Kearns-Sayre

    4. Stroke   D. All of the above

    5. Pes cavus   E. None of the above

6. Optic atrophy

7. Diabetes mellitus

8. Short stature

9. Bone cysts

10. Retinopathy

21. All of the following are associated with acute ataxia EXCEPT

    A. acute alcohol ingestion

    B. acute phenytoin overdose

    C. acute acetaminophen overdose

    D. postvaricella syndrome

    E. labyrinthitis

22. A 19-year-old Hmong female who emigrated to the United States 2 years ago presents with a 12-month history of personality changes, aggressive behavior, and reduced school performance. Two months ago, myoclonic seizures developed. The EEG demonstrates bursts of high-voltage slow waves interspersed with a normal background. Past medical history is unremarkable and includes the usual childhood viral illnesses. The most appropriate test is

    A. head ultrasonography

    B. cerebral angiography

    C. serum viral titers

    D. a lumbar puncture

    E. a Stanford-Binet test

23. A 12-year-old female develops acute monocular blindness of 2 days' duration. Past medical history reveals that she has had headaches for the past 3 years that she cannot characterize, one brief episode of diplopia, and one episode of paresthesias of the feet. These episodes were not related in time, did not occur in immediate proximity to the headache, and resolved spontaneously. Physical examination, other than reduced visual acuity, is unremarkable, including the funduscopic examination. The most important diagnostic step is to perform a

    A. CT

    B. MRI

    C. an electroencephalogram

    D. peripheral nerve conduction tests

    E. a nerve biopsy

24. **Matching:**

    1. Tay-Sachs disease

    2. Optic atrophy and peripheral neuropathy

    3. Hurler-like facies

    4. Optic atrophy and brown retina

    5. Academic deterioration and gait disturbance

    6. Marked startle response

    7. Spasticity with delayed nerve conduction

    8. Increased caudate densities

    9. Tan skin pigmentation

    10. Unexplained hyperpyrexia

    11. Arylsulfatase A deficiency

    12. Macroglossia

    A. GM_1 gangliosidosis

    B. GM_2 gangliosidosis

    C. Krabbe disease

    D. Metachromatic leukodystrophy

    E. Neuronal ceroid lipofuscinosis

    F. Adrenoleuko-dystrophy

25. A 13-year-old complains of headache and poor vision. In addition, the patient has noted increased thirst and urination. There are also no signs of puberty. The most likely diagnosis is

    A. diabetes mellitus

    B. craniopharyngioma

    C. cerebellar astrocytoma

    D. neurofibromatosis

    E. diencephalic syndrome

26. A 6-year-old complains of headaches on arising in the morning before school for 2 months. In addition, for the past 2 days the patient demonstrates head tilt. Physical examination reveals past pointing and difficulty in performing rapid alternating hand movements. The fundi are difficult to visualize. The next part of the evaluation should be

    A. an EEG

    B. a visit to the school psychologist

    C. a CT scan

    D. lumbar puncture

    E. a vision test

27. All of the following are associated with brain abscesses EXCEPT
    A. cyanotic heart disease
    B. sinusitis
    C. birth asphyxia
    D. trauma
    E. mastoiditis

28. A 7-year-old with poor dentition has persistent frontal headaches, fever, and irritability of 5 weeks' duration. A lumbar puncture reveals an opening pressure of 250 mm Hg, a white blood cell count of 120 with 75% leukocytes, a glucose level of 80 mg/dL, and a protein level of 95 mg/dL. Results of a Gram stain and culture are negative. The next appropriate step is
    A. a CSF culture for tuberculosis
    B. cryptococcal antigen determination
    C. an EEG
    D. a CT scan
    E. a dental consultation

29. All of the following are associated with intracranial bleeding EXCEPT
    A. thrombocytopenia
    B. hemophilia A
    C. trauma
    D. aspirin
    E. polycystic renal disease
    F. L-asparaginase

30. A 12-year-old presents with a severe headache, a grand mal seizure, and sudden collapse with unresponsive flaccid coma. The patient had a history of intermittent right-sided headaches without an aura and at times without relief with rest. In addition to coma on physical examination, the patient is afebrile and has nuchal rigidity. The most likely diagnosis is
    A. bacterial meningitis
    B. tuberculous meningitis
    C. brain tumor
    D. arteriovenous malformation
    E. Pott puffy tumor

31. All of the following are associated with permanent hemiplegia EXCEPT

A. sickle cell anemia
B. cyanotic heart disease
C. protein C deficiency
D. moyamoya disease
E. maple syrup urine disease
F. systemic lupus erythematosus
G. neurofibromatosis
H. homocystinuria

32. A mother describes her 5-year-old daughter as being "intelligent" but says she has occasional "lapses" during which she is "not here" and "drops things." What is the most likely diagnosis?
    A. Grand mal seizures
    B. Petit mal seizures
    C. Focal seizures
    D. Myoclonic seizures
    E. Psychomotor seizures

33. *Matching:* For each disorder listed, select the most likely neurologic findings for a patient in a coma.

    1. Arteriovenous malformation
    2. Lead poisoning
    3. Drug intoxication
    4. Reye syndrome
    5. Brain tumor (left parietal)
    6. Subdural hemorrhage (in an infant)
    7. Hydrocephalus

    A. No focal signs, normal intracranial pressure (ICP)
    B. No focal signs, increased ICP
    C. Focal signs, normal ICP
    D. Focal signs, increased ICP

34. Cerebellar ataxia, spastic weakness, optic neuritis, and diplopia are common presenting symptoms of which one of the following?
    A. Schilder disease
    B. Neuromyelitis optica
    C. Metachromatic leukodystrophy
    D. Multiple sclerosis
    E. Muscular dystrophy

28 Neuromuscular Disorders

The differential diagnosis of hypotonia is extensive and intimidating, but if approached in a systematic manner, it is educationally rewarding. This *part* focuses on the peripheral nervous system and includes the ever-expanding field of myopathies (inherited, endocrine, lipid, glycogenosis, mitochondrial, vitamin deficiency).

The ability to respond to the questions in this *part* of the *Nelson Review* will test your patience and differential diagnostic abilities.

1. A 12-year-old female developed diarrhea that lasted for 3 days, 2 weeks before manifesting progressive weakness and inability to walk. She has intermittent tingling of her fingers and toes. Physical examination reveals marked peripheral muscle weakness without atrophy or fasciculations. The deep tendon reflexes are absent in her ankles and 1+ at her knees. Findings on the sensory examination are normal. Motor involvement is symmetric. The most likely diagnosis is

   A. transverse myelitis

   B. Guillain-Barré syndrome

   C. polio

   D. myasthenia gravis

   E. mononeuritis multiplex

2. The patient described in Question 1 is admitted to the hospital and now develops progressive weakness and areflexia of the knee and ankle reflexes. An important test to perform is

   A. urine specific gravity

   B. an electrocardiogram (ECG)

   C. serum CPK determination

   D. muscle biopsy

   E. a pulmonary function test

3. A 5-month-old female manifests weakness and hypotonia that began 1 month before admission. Physical examination reveals an alert, smiling, interactive infant with weakness, absent deep tendon reflexes, and fasciculations of the tongue. Her serum CPK level is 500 IU/mL. The most likely diagnosis is

   A. myasthenia gravis

   B. spinal muscular atrophy

   C. polio

   D. Guillain-Barré syndrome

   E. muscular dystrophy

4. A 15-year-old male has lost his ability to walk. On physical examination, his ankle and knee deep tendon reflexes are noted to be diminished. The weakness is greatest in peripheral muscles. Cranial nerves all are normal. One week before these symptoms, he returned from a camping trip. The most likely diagnosis is

   A. myasthenia gravis

   B. organophosphate poisoning

   C. spinal muscular atrophy

   D. botulism

   E. tick paralysis

5. *Matching:* Neuromuscular disorders

1. Absent deep tendon reflexes	A. Polyneuropathy
2. Proximal weakness	B. Myopathy
3. Spasticity	C. Neuromuscular junction defect
4. Fatigable weakness	D. Upper motor neuron defect
5. Paresthesias	

6. A 2.7-kg white male presents at birth with severe hypotonia and weakness. Respiratory arrest necessitates mechanical ventilation. The infant has bilateral undescended testes but normal facies. His tongue is small and without fasciculations. The mother reports a history of decreased fetal movements. The infant's chest radiograph reveals a normal heart size but thin ribs. The serum creatine phosphokinase (CPK) level of both the mother and infant is normal. The most likely diagnosis is

   A. Pompe disease

   B. myotubular myopathy

C. Werdnig-Hoffmann syndrome

D. spinal cord transection

E. congenital muscular dystrophy

7. A 3-year-old female with nonprogressive muscle weakness undergoes surgery for congenital dislocated hips. Results of preoperative laboratory studies all are normal, including a normal serum CPK level. During the operation, she develops a combined respiratory and metabolic acidosis, and her temperature increases from 37.5°C to 39.5°C in 30 minutes. The most likely diagnosis is

A. endotracheal tube obstruction

B. anaphylaxis to latex

C. hemorrhagic shock

D. malignant hyperthermia

E. septic shock

8. In the patient described in Question 7, the most appropriate treatment is to administer

A. diazepam

B. lidocaine

C. whole blood

D. morphine

E. dantrolene

9. A 3-year-old white male with a waddling gait is brought to an orthopedic surgeon. He has proximal muscle weakness but normal deep tendon reflexes. On standing from a supine position, he uses his arms to push off his thighs to assume a vertical posture, which demonstrates a marked lordosis. He walked at 12 months of age, but he appears to be slightly behind his siblings in cognitive function. A diagnostically useful screening test is

A. capillary blood gas determination

B. serum lactate determination

C. serum CPK determination

D. an electrocardiogram

E. the Stanford-Binet test

F. a lumbar puncture

10. The most likely diagnosis in the patient described in Question 9 is

A. myotonic dystrophy

B. central core disease

C. Werdnig-Hoffmann syndrome

D. muscular dystrophy

E. myotonia congenita

11. A 2.9-kg white male presents at birth with severe hypotonia and weakness. He needs respiratory support with mechanical ventilation and subsequently needs gavage feedings. His mother has a history of mild muscle weakness but no myalgias or muscle spasm. She has a long face with concavities in the areas of her temporalis muscle. The mother's deep tendon reflexes are normal, but her muscles relax slowly after a contraction. Both the child and mother most likely have

A. myasthenia gravis

B. muscular dystrophy

C. spinal muscular atrophy

D. myotonic muscular dystrophy

E. amyotonia congenita

12. **Matching:** Endocrine and metabolic myopathies

1. Kocher-Debré-Sémélaigne syndrome	A. Hypokalemia
	B. Pompe disease
2. Myasthenia gravis–like syndrome	C. McArdle disease
	D. Hypothyroidism
3. Episodic paralysis	E. MELAS
4. Cardiomegaly	F. Hyperthyroidism
5. Exercise-induced rhabdomyolysis	G. Kearns-Sayre syndrome
6. External ophthalmoplegia	
7. Cerebrovascular accidents	

13. A 10-year-old female has had diplopia and ptosis and weakness of her neck flexors for 2 months. Symptoms are worse in the evening and are usually partially improved on awakening in the morning. She has no fasciculations or myalgias, and her deep tendon reflexes are 1 to 2+. The most likely diagnosis is

A. hysterical weakness

B. muscular dystrophy

C. spinal muscular atrophy

D. botulism

E. myasthenia gravis

14. The noninvasive test most useful in helping to make an immediate diagnosis of the condition described in Question 13 is

A. serum CPK determination

B. the Tensilon test

C. antimyelin antibody determination

D. serum pseudocholinesterase measurement

E. the histamine test

15. Fifteen years later, the patient described in Questions 13 and 14 becomes pregnant and delivers a full-term baby with Apgar scores of 2 and 3 at 1 and 5 minutes, respectively. The child has a weak cry and poor respiratory effort. The most important step in the treatment of the infant is to

A. administer epinephrine

B. administer bicarbonate

C. provide endotracheal intubation

D. administer edrophonium

E. provide CPAP

16. The mechanism of congenital disease in infants of mothers with myasthenia gravis is

A. steroid myopathy

B. genetic anticipation

C. overexpression of trinucleotide repeats

D. maternal antiacetylcholine receptor IgG

E. general anesthesia for the cesarean section

17. A 4-year-old child has difficulty in climbing stairs, slow motor development, and hypertrophied calf muscles. The most likely diagnosis is

A. myasthenia gravis

B. myotonia congenita

C. Duchenne muscular dystrophy

D. hypokalemic periodic paralysis

E. central core disease

29 Disorders of the Eye

Ocular manifestations of systemic illnesses often provide clues to the underlying disease. Of equal importance are primary ophthalmologic problems that are congenital, inherited, or acquired and that affect the vision of children. This *part* appropriately emphasizes early detection and treatment to avoid poor vision.

Questions in this part of the *Nelson Review* reinforce the concepts of early detection and treatment to prevent blindness. Nonetheless, answering these questions will not enable you to decipher the many Latin-based notations of our ophthalmology colleagues.

1. ***Matching:*** Pupils

   1. Abnormal pupil position
   2. Inequality of pupil size
   3. Abnormal pupil shape
   4. Absence of dilator pupillae muscle
   5. Ocular trauma

   A. Dyscoria
   B. Corectopia
   C. Anisocoria
   D. Fixed, dilated pupil
   E. Microcoria

2. The patient shown in Figure 29–1 demonstrates

   A. strabismus
   B. leukocoria
   C. amblyopia
   D. dyscoria
   E. aniridia

3. The best appropriate approach to the patient described in Question 2 is

   A. evaluation by an ophthalmologist
   B. CT scan
   C. to detect urine-reducing substances
   D. to measure intraocular pressure
   E. ultrasonography

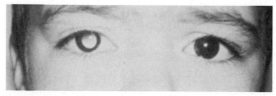

Figure 29-1

4. The differential diagnosis of leukokoria includes all of the following EXCEPT

   A. retinoblastoma
   B. endophthalmitis
   C. larval granulomatosis
   D. cataract
   E. retinal artery occlusion
   F. Coats disease
   G. persistent hyperplastic primary vitreous
   H. retinal detachment

5. A 1½-year-old child has begun to squint or to occlude her right eye with her hand. In addition, she complains of headache, demonstrates head tilting behavior, and is clumsy. The most likely visual problem is

   A. diplopia
   B. nystagmus
   C. cataract
   D. nyctalopia
   E. psychogenic hysteria

6. The most likely diagnosis in the patient described in Question 5 is

   A. psychologic stress
   B. brain tumor
   C. hyperthyroidism
   D. amblyopia
   E. amaurosis

7. Delayed removal of a congenital and complete unilateral cataract may lead to

   A. amblyopia
   B. glaucoma

C. uveitis

D. strabismus

E. nyctalopia

8. Myopia is associated with all of the following EXCEPT

A. prematurity

B. retinopathy of prematurity

C. myopic parents

D. onset at age 1 year

E. keratoconus

F. glaucoma

9. *Matching:* Strabismus

1. Inward deviation
2. Latent tendency to malalignment
3. Outward deviation
4. Misalignment at all times
5. Downward deviation
6. Upward deviation

A. Heterophoria
B. Heterotropia
C. Esophoria
D. Exophoria
E. Hyperdeviation
F. Hypodeviation

10. *Matching:* Papilledema—optic neuritis

1. Blurring of optic disk margin
2. Acute vision loss
3. Chronic vision loss
4. Elevation of optic nerve head
5. Engorgement of optic nerve veins
6. May be unilateral
7. Nerve fiber layer hemorrhage
8. Pain on movement of globe
9. Normal-appearing nerve head
10. Seen after an epileptic seizure

A. Papilledema
B. Optic neuritis
C. Neither A nor B
D. Both A and B

11. A 7-year-old male with a history of swollen joints, a limp, and fevers now manifests a red eye. He has pain, photophobia, and perilimbal erythema. The most likely acute problem is

A. congenital syphilis

B. herpes keratitis

C. conjunctivitis

D. chorioretinitis

E. iridocyclitis

12. The most likely underlying disease in the patient described in Question 11 is

A. systemic lupus erythematosus

B. periarteritis nodosa

C. sarcoidosis

D. pauciarticular JRA

E. Kawasaki disease

13. Aniridia is associated with all of the following EXCEPT

A. cataracts

B. being an isolated defect

C. TORCH infections

D. Wilms tumor

E. cerebellar ataxia

F. mental retardation

G. macular hypoplasia

14. Cataracts are noted in all of the following EXCEPT

A. rubella (congenital)

B. galactosemia

C. galactokinase deficiency

D. neonatal hypoglycemia

E. hypocalcemia

F. Lowe syndrome

G. hyperoxygenation

H. steroid therapy

I. child abuse

15. Acquired ptosis may be seen in all of the following EXCEPT

A. botulism

B. myasthenia gravis

C. increased intracranial pressure

D. hyperthyroidism

E. inflammation of the lid

16. Congenital ptosis may be seen in all of the following EXCEPT

A. abnormal innervation of the levator muscle

B. Marcus Gunn jaw-winking syndrome

C. Horner syndrome

D. Wilms tumor

E. von Recklinghausen syndrome

F. Sturge-Weber syndrome

17. An 18-month-old manifests pendular nystagmus, head nodding, and torticollis. Findings on a cranial MRI scan are normal. This child most likely has

A. epilepsy

B. congenital blindness

C. neuroblastoma

D. dysmetria

E. spasmus nutans

18. A 2-month-old infant male manifests a small rudimentary iris and nystagmus bilaterally. Both optic nerves appear smaller than normal. There is no family history of similar ocular findings. What is the most appropriate next step in the systematic evaluation of this child?

A. CT scan of the head

B. Renal ultrasonography

C. Bone marrow sampling

D. Echocardiogram

E. Liver studies

19. A 6-month-old female manifests a large alternating esotropia. The child cross-fixates: When she looks to the right, she uses her left eye, and she uses her right eye when looking to the left. She is minimally farsighted. What is the most appropriate next step in treatment?

A. Patching the right eye

B. Glasses for the farsightedness

C. Eye muscle surgery

D. Eye exercises

E. Prism glasses

20. A 4-month-old male infant has intermittent tearing and discharge from both eyes. The conjunctivae remain white. Both corneas are of normal size and clarity. What is the most appropriate next step in management?

A. Proper massage and lid hygiene

B. Probing

C. Placement of tubes

D. Nasolacrimal duct irrigation

E. Intraocular pressure measurement

21. A 4-month-old female infant has had tearing and photophobia for the past 2 months. Her left cornea appears larger and not as clear as her right cornea. What is the most likely diagnosis?

A. Keratoconus

B. Interstitial keratitis

C. Wilson disease

D. Glaucoma

E. Cataract

22. A 7-year-old female develops fullness of the right upper eyelid and downward displacement of the eye over a 2-month period. The right eye also appears to be proptotic. What is the most likely diagnosis?

A. Myasthenia gravis

B. Right superior oblique palsy

C. Chalazion

D. Rhabdomyoscarcoma

E. Hypothyroidism

23. *Matching:* Match the disease or syndrome with the ophthalmologic manifestation.

1. Morquio syndrome
2. Tay-Sachs disease
3. Tuberous sclerosis
4. Wilson disease
5. Pierre Robin syndrome
6. Niemann-Pick disease
7. Seckel syndrome
8. Congenital rubella

A. Congenital glaucoma
B. Corneal clouding
C. Hypertelorism
D. Macular cherry-red spot
E. Retinal phakomata
F. Kayser-Fleischer ring

24. Leukocoria is the initial presentation of

A. chondrosarcoma

B. retinoblastoma

C. nasopharyngeal carcinoma

D. optic glioma

E. chronic lymphocytic leukemia

30 The Ear

Deafness and otitis media are two fundamentally important problems that affect children. Hearing loss has significant implications for the development of hearing-impaired children. Otitis media is an extremely common disorder with potentially serious acute and chronic sequelae. Expert pediatricians should never miss the diagnosis of either of these disorders.

Questions in this *part* are designed for general pediatricians and focus on important aspects of the ear.

1. Which of the following are associated with conductive hearing loss?

   A. Cholesteatoma

   B. Otosclerosis

   C. Otitis media with effusion

   D. Foreign body in the external canal

   E. Impacted cerumen

   F. All of the above

2. All of the following congenital syndromes are associated with hearing loss EXCEPT

   A. Pendred

   B. Usher

   C. Waardenburg

   D. Treacher Collins

   E. autosomal recessive deafness

3. All of the following problems of the neonatal period place infants at increased risk for hearing loss EXCEPT

   A. furosemide therapy

   B. primary pulmonary hypertension

   C. kernicterus

   D. hypocalcemia

   E. gentamicin therapy

   F. cytomegalovirus infection

4. Risk factors for acquired hearing loss include all of the following EXCEPT

   A. bacterial meningitis

   B. head trauma

   C. low birth weight

   D. TORCH infections

   E. epilepsy

5. A hearing deficit of moderate loss is associated with an average sound threshold of 41 to 65 dB and all of the following EXCEPT

   A. middle ear anomalies

   B. missing speech sounds at normal conversational levels

   C. language retardation

   D. missing unvoiced consonant sounds

   E. inattention

6. The etiology of external otitis includes all of the following pathogens EXCEPT

   A. herpes zoster virus

   B. *Pseudomonas aeruginosa*

   C. pneumococci

   D. *Proteus mirabilis*

   E. *Candida*

7. Common features of external otitis include all of the following EXCEPT

   A. itching

   B. edema

   C. green otorrhea

   D. perforation of the tympanic membrane

   E. regional lymphadenopathy

   F. pain on movement of the pinna and tragus

8. *Matching:*

   1. Bulging eardrum
   2. Pain on movement of auricle
   3. Lymphadenitis
   4. Periauricular edema
   5. Sinusitis
   6. Obliteration of posterior auricular fold

   A. External otitis
   B. Mastoiditis
   C. Both A and B
   D. Neither A nor B

7. Tenderness over
   mastoid antrum

9. Risk factors for otitis media include all of the
   following EXCEPT
   A. being male
   B. poverty
   C. being Native American
   D. cleft palate
   E. summer months

10. Manifestations of otitis media include all of
    the following EXCEPT
    A. fever in 90% of patients
    B. irritability
    C. diarrhea
    D. emesis
    E. otalgia

11. With appropriate treatment, manifestations
    (pain and fever) of acute otitis media should
    abate within
    A. 6 to 12 hours
    B. 12 to 18 hours
    C. 24 to 48 hours
    D. 5 days
    E. 10 days .

12. The best initial approach to middle ear
    effusion persisting for 4 weeks after otitis
    media is
    A. tympanocentesis
    B. oral antimicrobial therapy for 2 weeks
    C. intravenous antibiotics
    D. methylprednisolone
    E. intravenous immunoglobulin

13. Possible complications of otitis media include
    all of the following EXCEPT
    A. pseudotumor cerebri
    B. cerebellar abscess
    C. mastoiditis
    D. sinusitis
    E. facial nerve paralysis

14. Pathogens associated with otitis media include
    all of the following EXCEPT
    A. respiratory syncytial virus
    B. pneumococcus
    C. *Moraxella catarrhalis*
    D. *Haemophilus influenzae* type b
    E. *Streptococcus pyogenes*

31 The Skin

Most pediatricians are amateur dermatologists. Rashes are quite common at all ages. Rashes, because of their obvious appearance, often lead parents to bring their child to a pediatrician's office for evaluation. This *part* concentrates on diseases of the skin, hair, and nails that may be congenital, neoplastic, infectious, inflammatory, or of unknown cause. The treatments are well described.

Questions in this *part* enhance the amateur dermatologist in all of us and reinforce our diagnostic skills.

1. The patient shown Figure 31–1 probably has

   A. alopecia areata

   B. traction alopecia

   C. lupus erythematosus

   D. kerion

   E. Pott puffy tumor

2. The 2-week-old infant shown in Figure 31–2 is acutely ill with tender erythematous skin, fever, and irritability. A positive Nikolsky sign is noted. The most likely diagnosis is

   A. icthyosiform erythroderma

   B. epidermolysis bullosa

   C. staphylococcal scalded skin syndrome

   D. Kawasaki disease

   E. erythema multiforme minor

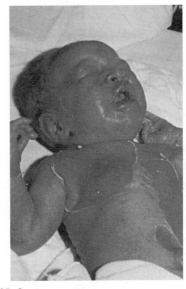

Figure 31–2

3. The lesions shown in Figure 31–3 most likely represent

   A. trichotillomania

   B. traction alopecia

   C. alopecia areata

   D. tinea

   E. none of the above

4. The lesions shown in Figure 31–4 are most typical of

   A. psoriasis

   B. pityriasis rosea

   C. atopic dermatitis

   D. lichen nitidus

   E. lichen planus

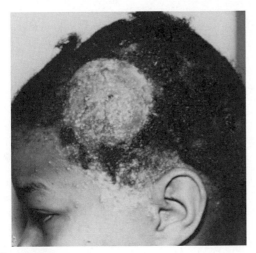

Figure 31–1

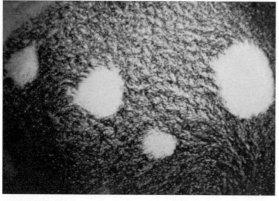

Figure 31-3

5. *Matching:*

1. Flat, nonpalpable change in skin color
2. Macule > 1 cm
3. Palpable lesion < 0.5 to 1 cm
4. Large nodule
5. Fluid-filled raised lesion < 0.5 cm
6. Vesicle > 0.5 cm
7. Papule > 1 cm

A. Macule
B. Tumor
C. Vesicle
D. Papule
E. Patch
F. Nodule
G. Bulla

6. The neonatal rash shown in Figure 31–5 is associated with all of the following EXCEPT

A. white race
B. evanescent superficial pustules
C. hyperpigmented macules
D. fine scales
E. onset at birth

7. The most likely diagnosis for the rash illustrated in Figure 31–5, Question 6 is

A. erythema toxicum
B. pustular melanosis
C. miliaria rubra
D. herpes simplex
E. none of the above

8. A solitary, noninflammatory, well-demarcated, ovoid ulcer of 1 to 2 cm on the scalp of a neonate (Fig. 31–6) is most probably

A. fat necrosis
B. an encephalocele
C. herpes simplex
D. cutis aplasia
E. congenital varicella

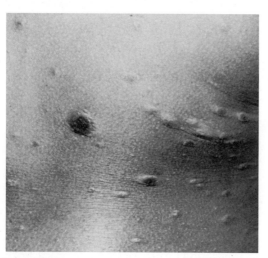

Figure 31-4

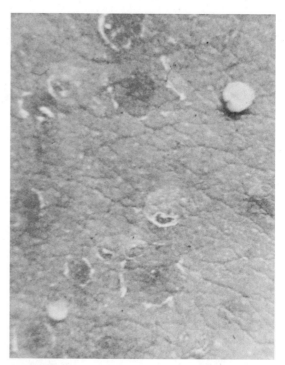

Figure 31-5

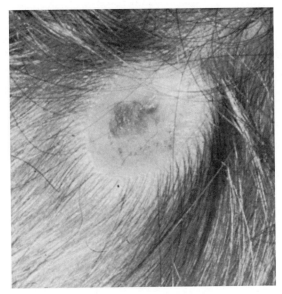

Figure 31-6

9. The treatment of choice for a port-wine stain is

   A. interferon

   B. prednisone

   C. YAG laser

   D. flashlamp pulsed dye laser

   E. none of the above

10. Giant congenital pigmented nevi are associated with all of the following EXCEPT

    A. an incidence of less than 1 in 20,000 births

    B. leptomeningeal involvement

    C. malignant melanoma

    D. hydrocephalus

    E. male predominance

11. Peutz-Jeghers syndrome is characterized by all of the following EXCEPT

    A. gastrointestinal polyposis

    B. lentigines

    C. ephelides

    D. nongastrointestinal tract malignancies

    E. gastrointestinal cancer

12. Incontinenta pigmenti is associated with all of the following EXCEPT

    A. lethality in females

    B. erythematous linear streaks and vesicles

    C. alopecia

    D. hypodontia

    E. microphthalmos

    F. seizures

13. Additional features of the disease illustrated in Figure 31–7 include all of the following EXCEPT

    A. mental retardation

    B. seizures

    C. autosomal dominant inheritance

    D. renal angiomyolipoma

    E. eighth-nerve deafness

    F. periungual fibroma

    G. cardiac rhabdomyoma

    H. ash leaf lesions

14. Stevens-Johnson syndrome (erythema multiforme major) is associated with all of the following EXCEPT

    A. a good response to prednisone

    B. involvement of two mucous membranes

    C. esophageal stricture

    D. corneal scarring

    E. infectious causes

    F. drug-related causes

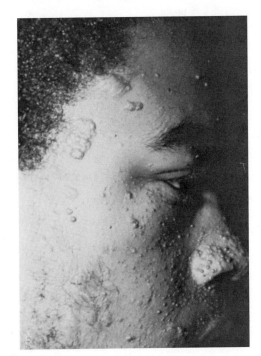

Figure 31-7

15. The Köbner (isomorphic) response is best described as

    A. cold urticaria

    B. herpetic lesions in thumb-sucking infants

    C. new lesions appearing at sites of trauma

    D. pinpoint bleeding after lifting a plaque

    E. none of the above

16. Hypopigmented, round, macular, slightly scaly lesions that have a poorly marginated border and do not itch are characteristic of which one of the following?

    A. Candidiasis

    B. Pityriasis alba

    C. Pityriasis rosea

    D. Lichen simplex chronicus

    E. Dyshidrotic eczema

17. Which one of the following begins with a herald patch and has a Christmas tree distribution?

    A. Guttate psoriasis

    B. Lichen spinulosus

    C. Keratosis pilaris

    D. Xeroderma pigmentosum

    E. Pityriasis rosea

32 Bones and Joints

Limps, bumps, pain, disuse, and poor function are common orthopedic problems of childhood. These are due to congenital, inherited, infectious, anatomic, inflammatory, and neoplastic lesions. This extensive *part* of the *Nelson Textbook* includes sections on general basic orthopedics (including fractures and sports medicine), genetic skeletal dysplasias, and metabolic bone disease.

These questions help clarify definitions (varus vs. valgus) and identify common bone and joint diseases.

1. An adolescent female who is a cheerleader comes to you with a painful bump below her right knee. She denies fever or trauma. Which is the most likely diagnosis?

    A. Legg-Calvé-Perthes disease

    B. Osteoid osteoma

    C. Osgood-Schlatter disease

    D. Osteochondritis dissecans

    E. Osteomyelitis of the tibial tubercle

2. The best treatment for the patient described in Question 1 is

    A. decreased activity of the knee

    B. antiinflammatory drugs

    C. antibiotics

    D. excisional biopsy

    E. casting for 6 to 8 weeks

3. Which of the following is the most severe form of flatfoot?

    A. Vertical talus

    B. Talus-calcaneus coalition

    C. Calcaneus-navicular coalition

    D. Talonavicular coalition

    E. Peroneal spastic flatfoot

4. Which is the best initial treatment for dislocated, unrelocatable, congenitally dysplastic hips first discovered at 7 months of age?

    A. Triple diapers

    B. von Rosen splint or other rigid device

    C. Plaster spica case

    D. Traction

    E. Open (surgical) reduction

5. An overweight adolescent male complains of pain in the medial aspect of his knee. He denies trauma, and he has not had a fever. The most likely diagnosis is

    A. toxic synovitis

    B. Legg-Calvé-Perthes disease

    C. medial collateral ligament (knee) strain

    D. slipped capital femoral epiphysis

    E. avulsion of the gastrocnemius muscle

6. A 2-year-old child is brought to you because he refuses to use his right arm. Any attempt to touch it is met with a cry, and the child will not hold objects in his right hand. The mother denies trauma, but she did pull the child by the arm recently when he refused to go into an elevator. The most likely diagnosis is

    A. nonaccidental trauma (child abuse)

    B. fracture of the radius

    C. muscle strain of the right pronator

    D. dislocated radial head

    E. osteomyelitis

7. Plans for the child described in Question 6 should include (choose one or more)

    A. roentgenogram of the arm, thin casting or splinting

    B. supination of the forearm

    C. antibiotics

    D. alerting the parents to the cause of the problem

    E. reporting the case to a child welfare agency

8. A 6-month-old infant has fever, irritability, and swelling of his mandible. Laboratory studies show anemia and an elevated

erythrocyte sedimentation rate (ESR). What is the most likely diagnosis?

A. Osteomyelitis

B. Rickets

C. Hypervitaminosis A

D. Chondrodysplasia punctata

E. Infantile cortical hyperostosis

9. **Matching:** Bone and joint orthopedic terminology

1. Angulation of the vertex of bone or joint toward midline

2. Plantar-flexed foot

3. Angulation of bone or joint away from midline

4. High-arched foot

5. Incision into a joint

   A. Varum

   B. Cavus

   C. Valgum

   D. Equinus

   E. Arthrotomy

10. A 12-year-old male sustains a nail puncture of his right foot through an old sneaker. Two days later, he limps and complains of pain and swelling of that area. The most likely diagnosis is

A. tetanus

B. osteochondritis

C. foreign body reaction

D. toxic shock syndrome

E. ecthyma gangrenosum

11. The most likely organisms causing the problem described in Question 10 include (choose one or more)

A. *Clostridium perfringens*

B. *Staphylococcus aureus*

C. *Staphylococcus epidermidis*

D. *Pseudomonas aeruginosa*

E. *Serratia marcescens*

12. The most appropriate important first therapeutic approach for the boy described in Questions 10 and 11 is

A. Timentin

B. ciprofloxacin

C. incision, drainage, debridement

D. tetanus toxoid

E. warm soaks

13. Internal tibial torsion is usually due to

A. femoral torsion

B. hypermobility syndrome

C. femoral retroversion

D. in utero positioning

E. rickets

14. **Matching:**

1. Talipes equinovarus

2. Congenital vertical talus

3. Flexible flatfeet

4. Tarsal coalition

5. Cavus feet

   A. Soft tissue surgical release required

   B. Usually painless

   C. Peripheral neuropathy

   D. Responds to serial casting

   E. Fusion or failure of segmentation

15. Metatarsus adductus is occasionally associated with

A. cerebral palsy

B. prematurity

C. developmental dysplasia of the hip

D. tethered cord

E. spina bifida occulta

16. Risk factors for developmental dysplasia of the hip include all of the following EXCEPT

A. female sex

B. first born

C. breech presentation

D. congenital torticollis

E. prematurity

17. A 3-year-old presents with a 2-day history of right leg pain and a limp. The pain is in the anterior thigh region. One week ago, the patient had a nonspecific upper respiratory tract infection. The physical examination reveals an afebrile, nontoxic-appearing child with normal range of motion of all lower extremity joints. The complete blood count and ESR are normal. The most likely diagnosis is

A. juvenile rheumatoid arthritis

B. rheumatic fever

C. toxic synovitis

D. slipped capital femoral epiphysis

E. septic arthritis

18. *Matching:*

    1. Osteonecrosis
    2. Obesity
    3. Tall, thin patient
    4. Males predominate
    5. Sickle cell trait
    6. Hypothyroidism
    7. Nontraumatic
    8. Onset before 10 years of age
    9. Onset after 10 years of age
    10. Delayed bone age

    A. Legg-Calvé-Perthes

    B. Slipped capital femoral epiphysis

    C. Both

    D. Neither

19. Danger signs in children with back pain include all of the following EXCEPT

    A. weight loss
    B. bladder dysfunction
    C. fever
    D. right scoliosis curvature
    E. lumbar sacral hairy cutaneous patch
    F. parental history of herniated disk

20. Children should be excluded from all vigorous sports if they have any of the following EXCEPT

    A. acute splenomegaly
    B. a single testicle
    C. fever
    D. diarrhea
    E. carditis

21. *Matching:*

    1. Lethal
    2. Hydrocephalus
    3. Immunodeficiency
    4. Fractures
    5. Curved bones
    6. Cervical spine dislocation

    A. Cartilage-hair hypoplasia

    B. Osteogenesis imperfecta

    C. Thanatophoric dysplasia

    D. Achondroplasia

    E. Larsen syndrome

    F. Camptomelic dysplasia

22. *Matching:*

    1. Ellis–van Creveld syndrome

    A. Blue sclera

    B. Encephalocele

    2. Osteogenesis imperfecta
    3. Dyssegmented dysplasia
    4. Saldino-Noonan syndrome
    5. Robinow syndrome
    6. Acrodysostosis

    C. Renal cysts

    D. Heart defects

    E. Hypoplastic nasal bridge

    F. Hypertelorism

23. A 14-month-old male infant has tibial bowing and a waddling gait. His forehead appears large and box shaped. Laboratory findings in this infant reveal serum levels of calcium of 9.1 mg/dL, phosphate 2.1 mg/dL, and alkaline phosphatase 79 IU/L and radiologic evidence of a widened metaphysis, metaphyseal fraying, and demineralization. No aminoaciduria is found. The most likely diagnosis is

    A. vitamin D deficiency rickets
    B. vitamin D dependence type 1
    C. X-linked hypophosphatemic rickets
    D. hepatic rickets
    E. oncogenous rickets

24. *Matching:* Match the disorder with the laboratory values.

    1. Hyperphosphatasia
    2. X-linked hypophosphatemic rickets
    3. Hypophosphatasia
    4. Vitamin D dependence rickets type 1
    5. Vitamin D deficiency rickets

Serum Chemistry Values

	Calcium (mg/dL)	Phosphate (mg/dL)	Alkaline Phosphatase (IU/L)	25(OH)D (ng/mL)	1,25(OH)$_2$D$_3$ (pg/mL)
A.	9.2	1.9	754	28	31
B.	12.2	4.5	74	28	31
C.	9.3	4.8	8700	28	43
D.	6.1	2.4	1070	3	21
E.	6.1	2.4	1070	28	4

25. The major body pool for the element calcium is

    A. plasma free calcium
    B. protein-bound calcium in the blood
    C. within the mitochondrial matrix
    D. in bone as hydroxyapatite
    E. in bone as calcium carbonate

26. ***Matching:***

   1. Juvenile renal osteodystrophy
   2. $1,25(OH)_2D_3$ therapy
   3. Osteitis fibrosa
   4. Aluminum overload
   5. Hyperphosphatemia

   A. Elevated intact parathyroid hormone
   B. Failure to grow
   C. GFR $\leq$ 30% of age-related normal values
   D. Hypercalcemia a common drug-induced side effect
   E. Low-turnover osteomalacia

27. A 14-month-old female has hypotonia, chronic constipation, and failure to thrive. She meets the biochemical criteria for the Fanconi syndrome and has a serum creatinine level of 0.7 mg/dL. Her leukocyte cystine content is 60 times normal. What is the most appropriate next step in this patient's treatment?

   A. Introduction of oral cysteamine
   B. Supplemental phosphate and alkali therapy administered by mouth
   C. Genetic counseling of the family
   D. A diagnostic workup on the parents and siblings
   E. A patient workup for hypothyroidism
   F. A slit-lamp examination of the patient

28. A 2-year-old male presents with failure to thrive, generalized aminoaciduria, renal glycosuria, and hypophosphatemia secondary to renal phosphate wasting. An appropriate diagnostic workup would include which of the following studies?

   A. Serum sodium level
   B. Complete blood count
   C. Ascertaining exposure to drugs and heavy metals
   D. Renal ultrasound examination
   E. Serum glucose level

33 Unclassified Diseases

This *part* includes sudden infant death syndrome (SIDS), sarcoidosis, progeria, histiocytic lesions, and chronic fatigue syndrome. Slowly but surely, these will eventually be reclassified into other chapters as their causes become more apparent. Nonetheless, other new diseases of unknown cause or classification are likely to appear soon and take their place.

Questions in this *part* help readers identify many of these unclassified disorders.

1. Prone sleep position has been identified as an apparently important epidemiologic risk factor for SIDS. Suggested likely mechanisms include an interaction with all of the following biologic risk factors EXCEPT

   A. impaired temperature regulation

   B. deficient ventilatory responsiveness

   C. impaired arousal responsiveness

   D. gastroesophageal reflux

   E. none of the above

2. Epidemiologic studies have shown an increased risk of SIDS to be associated with all of the following EXCEPT

   A. maternal smoking during pregnancy

   B. fetal cocaine exposure

   C. being large for gestational age

   D. colder season and climate

   E. postnatal growth failure

3. A 5-month-old infant is admitted to the hospital 15 minutes after being discovered apneic, blue, and limp by the baby sitter during an afternoon nap. The baby had been placed down for sleep in the supine position. The baby was seen in the emergency room 1 day previously for nasal congestion and a low-grade temperature; because no immunizations had yet been given, the first DPT and OPV were administered. Findings on physical examination on admission were normal. A five-channel cardiorespiratory recording performed during the first night in the hospital was unremarkable. The most likely diagnosis is

   A. DPT reaction

   B. sepsis and/or meningitis

   C. child abuse

   D. apnea of infancy

   E. congenital fatty acid metabolic abnormality

4. A 3-month-old infant dies suddenly and unexpectedly. Which of the following statements is most likely true?

   A. The infant is female.

   B. The infant is African-American.

   C. The mother smokes.

   D. The birth weight was <2500 g.

   E. None of the above is necessarily likely.

5. Autopsy studies of infants with SIDS have identified all of the following EXCEPT

   A. pulmonary edema

   B. persistent dendritic spines in the vagal nuclei

   C. decreased levels of hypoxanthine in vitreous humor

   D. tissue markers of asphyxia

   E. petechiae in the pleura or pericardium

6. The pathophysiology of SIDS is most likely related to which one of the following?

   A. Prematurity

   B. Impaired brainstem function

   C. Gastroesophageal reflux

   D. Medium-chain fatty acid deficiency

   E. Fatal child abuse

7. A 4-year-old female presents with severe failure to thrive; she weighs 18 pounds and is 30 inches tall. She has a high-pitched voice, a sclerodermatous appearance of the skin overlying her abdomen, nearly total alopecia, a small jaw and face relative to her head circumference, and normal mental and motor development. The most likely diagnosis is

A. cystic fibrosis

B. child abuse and malnutrition

C. Hutchinson-Gilford progeria syndrome

D. Marfan syndrome

E. Hallermann-Streiff syndrome

8. A 6-month-old child is diagnosed as having Langerhans cell histiocytosis by biopsy of a lesion and demonstration of Birbeck granules in the lesional cells. The disease is disseminated, involving skin, lymph nodes, bones, liver, and bone marrow. Treatment could include

A. radiation therapy

B. Adriamycin

C. etoposide

D. vincristine

9. A 6-month-old child presents with fever, irritability, and recent weight loss. Physical examination reveals hepatosplenomegaly. Laboratory studies demonstrate marked anemia. A sister died early in infancy, of "leukemia." A bone marrow examination reveals no malignant cells but marked hemophagocytosis by bone marrow macrophages, which are prominent. The most likely diagnosis is

A. Langerhans cell histiocytosis

B. infection-associated hemophagocytic syndrome

C. familial erythrophagocytic lymphohistiocytosis

D. congenital leukemia

10. The Langerhans cell, which constitutes a central cell in lesions of Langerhans cell histiocytosis, is positive by immunostaining for

A. CD1

B. CD3

C. CD4

D. CD8

11. A 12-year-old black male has fever and weight loss and tires easily. He has mild hepatosplenomegaly and peripheral adenopathy including a 2-cm cervical lymph node and 1-cm epitrochlear nodes bilaterally. His chest radiograph shows a diffuse interstitial infiltrate and hilar adenopathy. Which of the following study results confirms the diagnosis of sarcoidosis?

A. Elevated serum angiotensin-converting enzyme (ACE) level

B. Noncaseating granulomas in biopsy specimen of cervical node

C. Elevated serum calcium level

D. Positive (15-mm) reaction to Mantoux skin test

E. Predominantly lymphocytes in bronchoalveolar lavage fluid

12. A lymph node biopsy of the patient described in Question 11 confirms the diagnosis of sarcoidosis. Further evaluation should include

A. chest MRI

B. bone marrow aspirate

C. staging laparotomy

D. slit-lamp examination of the eye

E. lumbar puncture

13. A 6-year-old female is suffering from unilateral exophthalmos. Further evaluation reveals a lytic lesion of a rib but no other abnormalities. Langerhans cell histiocytosis is diagnosed by biopsy of the rib lesion. The characteristic Birbeck granules are detectable only by

A. light microscopy

B. electron microscopy

C. immunostaining

D. vital staining

34 Environmental Health Hazards

After this *part* the test is over. This *part* includes important chapters on the ever-increasing number of intoxicants or pollutants to which children are exposed. Their proper identification and their treatment are emphasized.

Questions in this *part* help identify the important aspects about environmental health hazards. Good luck with this test. We hope that you were appropriately challenged and that in being challenged you were able to continue to learn.

1. Risks to children born after fetal exposure to the atomic bomb in Japan include all of the following EXCEPT

   A. acute pancytopenia

   B. hypothyroidism

   C. breast cancer at age 35 to 45 years

   D. congenital neuroblastoma

   E. leukemia

2. *Matching:* Chemical pollutants

   1. Cerebral palsy
   2. Dark skin pigmentation (transient)
   3. Neuroblastoma
   4. Chloracne
   5. Hypocalcemia

   A. Polychlorinated biphenyls
   B. Methylmercury
   C. Dioxin
   D. Phenytoin
   E. Fluoride

3. Potential sources of mercury include all of the following EXCEPT

   A. swordfish

   B. old teething powders

   C. quicksilver

   D. milk

   E. pesticides

   F. latex paint

   G. folk remedies

4. Acute exposure to mercury vapor produces all of the following EXCEPT

   A. nephrotic syndrome

   B. myocarditis

   C. metallic taste

   D. cough

   E. stomatitis

   F. pulmonary edema

   G. fever

5. The most serious manifestation of lead intoxication is

   A. peripheral neuropathy

   B. mental retardation

   C. anemia

   D. cerebral edema

   E. lead lines

6. All of the following are direct manifestations of lead intoxication EXCEPT

   A. anemia

   B. encephalopathy

   C. colic

   D. peripheral neuropathy

   E. reduced IQ

7. A 2-year-old is noted to be drinking from a container filled with kerosene. He immediately coughs, becomes tachypneic, and is brought to the hospital. The best approach to his treatment is to

   A. induce emesis

   B. perform nasogastric tube lavage

   C. instill mineral oil

   D. administer steroids

   E. do none of the above

8. *Matching:* Drug intoxication—antidotes

   1. Carbon monoxide
   2. Cyanide

   A. Sodium nitrate and sodium thiosulfate

3. Heroin

4. Methemo-globinemia

5. Organophosphate insecticides

6. Ethylene glycol

7. Acetaminophen

B. Narcan

C. Oxygen

D. Atropine

E. Methylene blue

F. *N*-acetylcysteine

G. Ethanol

9. Acute, severe iron intoxication is best managed with

A. oral deferoxamine

B. induced emesis

C. saline lavage

D. activated charcoal

E. none of the above

10. A 2-year-old born to a mother with severe depression is brought to the emergency room with lethargy of 2 hours' duration. On examination, the child has tachycardia, dilated pupils, dry mucous membranes, and cutaneous flushing. An electrocardiogram reveals frequent premature ventricular contractions and a QRS complex of 0.18 second. The next important step in the management of this patient is to

A. administer sodium bicarbonate by vein

B. perform a drug toxicology test on urine and blood

C. administer physostigmine

D. perform a head CT scan

E. administer diazepam

11. The next most important step in the treatment of the child described in Question 10 is to administer

A. *N*-acetylcysteine

B. deferoxamine

C. ipecac

D. nasogastric lavage

E. activated charcoal

12. The patient described in Questions 10 and 11 has most likely ingested

A. an opiate

B. an organophosphate insecticide

C. a tricyclic antidepressant

D. acetaminophen

E. none of the above

13. *Matching:* Spider bites

1. Orange hourglass marking

2. Lives in dark, undisturbed areas

3. Neurotoxin

4. Bite may be unnoticed initially

5. Severe muscle spasms

6. Hypertension

7. Acute abdomen

8. Fiddle marking on back

9. Bite becomes hemorrhagic blister

10. Laryngospasm

11. Hemolysis

12. Disseminated intravascular coagulation

A. Black widow

B. Brown recluse

C. Both A and B

D. Neither A nor B

14. *Matching:* Plant intoxications

1. Dieffenbachia

2. Jimson weed

3. Castor bean

4. Foxglove

5. Hemlock

A. Atropine-like

B. Oxalates

C. Hyperkalemia

D. Hemolytic anemia

E. Similar to nicotine

15. Specific antivenin is available for the treatment of which one of the following?

A. Myiasis

B. Tick paralysis

C. Black widow spider bite

D. Honeybee sting

E. Scabies

16. Some people are concerned about adverse effects of fluoride added to the water supply to prevent dental caries. When parents ask about the risk, they should be told that

A. there is a very small risk of osteosarcoma

B. the risk is uncertain because of inadequate study

C. conjunctivitis may occasionally occur

D. congenital malformations are a theoretic possibility

E. there is no danger, but use only small

amounts of fluoridated toothpaste on the child's toothbrush

17. A child with which of the following diseases may suffer a severe acute reaction to radiotherapy?

   A. Chédiak-Higashi syndrome
   B. Neurofibromatosis
   C. Chronic mucocutaneous candidiasis
   D. Ataxia-telangiectasia
   E. Wiskott-Aldrich syndrome

18. In support of the concept of transplacental carcinogenesis, which one of the following cancers of the young has been related to maternal exposure during pregnancy?

   A. Mesothelioma after cigarette smoking
   B. Hepatoma after progestational compounds
   C. Vaginal cancer after diethylstilbestrol
   D. Nasopharyngeal carcinoma after immunosuppressive drugs
   E. Adenocarcinoma of the colon after cocaine abuse

19. Almost all environmental agents that cause cancer or birth defects in humans have first been identified by

   A. animal experimentation
   B. in vitro testing
   C. cohort studies
   D. alert practitioners
   E. academic physicians

20. The only clearly established effect of dioxin exposure on children is

   A. leukemia
   B. chloracne
   C. slowed nerve conduction velocity
   D. hepatomegaly
   E. behavioral disorders

21. Parents are planning to buy a house for themselves and their 7-year-old and 2-year-old daughters. They ask about testing for radon. Which of the following should you recommend?

   A. Call the state radon office to find out which neighborhoods have high radon emissions from the soil.
   B. Because homes with radon problems are

difficult to fix, even the most desirable house should be rejected.

   C. Pursue no testing, because epidemiologic and other studies of the risks are inconclusive.
   D. Rely on the results of tests done in the past, because indoor radon levels are constant over time.
   E. Request a state-certified radon tester to evaluate your prospective home using a short-term test.

22. The family described in Question 21 has located a home they like; however, it is next to a power line. They ask about the risks associated with power lines. Which of the following information will you provide?

   A. Epidemiologic findings of an association between electric and magnetic fields and cancer are inconclusive.
   B. They are causally associated with childhood leukemia and brain cancer.
   C. They are associated with spontaneous abortions in women.
   D. They are associated with birth defects.
   E. They are associated with behavioral changes in infants.

23. About 500 children have just been exposed to radiation from a nuclear power plant accident. The most appropriate first step in your treatment of these children should be to

   A. prescribe potassium iodide to protect the thyroid
   B. order thyroid function tests
   C. order complete blood counts (CBCs)
   D. do nothing acutely; evaluate in 4 to 6 weeks
   E. look for signs or symptoms of acute radiation sickness

24. With regard to x-ray exposures before 18 weeks of gestational age, which one of the following has been conclusively shown to occur after exposures of less than 20 cGy (rad)?

   A. Leukemia
   B. Small head size
   C. Severe mental retardation
   D. Aplastic anemia
   E. Somatic cell mutations

25. A 15-year-old male has been working in the garage and develops painful muscle spasms of his right arm. During the course of the next hour, these spread to his trunk and lower extremities. When he arrives at the emergency room, he is noted to be hypertensive and diaphoretic and to have severe abdominal pain. His most likely diagnosis is

    A. toxin ingestion

    B. appendicitis

    C. opiate withdrawal

    D. black widow bite

    E. renal colic

26. Antivenins should be considered in the treatment of all of the following EXCEPT

    A. rattlesnake envenomations

    B. scorpion envenomations

    C. black widow envenomations

    D. stonefish envenomations

    E. Hymenoptera envenomations

27. Emergency management of poisonous snakebites should always include

    A. administration of antivenin

    B. cryotherapy for the wound

    C. arterial tourniquet to the affected extremity

    D. pressure and immobilization of the affected extremity

    E. cruciate incision and oral suction of the wound

28. Solanine intoxication follows ingestion of

    A. mushrooms of the genus *Inocybe*

    B. mushrooms of the genus *Amanita*

    C. sprouted green potatoes

    D. oysters

    E. amberjack

29. A 2-year-old child is found playing with a can of crystalline drain cleaner. There are several crystals in the mouth, which you have the mother wash out. Treatment should be to

    A. have the mother administer lemon juice or orange juice to neutralize the alkaline crystals and come to your office

    B. have the mother administer water or milk and call you back in 2 hours

    C. have the mother administer water or milk and bring the child in for esophagoscopy

    D. simply observe the child because the crystals are so bitter that the child was trying to spit them out when the mother called, and therefore no problems should occur

    E. administer ipecac at home and bring the child in to see you

30. A 2-year-old patient presents with fever (40.2°C), tachypnea, dehydration of 7% to 10%, serum potassium level of 2.3 mEq/L, and confusion. The most likely cause of this is

    A. ibuprofen overdose

    B. acetaminophen overdose

    C. iron overdose

    D. aspirin overdose

    E. acid toilet bowl cleaner ingestion

31. A 16-year-old, 165-pound patient reports consuming 20 to 40 325-mg capsules containing acetaminophen 1 hour ago. You should

    A. measure the plasma level and determine potential toxicity from the level on the nomogram

    B. wait until 4 hours after ingestion to measure the plasma level and do nothing else

    C. administer activated charcoal immediately and measure the plasma level of acetaminophen 4 hours after ingestion

    D. send the patient home because an ingestion of this magnitude is not toxic

    E. administer *N*-acetylcysteine at a dose of 140 mg/kg

Answers

1 The Field of Pediatrics

1. B. Injuries, congenital anomalies, and malignancy are the three leading causes of death in children 1 to 4 years old. Homicide is the fourth most prevalent cause of death in this group. (See Chapter 1 in *Nelson Textbook of Pediatrics,* 15th ed.)

2. D. Injuries, homicide, and suicide all are potentially preventable. (See Chapter 1 in *Nelson Textbook of Pediatrics,* 15th ed.)

3. A. The sensitivity of a test is reflected in the answer to the question, "Of all patients with a disease, how many will have a positive test result?" (See Chapter 2 in *Nelson Textbook of Pediatrics,* 15th ed.)

4. D. According to the principle of autonomy, we must respect a competent patient's decision. For younger children, we must balance the parent's autonomy and what is in the best interest of the child, because the child may be too young to express or understand his or her autonomous beliefs. (See Chapter 3 in *Nelson Textbook of Pediatrics,* 15th ed.)

5. D. If a decision is based on reliable data and is in the best interest of a patient, the act of withholding life support is no different from withdrawing such futile therapy. (See Chapter 3 in *Nelson Textbook of Pediatrics,* 15th ed.)

6. D. Drug rehabilitation does not prevent drug misuse but follows it. (See Chapter 105 in *Nelson Textbook of Pediatrics,* 15th ed.)

7. 1. A
   2. B
   3. A
   4. B
   5. A
   6. C
   7. B
   (See Chapter 5 in *Nelson Textbook of Pediatrics,* 15th ed.)

8. D. DPT immunization is an example of primary prevention. Anticipatory guidance would be an explanation of what to expect after the immunization, such as fever or other symptoms. (See Chapter 5 in *Nelson Textbook of Pediatrics,* 15th ed.)

9. 1. C. Beneficence is doing what is in the best interest of a patient. Physicians use this principle to overcome parental objections when the outcome is judged to be for the benefit of the child. Surrogate autonomy (choice *A*) is also involved in these cases.

2. D. There is rarely a circumstance in which a physician should not tell the truth. Truthfulness is particularly important in relationships in which one person (the physician) is in a powerful position of trust.

3. B. Few disagree that children should participate in their health care decisions, but they must be developmentally and cognitively competent to do so. Autonomy (choice *A*) is also involved.

4. E. The principle of confidentiality of the physician-patient relationship is crucial, but there are clear exceptions when the information discloses a situation that is harmful to others.

5. F. Physicians may find themselves in situations in which the best interests of the child and family conflict. Intrafamilial abuse, "Baby Doe" situations, and contraceptive use by adolescents are some examples. Nonetheless, all cases of suspected child abuse must be reported; this is beneficence (choice *C,* doing what is in the best interest of the child). (See Chapter 112 in *Nelson Textbook of Pediatrics,* 15th ed.)

10. D. This convenience sample bears very little relationship to the target population, assuming that the investigator intended to identify all causes of diarrhea in children. Only the sickest children will make it to this tertiary care emergency department. Organisms causing mild diarrhea will be missed. This sampling bias will diminish the generalizability of the study. The investigator's vacation habits will result in sampling bias that makes the actual sample different from the intended sample of study subjects, a problem with internal reliability. This problem with internal reliability will result in systematic undercounting of causes of diarrhea that occur in the season of the investigator's vacation, giving an inaccurate result.

Assuming the laboratory is better at identifying causes of diarrhea than the investigator is at collecting samples, the precision of the results will not be a problem. (See Chapter 2 in *Nelson Textbook of Pediatrics,* 15th ed.)

11. D. Studies paid for by drug companies may be open to subtle forms of bias. Always look at sources of support when reading a study report. Selection bias is minimized if a random mechanism is used to assign subjects to drug A or drug B. Make sure that this was a randomized trial. Selection bias is also possible with the choice of the study site. If the study is performed in a private office on patients with mild otitis media, the new drug may perform better than in a sample of subjects with severe recurrent otitis media selected from the office of an otolaryngologist. The small size of this study population limits the power to show anything except an extremely large difference between the two therapies. In fact, the finding of no difference in this study is compatible with a separate study that might have shown a difference of 55% in the rate of cure in the two groups. (See Chapter 2 in *Nelson Textbook of Pediatrics,* 15th ed.)

12. C. Case-fatality rate is expressed as number of deaths in the numerator and number with disease in denominator and for this example would be 100/500,000. The mortality rate differs because the denominator has the number of persons at risk of death in the population. In this example, the mortality rate from diarrhea is 100/1,000,000. The risk of diarrhea in persons younger than 18 years is 150,000/300,000, or 50%. The risk in persons older than 60 years is 300,000/400,000, or 75%. The risk of diarrhea in the younger age group, relative to the risk in the older age group, is 0.5/0.75, or 0.67. A relative risk less than 1 implies the exposure (in this case age <18 years) is protective. The risk difference of diarrheal illness in persons younger than 18 compared with persons age 19 to 60 years is $(150,000/300,000) - (50,000/300,000) = 0.5 - 0.17 = 0.33$. Children had 33% more diarrhea than persons age 18 to 60. (See Chapter 2 in *Nelson Textbook of Pediatrics,* 15th ed.)

13. D. If a child is not initially crying, the cardiac examination is potentially the least disturbing to an infant and toddler. (See Chapter 7 in *Nelson Textbook of Pediatrics,* 15th ed.)

14. C. Ending note taking while sensitive information is being conveyed demonstrates your own respect and sensitivity to patients and creates a better physician-parent relationship. Continuing to take notes under such circumstances may create suspicion. (See Chapter 7 in *Nelson Textbook of Pediatrics,* 15th ed.)

15. A. Infants and toddlers should be observed initially in the parent's lap. They should be alert, consolable, and responsive to the parent's communication. Observation during sleep does not assess the level of consciousness. (See Chapter 7 in *Nelson Textbook of Pediatrics,* 15th ed.)

16. C. Visual attentiveness is most greatly influenced by development, as is the response to the parent's interaction. Verbalization also is an obvious indicator of developmental stage. (See Chapter 7 in *Nelson Textbook of Pediatrics,* 15th ed.)

17. D. At each stage of development, nutrition, accident prevention, and growth have different meaning. Discussions with parents must be directed toward both the developmental risks of that age and the developmental ability to modify the risks according to the child's understanding. (See Chapter 7 in *Nelson Textbook of Pediatrics,* 15th ed.)

18. D. Auscultation of the lungs and heart should be conducted when a child is asleep, distracted, or at rest. Do not attempt to perform auscultation after a potentially disturbing or threatening procedure such as otoscopy. (See Chapter 7 in *Nelson Textbook of Pediatrics,* 15th ed.)

19. D. Basic principles applied to any geographic region—urban, rural, or international—have helped improve child health in the United States and abroad. (See Chapter 6 in *Nelson Textbook of Pediatrics,* 15th ed.)

20. E. Although a laudable goal, establishing roads for emergency transport of ill children is not part of the goals established at the United Nations World Summit for Children. (See Chapter 6 in *Nelson Textbook of Pediatrics,* 15th ed.)

21. A. Breast-feeding is the best way to prevent various infectious and nutritional disorders in developing countries. (See Chapter 6 in *Nelson Textbook of Pediatrics,* 15th ed.)

22. E. Vitamin A has value for many problems of the developing world, including its nutritional and anti-infective properties. (See Chapter 6 in *Nelson Textbook of Pediatrics,* 15th ed.)

23. B. The American Academy of Pediatrics

recommends oral rehydration therapy for diarrhea in the United States. (See Chapter 56.1 in *Nelson Textbook of Pediatrics,* 15th ed.)

24. C. Diarrheal (*Escherichia,* rotavirus) illnesses plus vaccine-preventable illnesses such as measles, tetanus, and so on are common causes of death in the developing world. (See Chapter 6 in *Nelson Textbook of Pediatrics,* 15th ed.)

25. C. Children are often inappropriate intrepreters, partly because of the possibility of misunderstanding and the potentially sensitive nature of some information. (See Chapter 4 in *Nelson Textbook of Pediatrics,* 15th ed.)

26. D. Try to work with the culturally derived therapy and to add it to the standard treatment. This approach provides a reasonable compromise and does not alienate the family. (See Chapter 4 in *Nelson Textbook of Pediatrics,* 15th ed.)

27. E. Cultural aspects of any illness must be considered in the evaluation and treatment plan. Beware of home remedies, which are often medicinal but not considered by the family to be medicines. (See Chapter 4 in *Nelson Textbook of Pediatrics,* 15th ed.)

28. D. A patient's surname is a poor indicator of acculturation. (See Chapter 4 in *Nelson Textbook of Pediatrics,* 15th ed.)

29. C. Visual contact should be maintained as much as possible with the patient or the patient's family. (See Chapter 4 in *Nelson Textbook of Pediatrics,* 15th ed.)

2 Growth and Development

1. 1. C
   2. E
   3. D
   4. A
   5. B
   (See Chapter 8 in *Nelson Textbook of Pediatrics,* 15th ed.)

2. C. Birth weight is not affected by a doula but may be influenced by home visitation during the pregnancy. (See Chapter 9 in *Nelson Textbook of Pediatrics,* 15th ed.)

3. D. Newborn infants have six characteristic organizational behavioral states. (See Chapter 10 in *Nelson Textbook of Pediatrics,* 15th ed.)

4. B. The formula in choice *A* is used for 7- to 12-year-old children; *C,* for 3- to 12-month-old infants; *D,* for 1- to 6-year-olds in pounds; and *F,* for 7- to 12-year-

olds in pounds. (See Chapter 11 in *Nelson Textbook of Pediatrics,* 15th ed.)

5. D. Crying may or may not be in response to obvious stimuli (e.g., need for a diaper change). (See Chapter 10 in *Nelson Textbook of Pediatrics,* 15th ed.)

6. D. Demand feedings prevent periods of hunger and episodes of being fed while not being hungry for a child with an irregular rhythm. (See Chapter 10 in *Nelson Textbook of Pediatrics,* 15th ed.)

7. A. Out of sight, out of mind is the characteristic response of a 2-month-old. Object permanence appears at approximately 8 months of age. This is also called object constancy. (See Chapter 11 in *Nelson Textbook of Pediatrics,* 15th ed.)

8. C. Tooth eruption generally begins at age 6 to 8 months, usually with the central mandibular incisors. (See Chapter 11 in *Nelson Textbook of Pediatrics,* 15th ed.)

9. D. The pincer grasp, which is noted at age 8 to 9 months, along with increasing mobility, enables an infant to explore the environment. (See Chapter 11 in *Nelson Textbook of Pediatrics,* 15th ed.)

10. A. (See Table 11–3 in Chapter 11 in *Nelson Textbook of Pediatrics,* 15th ed.)

11. D. (See Table 11–3 in Chapter 11 in *Nelson Textbook of Pediatrics,* 15th ed.)

12. D. Transitional objects help toddlers (18 to 24 months) cope with separation (e.g., at nighttime for sleep, baby sitter, daycare). (See Chapter 12 in *Nelson Textbook of Pediatrics,* 15th ed.)

13. C. (See Table 12–1 in Chapter 12 in *Nelson Textbook of Pediatrics,* 15th ed.)

14. E. Handedness should not be attempted to be modified, because this leads to frustration. After 4 years of age, a spontaneous change in handedness should lead to the suspicion of a central nervous system lesion. (See Chapter 13 in *Nelson Textbook of Pediatrics,* 15th ed.)

15. E. Paranoia is not a normal developmental behavior. Choices *A* through *D* in the question are part of magical thinking. Animism is attributing motivations to inanimate objects or events. (See Chapter 13 in *Nelson Textbook of Pediatrics,* 15th ed.)

16. D. It is impossible to rationalize away a preschool child's fear of monsters. (See Chapter 13 in *Nelson Textbook of Pediatrics,* 15th ed.)

17. D. Handedness is not related to how a child responds to stimuli. Temperament is

considered innate in a child and resistant to changes. Parents must work in the framework of an individual child's temperament. Additional features of temperament include activity level, approach and withdrawal, threshold of responsiveness, and quality of mood. (See Chapter 11 in *Nelson Textbook of Pediatrics,* 15th ed.)

18. B. We are indebted to Dr. Brazelton and others who have taught us how better to understand the complex behavior of newborns. (See Chapter 10 in *Nelson Textbook of Pediatrics,* 15th ed.)

19. C. Waking up at night (if in fact the baby has already slept through the night) at 6 to 8 months is common behavior. Whether this is related to separation anxiety or something else (teething?) is not clear (edentulous babies wake up, too). Choice *A* would be highly unlikely, because 6½-month-old circumcised boys who have grown normally rarely contract urinary tract infections. Choice *B* would be unnecessary, because increased food intake does not improve night fussiness. *D* is wrong because DTP reactions occur 4 to 36 hours after the shot, not 2 weeks. (See Chapter 11 in *Nelson Textbook of Pediatrics,* 15th ed.)

20. C. The relationship of SMR to growth, strength, hematocrit, and so on is important and is useful when advising a family about the next stages of adolescent development. (See Chapter 15 in *Nelson Textbook of Pediatrics,* 15th ed.)

21. B. (See Chapter 15 in *Nelson Textbook of Pediatrics,* 15th ed.)

22. B. Newborns have been shown to fixate visually during the quiet, alert state. This state represents 10% of a 24-hour day. (See Chapter 10 in *Nelson Textbook of Pediatrics,* 15th ed.)

3 Psychologic Disorders

1. D. Common complications of neuroleptic antipsychotic agents include extrapyramidal symptoms (Parkinson-like syndrome), sedation, and anticholinergic symptoms. Neuroleptic malignant syndrome (malignant hyperthermia) and tardive dyskinesia are rarer complications. (See Chapter 30.2 in *Nelson Textbook of Pediatrics*, 15th ed.)

2. D. Autism is a disease of unknown cause and is more common in males. It is characterized by the symptoms noted in this patient, with onset usually before 30 months of age. (See Chapter 29.1 in *Nelson Textbook of Pediatrics*, 15th ed.)

3. 1. C
   2. B
   3. A
   4. D
   (See Chapter 28 in *Nelson Textbook of Pediatrics*, 15th ed.)

4. A. Ritalin is the stimulant drug most commonly used in the therapy of ADHD and is effective in 75% to 80% of patients. (See Chapter 27 in *Nelson Textbook of Pediatrics*, 15th ed.)

5. E. The soft neurologic signs listed in the question are not diagnostic of ADHD. They are inconsistently present and do not contribute to the diagnosis. (See Chapter 27 in *Nelson Textbook of Pediatrics*, 15th ed.)

6. A. The belief that choice *B* is correct leads to repeated attempts to "break" children (a distressing term and concept), probably in effect reinforcing the behavior. (See Chapter 22 in *Nelson Textbook of Pediatrics*, 15th ed.)

7. D. ADHD is characterized by poor ability to attend to a task, motoric overactivity, and impulsivity. Affected children are fidgety, have a difficult time remaining in their seats in school, and are easily distracted. Although no firm cause has been discovered, positron emission tomography scans have shown reduced glucose metabolism in premotor and superior prefrontal cortices in adults with ADHD. Epidemiologic studies suggest a varied prevalence; one study in England found only 2 hyperactive children in a group of 2000; studies in the United States suggest a prevalence rate of 1.5% to 4%. The syndrome is four to six times more likely to occur in males than females, and the age of onset is before 4 years in about half of the cases. A large percentage of children with ADHD also suffer with behavior disorders, anxiety disorders, and learning disabilities, especially reading disabilities. Both psychopharmacotherapy and behavioral management have proved efficacious in the treatment of this disorder. (See Chapter 27 in *Nelson Textbook of Pediatrics*, 15th ed.)

8. E. The prevalence of depressive disorders in childhood has been estimated to be between 0.15% and 2%. In the population with clinical problems, the prevalence has been estimated to be between 10% and

20%. The prevalence of major depression in prepubertal children has been reported as 1.8% and in adolescents between 3.5% and 5%. Girls report significantly more depressive symptoms than boys. Twin studies have shown a 76% concordance for depression among monozygotic twins reared together and a 67% concordance for monozygotic twins reared apart, compared with 19% for dizygotic twins reared together. Many studies have demonstrated an increased rate of depression (three to six times greater) in first-degree relatives of patients suffering with major affective disorder. (See Chapter 24 in *Nelson Textbook of Pediatrics*, 15th ed.)

9. A. Gilles de la Tourette syndrome, which has a lifetime prevalence rate of 0.5 per 1000 individuals, is a rare condition in children. It is characterized by multiple tics, compulsive barking, and shouting obscene words (coprolalia). It is more common in first-degree relatives of patients with Tourette syndrome than in the general population and affects boys three to four times more often than girls. The cause is uncertain, but research has shown that drugs that increase dopaminergic action precipitate or worsen both tics and Gilles de la Tourette syndrome. Many environmental precipitants have been noted to serve as emotional stress sources. The syndrome can be fairly well managed with haloperidol, a dopaminergic antagonist, and Orap, a powerful dopamine antagonist. Anecdotal reports in the literature suggest that the serotonin reuptake inhibitors are also efficacious in its treatment. (See Chapter 22 in *Nelson Textbook of Pediatrics*, 15th ed.)

10. D. Night terrors most commonly occur during stage IV, deep sleep. They do not occur with REM sleep. Neither the use of antipsychotic medication nor overeating after 7:00 P.M. has ever been shown to be associated with night terrors. They usually begin in the preschool years. A child having night terrors is confused and disoriented and shows signs of intense autonomic activity (labored breathing, dilated pupils, sweating, tachypnea, tachycardia). Sleepwalking may occur during night terrors and may put a child at risk for injury. The incidence of night terrors is said to be between 1% and 4% and is greater in boys. There is a familial pattern in the development of the symptoms, and febrile illnesses may serve

as precipitating factors. (See Chapter 21.5 in *Nelson Textbook of Pediatrics*, 15th ed.)

11. B. Infantile autism develops before 30 months of age and is characterized by a qualitative impairment in verbal and nonverbal communication, in imaginative activity, and in reciprocal social interactions. The prevalence is generally 3 to 4 per 10,000 children. This disorder is much more common in males than females and tends to be more common in siblings of autistic children than in the general population. The cause of autism is speculative. Theories have centered on various possibilities including brain injury, constitutional vulnerability, deficits in the reticular activating system, an interplay between psychogenic and neurodevelopmental factors, and structural cerebral changes. Contrary to notions invoked in the past, autism is not induced by parents. The prognosis is guarded. Some children, especially those with some speech, may grow up to live marginal, self-sufficient, albeit isolated lives in the community. For most, however, long-term placement in institutions is the ultimate outcome. (See Chapter 29.1 in *Nelson Textbook of Pediatrics*, 15th ed.)

12. C. Separation anxiety disorder is characterized by unrealistic and persistent worries of possible harm befalling primary caregivers, reluctance to go to school or to sleep without being near the parents, persistent avoidance of being alone, nightmares involving themes of separation, and numerous somatic symptoms and complaints of subjective distress. Affected children come from middle and lower socioeconomic classes. The first clinical sign of the disorder often does not appear until third or fourth grade, typically after the Christmas holidays or after a period in which the child has been absent from school because of an illness. Slightly more girls than boys are affected; 80% of the affected children are Caucasian. The majority of older children with separation anxiety disorder are also said to suffer with an affective disorder. Treatment includes a supportive understanding of the child's fear, liaison work with the school to help reintroduce the child to the classroom, and family work, especially helping parents learn how not to reinforce the symptoms. Benzodiazepines and tricyclics have also been shown to be quite efficacious in reducing symptoms

sufficiently to allow a child to return to school. (See Chapter 23 in *Nelson Textbook of Pediatrics*, 15th ed.)

13. B. The prevalence of enuresis at age 5 years is 7% for boys and 3% for girls; at age 10 it is 3% for boys and 2% for girls; and at age 18 it is 1% for males and extremely rare for females. Twin studies show a familial pattern for this symptom. Bed-wetting may be divided into the primary type, in which a child has never had a dry night, and the regressive type, in which a previously continent child begins to wet the bed again. Persistent nocturnal enuresis is often a result of inadequate or inappropriate toilet training. Chronic psychologic stress can also affect the occurrence of this symptom. A number of behavioral techniques have been shown to be quite efficacious in the treatment of enuresis. In addition, imipramine has been shown to be useful; it must be continued for several months after the remission of symptoms for successful treatment of this disorder. (See Chapter 21.3 in *Nelson Textbook of Pediatrics*, 15th ed.)

14. A. Carbamazepine, a tricyclic antidepressant-like agent, is traditionally used to treat complex partial seizures but has also been shown to be efficacious in the treatment of bipolar disorder and as an adjunct in the treatment of refractory manic-depressive disorder. Side effects include bone marrow suppression, which requires baseline measurements and close monitoring of blood cell counts, dizziness, drowsiness, rashes, nausea, and (uncommonly) liver toxicity. Daily doses vary between 10 and 20 mg/kg/day, but medication use should be monitored with serial blood level measurements until the therapeutic range has been achieved. Anecdotal reports have described carbamazepine as also useful in treating self-injurious behavior in organically impaired children and adolescents. (See Chapter 24 in *Nelson Textbook of Pediatrics*, 15th ed.)

15. B. Methylphenidate is the most commonly used pharmacotherapeutic agent for the treatment of ADHD. It is said to be efficacious in more than 70% of cases. Dextroamphetamine is the second most used agent, and its efficacy is slightly less than that of methylphenidate. Clonidine, an antihypertensive, has also shown efficacy, especially with the overactivity component of ADHD. Desipramine, a tricyclic antidepressant, has been shown to be efficacious in about 65% of children treated for ADHD. Thiothixene, an antipsychotic agent, is not appropriate for the treatment of this disorder. (See Chapter 27 in *Nelson Textbook of Pediatrics*, 15th ed.)

16. E. Conduct disorder is a distinct clinical entity manifested by several different antisocial behaviors: stealing, lying, fire setting, truancy, property destruction, cruelty to animals, rape, use of weapons while fighting, armed robbery, physical cruelty to others, and repeated attempts to run away from home. Many argue that conduct disorder is not a unitary illness but instead comprises three different syndromes characterized primarily by aggression, intermittent antisocial behaviors, and delinquency. Little is known about the antecedents of each of these subtypes or the outcome of patients suffering from them. Risk factors associated with the development of conduct disorders include antisocial behavior within family members, criminality in the father, physical abuse within the home, and marital discord within the home. Many different approaches have been used in the treatment of children and adolescents with aggressive behavior, antisocial behavior, and delinquency. The most effective results have been obtained with parent training management in which parents are trained directly to promote prosocial behaviors within the home and to place reasonable limits on unwanted, destructive behaviors. (See Chapter 26 in *Nelson Textbook of Pediatrics*, 15th ed.)

17. D. Encopresis, which is the passage of feces in inappropriate places at an age after bowel control should have been established, is predominantly a male disorder affecting about 1% of 5-year-olds. It more commonly affects children from lower socioeconomic backgrounds. Organic defects are rarely found. This symptom usually indicates a more serious emotional disturbance than enuresis. It is often encountered in boys who are angry. School performance and attendance may be affected as the child becomes a target of scorn and derision by schoolmates because of the offensive odor. (See Chapter 26 in *Nelson Textbook of Pediatrics*, 15th ed.)

18. E. Previous suicide attempts, substance abuse, easy access to firearms, and a family

history of depression and suicide all are closely related to both suicide attempts and completed suicides in both children and adolescents. Fifteen to 40% of completed suicides are preceded by other suicide attempts. In more than one third of suicides, a parent, a sibling, or another first-degree relative has previously shown overt suicidal behavior. Firearms served as the major method of death in adolescent suicide. Among preadolescents, jumping from heights is the most common method. Although perfectionism in the classroom has been shown to be associated with specific types of anxiety, no correlation has been shown between perfectionism and suicidal ideation or suicidal behavior. (See Chapter 25 in *Nelson Textbook of Pediatrics*, 15th ed.)

19. C. Math and writing require an active working memory process. (See Chapter 31 in *Nelson Textbook of Pediatrics*, 15th ed.)

20. A. Social skill training helps provide the feedback and possible insight needed in the situation described in the question. Pro-social behaviors will help this child. (See Chapter 31 in *Nelson Textbook of Pediatrics*, 15th ed.)

21. C. The question offers a classic example of a language problem, particularly a child with partial understanding. Many children or parents will not admit to this problem. (See Chapter 31 in *Nelson Textbook of Pediatrics*, 15th ed.)

22. C. Additional neurodevelopmental problems should be determined by careful evaluation in all children with attentional problems. (See Chapter 31 in *Nelson Textbook of Pediatrics*, 15th ed.)

23. E. Simultaneous retrieval memory defects are depicted by the history of the child described in the question. (See Chapter 31 in *Nelson Textbook of Pediatrics*, 15th ed.)

24. B. Phonologic skills are critical to the development of reading decoding and must be evaluated in the child described in the question. (See Chapter 31 in *Nelson Textbook of Pediatrics*, 15th ed.)

25. 1. C
    2. D
    3. A
    4. B
    (See Chapter 31 in *Nelson Textbook of Pediatrics*, 15th ed.)

26. B. Asthma may be exacerbated by psychologic factors and is therefore a psychophysiologic disorder. (See Chapter

20 in *Nelson Textbook of Pediatrics*, 15th ed.)

27. C. In the Munchausen by proxy syndrome, patients' symptoms disappear if the parent goes home. Manifestations reappear when the involved parent returns to the hospital. (See Chapter 20 in *Nelson Textbook of Pediatrics*, 15th ed.)

28. C. Urinary tract infections may complicate enuresis in children. Alternatively, secondary enuresis may be due to cystitis or pyelonephritis. (See Chapter 21.3 in *Nelson Textbook of Pediatrics*, 15th ed.)

29. 1. A
    2. B
    3. C
    4. C
    5. A
    6. B
    7. C
    (See Chapter 21.5 in *Nelson Textbook of Pediatrics*, 15th ed.)

30. E. Excessive physical activity is not characteristic of major depression. Loss of energy is characteristic. (See Chapter 24.1 in *Nelson Textbook of Pediatrics*, 15th ed.)

31. A. Delusions are characteristic of major depression but not of the more chronic but less severe dysthymic disorder. (See Chapter 24.2 in *Nelson Textbook of Pediatrics*, 15th ed.)

32. E. Choices *A* to *D* list methods more frequently used by younger children in suicide attempts, whereas firearms lead the list in adolescent males. (See Chapter 25 in *Nelson Textbook of Pediatrics*, 15th ed.)

33. C. In 2- to 4-year-olds, lying is similar to playing with language and testing parental reactions. (See Chapter 26 in *Nelson Textbook of Pediatrics*, 15th ed.)

34. E. Truancy and runaway behavior are never developmentally normal. (See Chapter 26 in *Nelson Textbook of Pediatrics*, 15th ed.)

35. 1. A
    2. B
    3. A
    4. B
    5. A
    6. A
    7. D
    8. C
    (See Chapter 26 in *Nelson Textbook of Pediatrics*, 15th ed.)

4 Social Issues

1. D. HSV type 1 may be autoinoculated from a patient's oral secretions. HSV type 2 is

diagnostic of abuse, as would be pregnancy. (See Chapter 38 in *Nelson Textbook of Pediatrics,* 15th ed.)

2. F. Children vulnerable to pedophiles are often mentally or physically handicapped, unwanted or unloved, previously abused, children of divorced or single parents, poor achievers, or those with low self-esteem. (See Chapter 38 in *Nelson Textbook of Pediatrics,* 15th ed.)

3. E. In the classic shaken baby syndrome, a computed tomography scan of the head reveals diffuse cerebral edema and hemorrhage. CPR in young children does not usually produce retinal hemorrhages and rarely, if ever, produces rib fractures. (See Chapter 38 in *Nelson Textbook of Pediatrics,* 15th ed.)

4. 1. B
   2. C
   3. A
   4. E
   5. D
   (See Chapter 38 in *Nelson Textbook of Pediatrics,* 15th ed.)

5. E. Fractures of the tibia in toddlers are produced by torsional forces from a fall or twisting motion when the foot is caught in a fixed position. The fracture presents with refusal to walk and is a hairline fracture with periosteal new bone formation. (See Chapter 38 in *Nelson Textbook of Pediatrics,* 15th ed.)

6. 1. C
   2. E
   3. B
   4. D
   5. A
   (See Chapter 38 in *Nelson Textbook of Pediatrics,* 15th ed.)

7. D. More than 90% of abusing adults are neither criminals nor psychotic. (See Chapter 38 in *Nelson Textbook of Pediatrics,* 15th ed.)

8. D. Almost 50% of children comment about their fears of violence to themselves or their family members or friends. (See Chapter 38 in *Nelson Textbook of Pediatrics,* 15th ed.)

9. B. Many young children continue in the daily activities and use denial and magical wishful thoughts for reunion and reappearance. (See Chapter 36 in *Nelson Textbook of Pediatrics,* 15th ed.)

10. C. Statements such as "stop it or you'll give me a headache" may cause a child to suffer significant and unrealistic guilt, especially if the parent leaves for some time or is hospitalized. (See Chapter 36 in *Nelson Textbook of Pediatrics,* 15th ed.)

11. A. Children should be told of their adoption by 3 to 4 years of age or when they have reasonably good verbal facility and comprehension. (See Chapter 32 in *Nelson Textbook of Pediatrics,* 15th ed.)

12. D. Children usually suffer no sequelae of childcare. Many are more interactive with children and more self-confident. (See Chapter 35 in *Nelson Textbook of Pediatrics,* 15th ed.)

13. C. In-home care provides a continued familiar environment for a child. (See Chapter 35 in *Nelson Textbook of Pediatrics,* 15th ed.)

5 Children with Special Needs

1. B. The pattern of abnormalities described in the question is most compatible with a congenital TORCH (toxoplasmosis, other, rubella, cytomegalovirus, herpes simplex 2) infection. In addition, intrauterine and postnatal growth retardation may be evident. (See Chapter 40.2 in *Nelson Textbook of Pediatrics,* 15th ed.)

2. B. The Denver developmental test is a screening test that requires confirmation by one of the other (choices *A, C, D*) more valid and reliable standard diagnostic measures. (See Chapter 40.2 in *Nelson Textbook of Pediatrics,* 15th ed.)

3. E. As a result of rubella immunization, cases of rubella during pregnancy and hence fetal rubella syndrome are quite rare in the United States. (See Chapter 207 in *Nelson Textbook of Pediatrics,* 15th ed.)

4. E. Many children with the common chronic diseases of childhood (asthma, seizures, diabetes, arthritis, cystic fibrosis, sickle cell anemia, and others) attend high school and graduate. (See Chapter 40.1 in *Nelson Textbook of Pediatrics,* 15th ed.)

5. E. Cystic fibrosis is not among the five most common chronic childhood illnesses (incidence 0.2 per 1000). The order of prevalence of these illnesses is asthma (10 per 1000), congenital heart disease (7 per 1000), seizures (3.5 per 1000), arthritis (2.2 per 1000) and diabetes (1.8 per 1000). (See Chapter 40.1 in *Nelson Textbook of Pediatrics,* 15th ed.)

6. C. Parents who are not able to see their deformed neonate may greatly exaggerate the severity of any anomaly and may have excessive feelings of guilt. Most parents benefit from seeing their child with anomalies and often identify aspects of

beauty or normalcy with the help of a nurse or physician. (See Chapter 41 in *Nelson Textbook of Pediatrics,* 15th ed.)

7. D. Magic thinking of young children often involves illusions that if they think about harming a person it could actually happen. (See Chapter 41 in *Nelson Textbook of Pediatrics,* 15th ed.)

8. C. This is a good open-ended question that may better determine the motive for the 10-year-old's initial question. She may be truly aware of the grave prognosis or may be concerned about a less significant (but important to her) issue. (See Chapter 41 in *Nelson Textbook of Pediatrics,* 15th ed.)

9. E. Most parents undergo various stages of disbelief, anger, guilt, fear, and resignation when they first hear that their child has a fatal illness. Denial or disbelief is a usual first response, as is anger. (See Chapter 41 in *Nelson Textbook of Pediatrics,* 15th ed.)

10. D. The child described in the question demonstrates important educational and social milestones that are partially predictive of future achievements. (See Chapter 40.2 in *Nelson Textbook of Pediatrics,* 15th ed.)

11. B. Neurogenic bladder is not typically encountered in Down syndrome, but Hirschsprung disease may occur. (See Chapter 40.2 in *Nelson Textbook of Pediatrics,* 15th ed.)

12. C. Cranial computed tomography is not indicated until other evaluations are completed unless a patient has macrocephaly, microcephaly, abnormal neurologic signs, or significant dysmorphology. (See Chapter 40.2 in *Nelson Textbook of Pediatrics,* 15th ed.)

13. D. In the eighth grade, most schools begin formal educational instruction in biology, anatomy, and physiology. (See Chapter 41 in *Nelson Textbook of Pediatrics,* 15th ed.)

14. D. WIC provides nutritional support to infants and is not targeted to those with chronic illness. (See Chapter 40.1 in *Nelson Textbook of Pediatrics,* 15th ed.)

15. C. Chronic childhood diseases are now challenging our internal medicine colleagues as children with congenital heart disease, diabetes mellitus, asthma, cystic fibrosis, and sickle cell anemia now survive to adulthood. (See Chapter 40.1 in *Nelson Textbook of Pediatrics,* 15th ed.)

16. D. In children, in contrast to adults, hypertension is not a chronic illness, even among adolescents. (See Chapter 40.1 in *Nelson Textbook of Pediatrics,* 15th ed.)

17. C. Forced feeding exacerbates abnormal psychosocial tension between a child and his or her caregiver. (See Chapter 39 in *Nelson Textbook of Pediatrics,* 15th ed.)

18. B. Minor infections can be managed on an outpatient basis with oral antibiotics together with appropriate nutritional rehabilitation. (See Chapter 39 in *Nelson Textbook of Pediatrics,* 15th ed.)

19. E. Amino acid screens are indicated if an inborn error of metabolism is suspected (acidosis, hypoglycemia, coma, seizures, developmental delay, unusual odor) or if results of routine screens are normal and other clues (such as those just mentioned) become evident with further evaluation. (See Chapter 39 in *Nelson Textbook of Pediatrics,* 15th ed.)

6 Nutrition

1. C. A strict vegan diet contains no eggs, meat, or milk products and is thus deficient in vitamin B_{12}. (See Chapter 44.5 in *Nelson Textbook of Pediatrics*, 15th ed.)

2. B. (See Chapter 45.2 in *Nelson Textbook of Pediatrics*, 15th ed.)

3. C. Weight loss in a seriously obese child with pickwickian syndrome is the most effective but most difficult treatment to achieve. (See Chapter 45.2 in *Nelson Textbook of Pediatrics*, 15th ed.)

4. 1. C
   2. A
   3. D
   4. E
   5. C
   6. D
   7. B or E
   8. F
   9. G
   10. H
   11. I
   (See Chapter 45.3 in *Nelson Textbook of Pediatrics*, 15th ed.)

5. 1. B
   2. D
   3. A
   4. C
   5. F
   6. A
   7. E
   8. H
   9. G
   (See Chapter 43.6 in *Nelson Textbook of Pediatrics*, 15th ed.)

6. 1. B
   2. D

3. A
4. C
5. E
(See Chapter 45.3 in *Nelson Textbook of Pediatrics*, 15th ed.)

7. D. HIV is most definitely transmitted in human milk, and breast-feeding by women in the United States who are HIV positive is contraindicated. In less-developed countries, unless clean water and safe formula alternatives are available, breast-feeding by HIV-positive women is not contraindicated. In these circumstances, human milk is safer than no milk or contaminated artificial formula. (See Chapter 44.1 in *Nelson Textbook of Pediatrics*, 15th ed.)

8. 1. D
   2. E
   3. F
   4. C
   Pyridoxine deficiency is part of the differential diagnosis of neonatal seizures; pseudoparalysis occurs secondary to painful bone lesions; the rachitic rosary is equivalent to enlarged costochondral junctions; the classic triad of pellagra is dermatitis, diarrhea, and dementia. (See Chapter 45.3 in *Nelson Textbook of Pediatrics*, 15th ed.)

9. 1. C
   2. A
   3. C
   4. A
   5. B
   6. A
   7. A
   8. A
   The bottom line is that breast milk is for babies, and except in unusual circumstances, cow's milk should be reserved for calves. (See Chapter 44 in *Nelson Textbook of Pediatrics*, 15th ed.)

10. D. Although breast milk contains relatively less iron by weight, the iron is more bioavailable than the iron in cereals. Fruits, yellow vegetables, and cow's milk are poor sources of iron. (See Chapter 44.1 in *Nelson Textbook of Pediatrics*, 15th ed.)

11. 1. C
    2. E
    3. F
    4. D
    5. A
    These deficiency diseases are rare in the United States among families with traditional diets but occur in developing countries and in families adhering to some fad diets. (See Chapter 45.3 in *Nelson Textbook of Pediatrics*, 15th ed.)

12. B. In rickets, parathyroid hormone level is elevated and results in low serum phosphate levels. Low serum phosphate levels result in abnormal osteoblastic activity, which may result in craniotabes and a rachitic rosary with enlargement at the costochondral junctions. Even though osteoid of the legs is uncalcified, bowing does not occur until weight is borne on the legs. (See Chapter 45.3 in *Nelson Textbook of Pediatrics*, 15th ed.)

13. B. Deficiency of any essential nutrient may result in failure to thrive and accompanying lack of protection against infection. However, infections are more common in children deficient in vitamin A, iron, or zinc. Infections in those deficient in vitamin D are not more frequent than in controls. (See Chapter 45.3 in *Nelson Textbook of Pediatrics*, 15th ed.)

14. D. The breast milk of a well-fed mother contains sufficient water-soluble vitamins for her infant and all of the fat-soluble vitamins except vitamins D and particularly K. The milk of a cow fed on pasture contains sufficient vitamins except vitamin D. Human milk contains about 2 μg/L vitamin K, compared with about 34 μg/L in cow's milk. A breast-fed infant with any form of malabsorption requires supplemental vitamin K. (See Chapter 44 in *Nelson Textbook of Pediatrics*, 15th ed.)

7 Pathophysiology of Body Fluids and Fluid Therapy

1. E. Adrenal deficiency may cause renal salt wasting and usually does not affect free water excretion. (See Chapter 46 in *Nelson Textbook of Pediatrics*, 15th ed.)

2. A. Normally 1% of the filtered sodium is excreted. High-sodium diets, adrenal insufficiency, and renal tubular injury result in a higher fractional excretion of sodium. (See Chapter 47 in *Nelson Textbook of Pediatrics*, 15th ed.)

3. E. Nephrogenic diabetes insipidus is a sex-linked recessive disorder due to deficient binding of ADH to the renal tubular cell. Exogenous administration of ADH is therefore ineffective. (See Chapter 47 in *Nelson Textbook of Pediatrics*, 15th ed.)

4. B. Hyponatremia due to feeding diluted formula or excessive amounts of sodium-free fluids (especially water) is relatively and unfortunately common among poor

families who run out of formula. (See Chapter 47 in *Nelson Textbook of Pediatrics,* 15th ed.)

5. D. Hypoglycemia is not usually associated with hyperkalemia. Transcellular buffering of H$^+$ during acidosis shifts K$^+$ out of the cell during intracellular H$^+$ buffering. (See Chapter 48 in *Nelson Textbook of Pediatrics,* 15th ed.)

6. E. Metabolic alkalosis produces hypokalemia. (See Chapter 48 in *Nelson Textbook of Pediatrics,* 15th ed.)

7. D. Hypokalemia usually causes hypotension if the blood pressure is affected at all. Muscle weakness is one of the most common manifestations of hypokalemia. (See Chapter 48 in *Nelson Textbook of Pediatrics,* 15th ed.)

8. B. Renal tubular acidosis with renal bicarbonate loss or diarrhea induced stool losses of bicarbonate are the common causes of a normal anion gap acidosis. (See Chapter 49 in *Nelson Textbook of Pediatrics,* 15th ed.)

9. D. Sarcoidosis is also associated with hypercalcemia. (See Chapter 50 in *Nelson Textbook of Pediatrics,* 15th ed.)

10. E. Trisomy 21 is not usually associated with hypercalcemia. (See Chapter 50 in *Nelson Textbook of Pediatrics,* 15th ed.)

11. A. Hyporeflexia usually precedes apnea and coma. (See Chapter 51 in *Nelson Textbook of Pediatrics,* 15th ed.)

12. C. Dehydration of 6% to 9% represents moderate dehydration and early shock. Tachycardia reflects the intravascular volume loss, and deep respirations represent the pulmonary response to metabolic acidosis. (See Chapter 54 in *Nelson Textbook of Pediatrics,* 15th ed.)

13. B. Cerebral edema occurs if free water is given in excessive amounts, if the serum sodium falls more than 10 mEq/L/day, and if idiogenic osmols remain in neurons during rehydration. (See Chapter 55 in *Nelson Textbook of Pediatrics,* 15th ed.)

14. A. Tetany with laryngospasm and carpopedal spasm is encountered with hypocalcemia, hypomagnesemia, or alkalosis. (See Chapter 56.9 in *Nelson Textbook of Pediatrics,* 15th ed.)

15. A. Pulmonary and skin (not sweat) evaporation losses are considered insensible. (See Chapter 46 in *Nelson Textbook of Pediatrics,* 15th ed.)

16. D. Severe dehydration may produce renal parenchymal damage (acute tubular necrosis), whereas extreme

hyperosmolality is a strong stimulus for ADH secretion. (See Chapter 55 in *Nelson Textbook of Pediatrics,* 15th ed.)

17. E. Kayexalate, a potassium-binding resin, and dialysis are the only methods to remove potassium from the body. Other methods shift potassium from the extracellular to the intracellular space. (See Chapter 56.8 in *Nelson Textbook of Pediatrics,* 15th ed.)

18. D. Captopril, an angiotensin-converting enzyme inhibitor, may by this action actually raise serum potassium levels. (See Chapter 56.8 in *Nelson Textbook of Pediatrics,* 15th ed.)

19. D. Owing to the hypertonic-hyperosmolar state, the intravascular volume is relatively preserved. Therefore, the pulse and blood pressure may be less severely altered in hypernatremic dehydration. (See Chapter 54 in *Nelson Textbook of Pediatrics,* 15th ed.)

20. B. Marked potassium depletion is more likely, although laboratory error is possible. When in doubt, repeat laboratory tests, but such a repeat in this case would confirm the finding. (See Chapter 53 in *Nelson Textbook of Pediatrics,* 15th ed.)

21. B. All other responses are associated with hypoventilation and therefore with respiratory acidosis. (See Chapter 53 in *Nelson Textbook of Pediatrics,* 15th ed.)

22. C. Inability to draw blood is a good indication of poor intravascular volume and low venous pressure. Do not persist too long in such efforts. Start fluids by intraosseous line if necessary, and the veins will soon be more acccessible. (See Chapter 55 in *Nelson Textbook of Pediatrics,* 15th ed.)

23. C. Choice *A* is normal, *B* is hypernatremic, and *D* is highly unlikely. (See Chapter 55 in *Nelson Textbook of Pediatrics,* 15th ed.)

24. B. Boiled skim milk should never be prescribed for diarrhea because of the high association with hypernatremia. (See Chapter 55 in *Nelson Textbook of Pediatrics,* 15th ed.)

25. B. Urinary output initially and weight gain over the longer term are the ways to monitor improvement. In a child who is 10% dehydrated, a central venous pressure line is rarely necessary, and the blood pressure is usually normal. (See Chapter 55 in *Nelson Textbook of Pediatrics,* 15th ed.)

8 The Acutely Ill Child

1. E. Lack of immunization against tetanus may be managed with tetanus toxoid and, if a

wound is large or dirty, with tetanus immune globulin. The other responses are high risk and require hospitalization. (See Chapter 60.5 in *Nelson Textbook of Pediatrics,* 15th ed.)

2. C. All the other statements in the question are serious misconceptions. (See Chapter 62 in *Nelson Textbook of Pediatrics,* 15th ed.)

3. D. Tachycardia is not part of the pediatric trauma score scale, which assesses weight, airway stability, systolic blood pressure, level of consciousness, wounds, and fractures. (See Chapter 59 in *Nelson Textbook of Pediatrics,* 15th ed.)

4. E. Age is usually not as predictive of the prognosis after near-drowning as the other risk factors listed in the question. The best predictive factors are the initial signs of improvement within 24 hours of the episode. In addition, normal cardiopulmonary function and alertness at the scene are favorable prognostic features. (See Chapter 60.4 in *Nelson Textbook of Pediatrics,* 15th ed.)

5. A. Control of the airway is essential in the gravely ill and unstable patient described in the question. Prevention of hypoxia and hypercarbia is critical to avoid secondary injury to vital tissues. (See Chapter 60.2 in *Nelson Textbook of Pediatrics,* 15th ed.)

6. A. Hyperventilation is the fastest method to relieve intracranial hypertension (increased intracranial pressure), which in this patient may be due to cerebral edema or a bleed. Dexamethasone is ineffective in treating this type of cerebral edema, and furosemide may acutely reduce central nervous system perfusion. (See Chapter 60.1 in *Nelson Textbook of Pediatrics,* 15th ed.)

7. B. Now is the time to perform a head CT scan. After this patient was stabilized, the CT scan revealed an epidural hematoma, which was surgically evacuated. (See Chapter 60.1 in *Nelson Textbook of Pediatrics,* 15th ed.)

8. B. (See Table 59–5 in Chapter 59 in *Nelson Textbook of Pediatrics,* 15th ed.)

9. 1. E
   2. A
   3. B
   4. C
   5. D
   (See Chapter 60.6 in *Nelson Textbook of Pediatrics,* 15th ed.)

10. D. Multiple organ involvement in addition to the normal-pressure pulmonary edema augurs a poor prognosis. Such involvement

includes coma, hemorrhage, jaundice, ileus, pancreatitis, and anuria reflecting central nervous system, hematologic, hepatic, intestinal, pancreatic, and renal dysfunction. The systemic inflammatory response syndrome is usually present in patients with multisystem organ dysfunction. (See Chapter 60.7 in *Nelson Textbook of Pediatrics,* 15th ed.)

11. D. Bradycardia or any dysrhythmia during anesthesia is due to hypoxia until proved otherwise. (See Chapter 61 in *Nelson Textbook of Pediatrics,* 15th ed.)

12. 1. B
    2. C
    3. A
    4. E
    5. G
    6. D
    7. F
    (See Chapter 61 in *Nelson Textbook of Pediatrics,* 15th ed.)

13. C. Apnea does not respond to any drug (other than the reversal of opioid overdose by naloxone). Apnea is treated with bag and mask, mouth-to-mouth ventilation, or endotracheal intubation and mechanical ventilation. (See Chapter 60 in *Nelson Textbook of Pediatrics,* 15th ed.)

14. D. Restrictive lung disease classically produces shallow but rapid respiration. (See Chapter 60 in *Nelson Textbook of Pediatrics,* 15th ed.)

15. C. Motor vehicle accidents are the leading cause of death among children 4 to 15 years old, although firearm-related injury and death are becoming increasingly common in childhood and adolescence. (See Chapter 58 in *Nelson Textbook of Pediatrics,* 15th ed.)

16. 1. D
    2. A
    3. C
    4. B
    5. E
    (See Chapter 58 in *Nelson Textbook of Pediatrics,* 15th ed.)

17. A. Most nonintentional firearm injuries occur at home. (See Chapter 58 in *Nelson Textbook of Pediatrics,* 15th ed.)

18. C. Checking the carotid pulse is not recommended for infants younger than 1 year. Use the femoral or brachial artery. (See Chapter 60.2 in *Nelson Textbook of Pediatrics,* 15th ed.)

19. D. Placement of an intraosseous line is indicated in the emergency situation described in the question. If the child is in

cardiopulmonary arrest, certain medications (epinephrine, lidocaine) may be given by the endotracheal route. This patient requires fluid and blood replacement, which must be given by intraosseus line at this time. (See Chapter 59 in *Nelson Textbook of Pediatrics,* 15th ed.)

20. D. Pneumothorax in this case most likely resulted from a fractured rib that punctured the lung. Treatment is with immediate needle aspiration. (See Chapter 59 in *Nelson Textbook of Pediatrics,* 15th ed.)

21. C. Camp pools usually are enclosed in a fenced-in area. All swimmers are closely supervised and have their skills tested. (See Chapter 58 in *Nelson Textbook of Pediatrics,* 15th ed.)

22. A. Hyperglycemia is a risk factor for poor outcome in drowning and has traditionally been managed conservatively with normal saline and not insulin. (See Chapter 60.4 in *Nelson Textbook of Pediatrics,* 15th ed.)

23. D. A bulging fontanel is not part of the observational scale but nonetheless must be part of a physical examination in an acutely ill febrile child. (See Chapter 57 in *Nelson Textbook of Pediatrics,* 15th ed.)

24. 1. C
    2. A
    3. B
    4. C
    5. D
    6. C
    7. B
    (See Chapter 60.4 in *Nelson Textbook of Pediatrics,* 15th ed.)

25. C. Home ownership of guns poses a greater threat to members of the family or to friends than to any unlawful intruder. (See Chapter 58 in *Nelson Textbook of Pediatrics,* 15th ed.)

26. C. Hot food or drinks from the microwave or more often from pots and pans that extend over the top of stoves are the most common causes of burn injury resulting in hospitalization in young children. Beware of the possible telltale signs of child abuse or neglect. (See Chapter 58 in *Nelson Textbook of Pediatrics,* 15th ed.)

27. B. Unfortunately, driver education programs do not decrease the high rate of motor vehicle injuries among teenage drivers. (See Chapter 58 in *Nelson Textbook of Pediatrics,* 15th ed.)

28. A. Passive intervention (such as air bags), which requires no effort on the part of a child or adolescent, is more effective than active prevention requiring the active use of a product (seat belt). (It is extremely difficult to identify injury-prone children, let alone prevent such accidents.) (See Chapter 58 in *Nelson Textbook of Pediatrics,* 15th ed.)

29. C. Suicide rates have actually increased, partly because of access to handguns. (See Chapter 58 in *Nelson Textbook of Pediatrics,* 15th ed.)

30. A. Anaphylaxis significantly reduces systemic vascular resistance, thus removing this sign as a reliable indicator of perfusion. (See Chapter 60.3 in *Nelson Textbook of Pediatrics,* 15th ed.)

31. B. Oxygen delivery is reduced in shock, and oxygen therapy is indicated. Nonetheless, in hypovolemic shock, isotonic fluids such as normal saline or lactated Ringer solution are the first line of therapy. It is not necessary to wait for laboratory results to administer these isotonic solutions. (See Chapter 60.3 in *Nelson Textbook of Pediatrics,* 15th ed.)

32. E. Once cold shock is present, compensatory measures fail to maintain the cardiac index but significantly reduce peripheral perfusion by an increase in the SVR. (See Chapter 60.3 in *Nelson Textbook of Pediatrics,* 15th ed.)

33. C. Isoproterenol, with its beta effect, further reduces SVR. Epinephrine is the agent of choice for anaphylactic shock. (See Chapter 60.3 in *Nelson Textbook of Pediatrics,* 15th ed.)

34. B. Electric burns on the mouth are usually minor but do require anticipatory guidance and raise a suspicion that the child may not be well supervised. (See Chapter 60.5 in *Nelson Textbook of Pediatrics,* 15th ed.)

35. D. Because of large third-space losses in burn victims, urine output as an assessment of intravascular volume and cardiac output is the best determinant of adequate fluid resuscitation. (See Chapter 60.5 in *Nelson Textbook of Pediatrics,* 15th ed.)

36. C. Burns on both hands and wrists in a glove distribution suggest that the child has been forcibly placed in hot water (bathtub). Most children jump out or do not enter a hot bathtub. (See Chapter 60.5 in *Nelson Textbook of Pediatrics,* 15th ed.)

37. A and D. The other choices are not immediate life-threatening emergencies. (See Chapter 59 in *Nelson Textbook of Pediatrics,* 15th ed.)

38. C. Stabilization of cardiopulmonary function

is needed before transfer. (See Chapter 59 in *Nelson Textbook of Pediatrics,* 15th ed.)

39. D. Patients such as the child described in the question are in shock and have decreased oxygen delivery to tissues. The next step is fluid resuscitation. (See Chapter 59 in *Nelson Textbook of Pediatrics,* 15th ed.)

40. G. Choices *A* through *F* are high-risk situations for an associated cervical spine injury. (See Chapter 59 in *Nelson Textbook of Pediatrics,* 15th ed.)

41. B. The child described in the question is severely ill and may suffer an arrest at any moment. (See Chapter 59 in *Nelson Textbook of Pediatrics,* 15th ed.)

42. D. The bone may not be reused during resuscitation, because the previous holes allow extravasation of fluid or medication administered into the marrow space. (See Chapter 59 in *Nelson Textbook of Pediatrics,* 15th ed.)

43. D. Intraosseous infusion is preferable to intratracheal administration of medication, because absorption through the intratracheal route is erratic. The recommended second dose of epinephrine is 0.1 mg/kg, 10 times the initial dose, and is best delivered using the more concentrated (1:1000) epinephrine solution. (See Chapter 60.2 in *Nelson Textbook of Pediatrics,* 15th ed.)

44. A. Oropharyngeal airways are recommended only for unconscious patients, because they may cause gagging and vomiting in conscious patients. (See Chapter 60.2 in *Nelson Textbook of Pediatrics,* 15th ed.)

45. C. The preferred method for opening the airway in a potentially traumatized victim is the jaw thrust, which results in less movement of the cervical spine. (See Chapter 60.2 in *Nelson Textbook of Pediatrics,* 15th ed.)

46. D. Repeating the examination is helpful in determining the effects of fever or those of the underlying illness. (See Chapter 57 in *Nelson Textbook of Pediatrics,* 15th ed.)

47. D. Each of these is vital in determining the primary (pneumonia and cyanosis or respiratory effort) or secondary (dehydration) cause of an illness. Nonetheless, a child's response to stimuli is most critical. (See Chapter 47 in *Nelson Textbook of Pediatrics,* 15th ed.)

48. A. Tachypnea, retractions, and rarely cyanosis are important clues to the need for a chest radiograph, because rales are inconsistently demonstrated. (See Chapter 47 in *Nelson Textbook of Pediatrics,* 15th ed.)

49. E. Group B streptococcal meningitis followed by bacteremia, osteomyelitis, septic arthritis, and cellulitis is the most common of the bacterial infections encountered in the first few months of life. Also consider *Escherichia coli* in the context of pyelonephritis. Nonetheless, many febrile episodes during this age period are viral. Unfortunately, it is frequently difficult to differentiate viral from serious bacterial illnesses in infants between birth and 2 months of age. (See Chapter 47 in *Nelson Textbook of Pediatrics,* 15th ed.)

9 Human Genetics

1. E. Fragile X is a common chromosomal cause of mental retardation in boys. Affected boys have an allelic expansion of trinucleotide repeats to over 200 (normal is 6 to 54). (See Chapter 67 in *Nelson Textbook of Pediatrics*, 15th ed.)

2. D. Y chromosome material is present in 5% to 10% of girls with Turner syndrome. Gonadoblastoma may develop in the ovary, thus necessitating bilateral oophorectomy as a preventive measure. (See Chapter 67 in *Nelson Textbook of Pediatrics*, 15th ed.)

3. C. The woman described in the question can have three types of *viable* offspring: normal phenotype and karyotype, phenotypically normal translocation carrier like the mother, and a translocation trisomy 21. (See Chapter 66 in *Nelson Textbook of Pediatrics*, 15th ed.)

4. 1. A
   2. B
   3. A
   4. D
   5. C
   6. D
   7. C
   8. E
   9. C
   10. C
   (See Chapter 67 in *Nelson Textbook of Pediatrics*, 15th ed.)

5. A. Uniparental disomy in Prader-Willi syndrome results from the inheritance of two copies of the *maternal* chromosome 15. (See Chapter 66 in *Nelson Textbook of Pediatrics*, 15th ed.)

6. B. Mitochondrial inheritance of the diseases listed in the question involves mutation of the mitochondrial genome, which originated solely from the ovum. (See Chapter 66 in *Nelson Textbook of Pediatrics*, 15th ed.)

7. 1. B
    2. A
    3. D
    4. E
    5. C
    (See Chapter 65 in *Nelson Textbook of Pediatrics*, 15th ed.)

8. 1. B
    2. C
    3. D
    4. E
    5. A
    (See Chapter 64 in *Nelson Textbook of Pediatrics*, 15th ed.)

9. B. Approximately 0.5% of newborns have an inborn error of metabolism or sex chromosome abnormality that causes no physical abnormality and can be detected by laboratory test only. (See Chapter 65 in *Nelson Textbook of Pediatrics*, 15th ed.)

10. A. *B* defines a gene locus, *C* a dominant gene, and *D* a recessive gene. (See Chapter 66 in *Nelson Textbook of Pediatrics*, 15th ed.)

11. 1. B
    2. A
    3. A
    4. C
    5. C
    6. B
    7. D
    8. B
    9. A
    10. C
    11. C
    12. C
    (See Chapter 66 in *Nelson Textbook of Pediatrics*, 15th ed.)

10 Metabolic Diseases

1. 1. C
    2. E
    3. A
    4. D
    5. B
    6. F
    (See Chapter 71 in *Nelson Textbook of Pediatrics*, 15th ed.)

2. C. Propionic acidemia presents as pernicious vomiting and acidosis with a high anion gap. (See Chapter 71.6 in *Nelson Textbook of Pediatrics*, 15th ed.)

3. B. The mechanism for this self-destructive behavior is unknown but is not necessarily thought to be an inability to feel pain. (See Chapter 75 in *Nelson Textbook of Pediatrics*, 15th ed.)

4. B. The combination of hypoglycemia, jaundice, elevated liver enzyme values, and *Escherichia coli* sepsis is classic for early-onset severe galactosemia. A white blood cell defect may predispose to *E. coli* sepsis, and the toxic effects of galactose-1-phosphate explain the hepatotoxicity. In this child, who was fed cow's milk–based formula, the urine reducing substances (galactose) were positive. (See Chapter 73.2 in *Nelson Textbook of Pediatrics*, 15th ed.)

5. D. The acute or subacute presentation of hereditary fructose intolerance is very similar to that of galactosemia. The inability to metabolize fructose can produce shock, hypoglycemia, hepatic dysfunction, and emesis. In the child described in the question, the urine reducing substance was fructose. Before the initiation of fructose (sucrose)-containing foods (e.g., fruit juices), such a child will be asymptomatic. (See Chapter 73.3 in *Nelson Textbook of Pediatrics*, 15th ed.)

6. C. Biotinidase levels may reflect enzymatic deficiencies affecting carbohydrate and amino acid (organic acid) metabolism. Both enzymatic pathways require biotinidase; deficiencies produce manifestations as noted in this case. Treatment with oral biotin may overcome this defect in some affected patients. (See Chapter 73.4 in *Nelson Textbook of Pediatrics*, 15th ed.)

7. 1. A
    2. D
    3. E
    4. F
    5. B
    6. C
    (See Chapter 73.5 in *Nelson Textbook of Pediatrics*, 15th ed.)

8. D. Muscle biopsy may confirm the diagnosis of Pompe disease (glycogen storage disease type II). Deficiency of acid α-glucosidase results in marked lysosomal glycogen accumulation and primarily affects the heart and skeletal muscle. Death in the infantile form is due to respiratory muscle failure. (See Chapter 73.5 in *Nelson Textbook of Pediatrics*, 15th ed.)

9. D. All the diseases listed in the question are associated with an enlarged head. The finding of white matter disease on MRI rules out Tay-Sachs, because this is a gray matter disease. The other diseases can

have white matter involvement in the disease process. Diffuse white matter involvement on MRI is more typical of MLD or Canavan disease. The biochemical finding of NAA is characteristic only of Canavan disease. (See Chapter 71.13 in *Nelson Textbook of Pediatrics*, 15th ed.)

10. A. The mode of inheritance and resemblance to maternal uncles suggests X-linked disease. Dysostosis multiplex suggests a mucopolysaccharidosis. Although Fabry disease is sex linked, it is not a mucopolysaccharide storage disorder. No dysostosis multiplex, developmental delay, or coarse features are noted in Fabry disease. Farber disease is associated with lipogranulomatosis, which this child does not have. Farber disease is an autosomal recessive disorder and is not sex linked. Disorders of mucopolysaccharides in this group are Hunter, Sanfilippo A, and Maroteaux-Lamy. Only Hunter disease is sex linked. The others are autosomal recessive; therefore, Hunter disease is the most likely diagnosis. (See Chapter 74 in *Nelson Textbook of Pediatrics*, 15th ed.)

11. 1. E
    2. A
    3. D
    4. C
    5. B
    (See Chapters 72 and 74 in *Nelson Textbook of Pediatrics*, 15th ed.)

12. E. Developmental delay would not be found in Morquio disease. Corneal clouding can be seen in Hurler and Morquio disease. The developmental delay should lead to the suspicion of Hurler disease. Noisy breathing, chronic rhinitis, and gibbus are also typical of Hurler disease. Hepatomegaly is not found in Krabbe or Tay-Sachs disease. In Gaucher disease, one can find hepatomegaly, but no corneal clouding, chronic rhinitis, noisy breathing, or gibbus is noted. (See Chapter 74 in *Nelson Textbook of Pediatrics*, 15th ed.)

13. C. All five diseases listed in the question are prevalent among Ashkenazi Jews. Niemann-Pick A and Gaucher type I are the only two diseases that present with a very large spleen. Children with Niemann-Pick A disease are likely to be retarded, but this patient is not. Anemia, leukopenia, and thrombocytopenia are typically found in Gaucher disease. Patients with Canavan disease, Tay-Sachs disease, and mucolipidosis IV are neurologically impaired, but this patient is not. (See

Chapter 72.3 in *Nelson Textbook of Pediatrics*, 15th ed.)

14. B. The treatment of choice for Gaucher type I disease is enzyme therapy with glucocerebrosidase infused intravenously, which has been found to be very effective. Spleen size returns to normal; osteopenia, bone marrow depression, and liver dysfunction subside in most cases after treatment. Splenectomy or partial splenectomy alleviates the leukopenia, thrombocytopenia, and anemia. Splenectomy is a temporary measure, but the effects may last for years. Bone marrow transplantation has been effective because normal donor cells have normal enzyme activity. However, this carries the risk of rejection (and graft vs. host) and has high mortality and morbidity rates. Therefore, the treatment of choice is enzyme therapy with glucocerebrosidase, not splenectomy or bone marrow transplantation, which were accepted treatments before the availability of enzyme replacement therapy. (See Chapter 72.3 in *Nelson Textbook of Pediatrics*, 15th ed.)

15. B. Frequent nutrient ingestion provides sufficient glucose to prevent hypoglycemia. With longer periods of fasting, normal patients begin to oxidize fat to spare glucose for central nervous system use. Patients with a deficiency of medium-chain acyl-CoA dehydrogenase (MCAD) cannot completely oxidize fatty acids, and thus they more readily utilize glucose (becoming hypoglycemic) and do not produce ketones. (See Chapter 72.1 in *Nelson Textbook of Pediatrics*, 15th ed.)

16. A. Nonketotic hypoglycemia with or without hyperammonemia in a patient of this age is often due to this relatively common cause. In addition to hypoglycemia, MCAD is associated with a Reye-like syndrome, and some cases are initially diagnosed as SIDS. (See Chapter 72.1 in *Nelson Textbook of Pediatrics*, 15th ed.)

17. B. Erythropoietic protoporphyria has normal urine porphyrins but increased stool and erythrocyte porphyrins. (See Chapter 76 in *Nelson Textbook of Pediatrics*, 15th ed.)

18. B. Erythropoietic protoporphyria presents in early childhood with photosensitivity. (See Chapter 76 in *Nelson Textbook of Pediatrics*, 15th ed.)

19. E. Congenital erythropoietic porphyria is an autosomal recessive disorder; the others are usually autosomal dominant. (See

Chapter 76 in *Nelson Textbook of Pediatrics*, 15th ed.)

20. C. Acute intermittent porphyria is characterized by neurovisceral symptoms but no photosensitivity reactions. (See Chapter 76 in *Nelson Textbook of Pediatrics*, 15th ed.)

21. C. Bone marrow transplantation may be indicated with a confirmed diagnosis and early in the symptomatic phase of the disease process. (See Chapter 72.2 in *Nelson Textbook of Pediatrics*, 15th ed.)

22. C. X-linked leukodystrophy demonstrates normal peroxisome structure and number but has characteristic lamellar cytoplasmic inclusions. (See Chapter 72.2 in *Nelson Textbook of Pediatrics*, 15th ed.)

23. A. Zellweger syndrome is the prototypic neonatal peroxisomal disorder. (See Chapter 72.2 in *Nelson Textbook of Pediatrics*, 15th ed.)

24. B. Unfortunately, the clinical course of ALD is not identical in severity in the same family. Some have only spinal involvement, but others may have both spinal and cerebral involvement. (See Chapter 72.2 in *Nelson Textbook of Pediatrics*, 15th ed.)

25. C. Given the history and physical findings, elevated levels of plasma very long-chain fatty acids confirm the diagnosis of X-linked ALD. (See Chapter 72.2 in *Nelson Textbook of Pediatrics*, 15th ed.)

26. B. In rhizomelic chondrodysplasia punctata, plasma levels of phytanic acid and erythrocyte plasmalogens are elevated. (See Chapter 72.2 in *Nelson Textbook of Pediatrics*, 15th ed.)

27. C. Poor cognitive function and behavioral changes often precede increased pigmentation (adrenal insufficiency) or peripheral neuropathy. (See Chapter 72.2 in *Nelson Textbook of Pediatrics*, 15th ed.)

28. A. The Prudent diet is the first approach to the management of children with risk factors for atherosclerotic heart disease. (See Chapter 72.4 in *Nelson Textbook of Pediatrics*, 15th ed.)

29. C. Failure to thrive is a possible complication of reduced nutrient intake from skim milk. The additional fat limitation from other foods may contribute to poor weight gain. (See Chapter 72.4 in *Nelson Textbook of Pediatrics*, 15th ed.)

30. C. Hypertriglyceridemia, in contrast to isolated hypercholesterolemia, is associated with recurrent pancreatitis. (See Chapter

72.4 in *Nelson Textbook of Pediatrics*, 15th ed.)

31. C. Familial combined hyperlipidemia is clearly the most common dominantly inherited hyperlipidemia. (See Chapter 72.4 in *Nelson Textbook of Pediatrics*, 15th ed.)

32. D. The Achilles tendon is a first site for the development of xanthomas, an area that most of us do not usually examine other than to test deep tendon reflexes. (See Chapter 72.4 in *Nelson Textbook of Pediatrics*, 15th ed.)

33. B. Elevated LDL cholesterol level is a possible risk factor that warrants follow-up and dietary therapy. (See Chapter 72.4 in *Nelson Textbook of Pediatrics*, 15th ed.)

11 The Fetus and Neonatal Infant

1. 1. C
   2. A
   3. E
   4. B
   5. D
   6. F
   7. F
   8. F
   (See Chapter 86 in *Nelson Textbook of Pediatrics*, 15th ed.)

2. 1. A
   2. C
   3. C
   4. A
   5. B
   6. B
   (See Chapter 86 in *Nelson Textbook of Pediatrics*, 15th ed.)

3. C. One point in the Apgar score is taken off for color. (See Chapter 79.3 in *Nelson Textbook of Pediatrics*, 15th ed.)

4. B. Fetal hemoglobin is alkali resistant. (See Part XXI, Section 1 in *Nelson Textbook of Pediatrics*, 15th ed.)

5. E. The definition of a cephalohematoma requires that it be confined to a bone, and thus it does not cross or obliterate a suture. Caput succedaneum, which is primarily edema fluid, crosses suture lines. (See Chapter 84.1 in *Nelson Textbook of Pediatrics*, 15th ed.)

6. A. Daily hexachlorophene bathing has been associated with neurotoxicity. A single bath suffices if there is a *Staphylococcus aureus* epidemic. (See Chapter 79.3 in *Nelson Textbook of Pediatrics*, 15th ed.)

7. B. Choanal atresia or any upper airway obstruction leads to the symptoms

described in the question. (See Chapter 85 in *Nelson Textbook of Pediatrics*, 15th ed.)

8. C. Unless persistent fetal circulation is accompanied by a diaphragmatic hernia, 85% to 90% of affected infants treated with ECMO survive. (See Chapter 87.7 in *Nelson Textbook of Pediatrics*, 15th ed.)

9. B. The other three choices listed in the question are pathologic, not physiologic. (See Chapter 88.3 in *Nelson Textbook of Pediatrics*, 15th ed.)

10. D. No treatment is necessary for the infant described in the question, assuming normal growth and development. (See Chapter 88.3 in *Nelson Textbook of Pediatrics*, 15th ed.)

11. E. (See Chapter 89.4 in *Nelson Textbook of Pediatrics*, 15th ed.)

12. E. (See Chapter 89.4 in *Nelson Textbook of Pediatrics*, 15th ed.)

13. C. (See Chapter 89.4 in *Nelson Textbook of Pediatrics*, 15th ed.)

14. A. The infant described in Questions 11 to 14 has a case of severe vitamin K deficiency—hemorrhagic disease of the newborn. The next most likely diagnosis is child abuse; most infants in coma with retinal hemorrhages have been shaken, and a skeletal survey thus is appropriate. The combination of home delivery (no AquaMEPHYTON administered), breast-feeding (low vitamin K content), and the amoxicillin treatment that eliminated normal intestinal bacterial synthesis of vitamin K led to the tragic demise of an otherwise normal infant. Of all possible preventive measures, administration of vitamin K at birth would have been the most effective. (See Chapter 89.4 in *Nelson Textbook of Pediatrics*, 15th ed.)

15. D. Hypoglycemia is common in infants who are small for gestational age (1500 g at 36 weeks' gestation is SGA). Breast-feeding twins is often difficult, and this SGA infant began life with diminished glycogen and fat stores. The poor nutrient intake and this metabolic predisposition resulted in hypoglycemia. The blood glucose was 25 mg/dL. The infant responded to 2 mL/kg of intravenous 10% dextrose. Polycythemia is possible, but if the twins are mono-ovular and monochorionic-diamnionic, the small twin is usually anemic. (See Chapter 93.2 in *Nelson Textbook of Pediatrics*, 15th ed.)

16. E. Intubate the trachea and apply negative-pressure suction to help clear residual meconium from the airway, preventing

meconium from moving more distally and initiating meconium aspiration pneumonia. Stimulating the infant to breathe is potentially dangerous if meconium is present in the airway. Administer epinephrine at a later time if the infant does not respond. Providing positive-pressure bag-and-mask ventilation is also dangerous if meconium is in the airway. Intubating the trachea and providing positive-pressure ventilation is dangerous for the same reason. (See Chapter 85 in *Nelson Textbook of Pediatrics*, 15th ed.)

17. D. The patient described in the question had a catastrophic acute intraventricular hemorrhage (IVH). Ultrasonography through the anterior fontanel demonstrated a grade IV hemorrhage. Serum coagulation profile is of no value because coagulopathy is not associated with IVH in premature infants. Complete blood count with platelet determination may be useful to determine how low the hematocrit will decline after IVH and in term infants with IVH to determine the presence of thrombocytopenia due mainly to in utero isoimmune sensitization of the mother to the father's antigens on fetal platelets (similar to ABO incompatibility). (See Chapter 84.2 in *Nelson Textbook of Pediatrics*, 15th ed.)

18. D. The infant described in the question had severe oligohydramnios, which may cause reduced fetal lung growth and may or may not be associated with renal anomalies (Potter syndrome). Pulmonary hypoplasia places the patient at increased risk for a pneumothorax after resuscitation and mechanical ventilation. IVH would be a consideration in a very premature infant (this patient is 36 weeks' gestation but is small for gestational age). Furthermore, IVH is unusual at 1 hour of age. (See Chapter 87.8 in *Nelson Textbook of Pediatrics*, 15th ed.)

19. D. Hypothyroidism was confirmed by the late arrival of the newborn screening results indicating high TSH and low T_4 levels. Treatment with thyroxine improved the jaundice and the other signs. The hyperbilirubinemia is indirect (unconjugated). Crigler-Najjar syndrome is a possibility and is either autosomal dominant or recessive (check the family history). However, there are signs other than jaundice that suggest another disease. Biliary atresia is always a concern in infants with delayed clearance of jaundice

or worsening jaundice after 2 weeks of life. The hyperbilirubinemia is predominantly direct (conjugated). Galactosemia should be considered, especially in the presence of hypoglycemia, direct reacting jaundice, hepatomegaly, or ascites. (See Chapter 93 in *Nelson Textbook of Pediatrics*, 15th ed.)

20. E. All infants with hyperbilirubinemia due to ABO incompatibility usually resolve their jaundice in the first week of life. Nonetheless, the hemolysis continues without evidence of jaundice because the liver can now excrete the bilirubin load. Late-onset anemia must be watched for and treated with a packed red blood cell transfusion if the infant is symptomatic. Hereditary spherocytosis is a possibility but is relatively rare. A well-taken family history and examination of the child's and parents' blood smear are helpful (most are inherited as an autosomal dominant trait). Sickle cell anemia hemolytic crisis is not encountered this early in life because a considerable amount of fetal hemoglobin remains; thus, there are few sickle β-chains to sickle. (See Chapter 89.2 in *Nelson Textbook of Pediatrics*, 15th ed.)

21. B. Echocardiography is used to detect the presence and degree of left-to-right shunting through a patent ductus arteriosus (PDA). Intravenous indomethacin is the treatment of choice if fluid restriction and diuresis do not improve the infant's condition. Also note the excessively high intravenous fluid administration rate (175 mL/kg/24 hours), which has been associated with a PDA. (See Chapter 87.3 in *Nelson Textbook of Pediatrics*, 15th ed.)

22. D. Exogenous artificial or bovine extracted surfactant (there is no apparent difference between the two) has improved the survival of all ages of infants with the respiratory distress syndrome. PDA usually does not present at 1 hour of age. Furthermore, indomethacin has various complications such as oliguria and intestinal perforation. Administration of intravenous dexamethasone is usually reserved to treat or rarely to prevent bronchopulmonary dysplasia (BPD). Considerable evidence suggests that BPD is, in part, an inflammatory process. Nonetheless, dexamethasone is not usually started at 1 hour of age. (See Chapter 87.3 in *Nelson Textbook of Pediatrics*, 15th ed.)

23. C. The fetus described in the question has been slowly losing blood by a chronic

fetal-maternal hemorrhage. The Kleihauer-Betke test detects fetal cells circulating in the mother's blood by identifying fetal erythrocytes in the blood smear. (See Chapter 89.1 in *Nelson Textbook of Pediatrics*, 15th ed.)

24. B. Percutaneous umbilical blood sampling (PUBS) offers the ability to evaluate the actual fetal hematocrit, blood type, Coombs test results, and acid-base status. Direct intravenous packed red blood cell transfusion is much more appropriate in a patient with hydrops than is an intraabdominal transfusion. Survival may be as high as 80% to 85% with intravascular transfusions in the presence of hydrops. Amniocentesis has traditionally been used to evaluate the severity of immune hydrops. Nonetheless, it is less useful than PUBS, especially in the presence of hydrops (effusions, ascites, edema). (See Chapter 89.2 in *Nelson Textbook of Pediatrics*, 15th ed.)

25. B. Hypocalcemia classically develops at 24 to 48 hours of life in infants of diabetic (including gestational diabetes) mothers. The infant responded to 2 mL/kg of 10% calcium gluconate. The serum calcium level was 6.5 mg/dL and the ionized calcium level was 1.6. Hypoglycemia is an important consideration, and an immediate Dextrostix–rapid glucose determination is indicated. However, it is unusual for hypoglycemia first to manifest at 30 hours of life in a well-fed infant. Hypomagnesemia should be considered in infants who have documented hypocalcemia and who do not respond to intravenous calcium. Hypomagnesemia often accompanies hypocalcemia. (See Chapters 50 and 56.9 in *Nelson Textbook of Pediatrics*, 15th ed.)

26. B. TORCH titers are overall not of great value in diagnosing a congenital infection. In addition, TORCH infections do not produce congenital heart disease except the PDA associated with congenital rubella syndrome (which does not produce a cleft palate or lip). (See Chapter 97 in *Nelson Textbook of Pediatrics*, 15th ed.)

27. C. Central nervous system anomalies are unusual or absent in most syndromes associated with a tracheoesophageal fistula. (See Chapter 265 in *Nelson Textbook of Pediatrics*, 15th ed.)

28. B. Cleft lip, a multifactorial disease with unknown and as yet undetermined genetic influences, has a recurrence rate of 2% to

5% with unaffected parents. (See Chapter 86 in *Nelson Textbook of Pediatrics*, 15th ed.)

29. C. Translocations such as 21/21 may occur from either parent. (See Chapter 67 in *Nelson Textbook of Pediatrics*, 15th ed.)

12 Infections in the Neonatal Infant

1. D. A tense fontanel, wide sutures, lethargy, apnea, and bradycardia suggest increased intracranial pressure. The CSF profile (other than a negative Gram stain) is suggestive of meningitis or persistent unresolved CSF blood and inflammation. Computed tomography or a head ultrasonogram will confirm the diagnosis. In most neonatal intensive care units, pending the initial results of the sepsis evaluation, this infant would receive broad-spectrum antibiotics. (See Chapter 95 in *Nelson Textbook of Pediatrics*, 15th ed.)

2. 1. G
   2. D
   3. A
   4. B
   5. C
   6. E
   7. F
   (See Chapter 97 in *Nelson Textbook of Pediatrics*, 15th ed.)

3. E. Cefotaxime and ceftriaxone are excellent agents to treat meningitis because they both achieve high CSF levels. Choices *A* to *D* are unfortunately correct, and therefore, ampicillin is always initially used with either of these cephalosporins. (See Chapter 95 in *Nelson Textbook of Pediatrics*, 15th ed.)

4. F. In addition to bacterial pathogens, one must be concerned that infections with viral agents (herpes simplex 2, enteroviruses) may mimic late-onset neonatal sepsis. (See Chapter 98 in *Nelson Textbook of Pediatrics*, 15th ed.)

5. D. *S. epidermidis* usually causes late-onset nosocomial infections in premature infants while they are in a neonatal intensive care unit. *H. influenzae*, either type b or nontypable, has been associated with early-onset neonatal sepsis. The same is true of pneumococci. (See Chapter 98.5 in *Nelson Textbook of Pediatrics*, 15th ed.)

6. B. After an arterial blood gas determination that demonstrates hypoxia on an FIO_2 of 1.0, surfactant should be administered by direct endotracheal installation, *not* by

aerosol. In addition, the patient described in the question demonstrates severe hypotension, which should be treated first with intravenous fluids such as normal saline and then by inotropic agents such as dopamine. (See Chapter 98 in *Nelson Textbook of Pediatrics*, 15th ed.)

7. C. Severe hypoxia, hypotension, prolonged rupture of the membranes, neutropenia, and thrombocytopenia suggest early-onset sepsis and congenital pneumonia. (See Chapter 98.1 in *Nelson Textbook of Pediatrics*, 15th ed.)

8. A. HSV-2 represents approximately 75% of cases; the remaining are due to HSV-1. (See Chapter 97.2 in *Nelson Textbook of Pediatrics*, 15th ed.)

9. A. Unfortunately, many women have an asymptomatic primary HSV infection and thus are not aware of HSV genital lesions. Nonetheless, if typical lesions are noted and the amniotic membranes are intact, delivery by cesarean section is recommended. (See Chapter 97.2 in *Nelson Textbook of Pediatrics*, 15th ed.)

10. B. Dermal erythropoiesis is necessary if TORCH (usually cytomegalovirus [CMV] or rubella) infection damages the bone marrow and traditional extramedullary sites of erythropoiesis (liver, spleen). (See Chapter 97 in *Nelson Textbook of Pediatrics*, 15th ed.)

11. A. Approximately 1% of all infants born in the United States have congenital CMV infection manifested by asymptomatic viral excretion. Of all congenitally CMV-infected infants, only 10% have the signs or symptoms of infection that are characteristic of a TORCH infection. The most common sequela of asymptomatic viruria is acquired hearing loss in approximately 20%. (See Chapter 97.1 in *Nelson Textbook of Pediatrics*, 15th ed.)

12. F. Storage diseases usually are not apparent at birth. Symptoms usually develop after the neonatal period. (See Chapter 98.1 in *Nelson Textbook of Pediatrics*, 15th ed.)

13. A. Currently there is no method to prevent CMV infection. The other diseases listed in the question are preventable by antibiotics *(B, D, F)*, vaccines *(C, E)*, and screening *(B, D, F)*. (See Chapter 97.1 in *Nelson Textbook of Pediatrics*, 15th ed.)

14. E. Intrauterine herpesvirus infection is extremely rare, especially in comparison with choices *A* to *D* and the more common perinatal acquisition of HSV during birth.

(See Chapter 212 in *Nelson Textbook of Pediatrics*, 15th ed.)

15. B. Coagulase-negative streptococci are the most common nosocomial cause of bacteremia in premature infants in many neonatal intensive care units. (See Chapter 98.5 in *Nelson Textbook of Pediatrics*, 15th ed.)

16. B. Congenital pneumonia may be indistinguishable from respiratory distress syndrome. The blood culture results are not always positive, and meningitis is less common than in late-onset disease. (See Chapter 98.3 in *Nelson Textbook of Pediatrics*, 15th ed.)

17. E. The neonate described in the question most probably has late-onset group B streptococcal meningitis and sepsis. Choices *A, B,* and *C* may be indicated, but a lumbar puncture should give immediate results and alter therapy appropriately to treat meningitis. (See Chapter 98.3 in *Nelson Textbook of Pediatrics*, 15th ed.)

18. E. Neonatal enterovirus infection should be suspected with the maternal history of fever and diarrhea in a summer month. Any neonate who has a sepsis-like picture and who does not improve while taking broad-spectrum antibiotics should be considered to have a life-threatening viral illness, such as enterovirus or HSV. (See Chapter 209 in *Nelson Textbook of Pediatrics*, 15th ed.)

13 Special Health Problems During Adolescence

1. D. Oral contraceptive agents in the available doses contain too little estrogen to close growth plates. In addition, most females use oral contraceptive agents after the adolescent growth spurt. Other complications of oral contraceptives are quite rare in adolescent patients, and thrombophlebitis or diabetes is very unusual. (See Chapter 109 in *Nelson Textbook of Pediatrics*, 15th ed.)

2. 1. C
   2. D
   3. A
   4. E
   5. B
   (See Chapter 109 in *Nelson Textbook of Pediatrics*, 15th ed.)

3. C. There is no evidence suggesting an increased risk of anomalies among infants conceived with an IUD in place. The newer, smaller IUDs have a lower risk of bleeding, dysmenorrhea, and expulsion, and with a single sexual partner, the risk of pelvic inflammatory disease is also lower than with older IUDs or with multiple partners. (See Chapter 109 in *Nelson Textbook of Pediatrics*, 15th ed.)

4. E. Although a positive VDRL result in the situation described in the question is suggestive of syphilis and some would treat empirically (with benzathine penicillin G, *not* ceftriaxone), it is recommended that all positive VDRL results be confirmed with a specific treponemal antibody test. Culturing this patient for gonorrhea and *Chlamydia* is also a good idea. (See Chapter 110 in *Nelson Textbook of Pediatrics*, 15th ed.)

5. F. All of the conditions listed in the question produce a false-positive result in the VDRL or other nontreponemal test for syphilis. This patient actually had systemic lupus erythematosus (SLE). (See Chapter 201.1 in *Nelson Textbook of Pediatrics*, 15th ed.)

6. B. The VDRL test result should decline and eventually become seronegative (nonreactive) within 1 year of therapy for primary syphilis while the fluorescent treponemal antibody–IgG value remains elevated. (See Chapters 110 and 201.1 in *Nelson Textbook of Pediatrics*, 15th ed.)

7. E. Mononucleosis rarely if ever produces a false-positive result for a treponemal titer. If you suspect a false-positive treponemal test result, perform a VDRL—it should be nonreactive. (See Chapter 110 in *Nelson Textbook of Pediatrics,* 15th ed.)

8. D. Bacterial vaginosis due to *G. vaginalis* or other pathogens typically is associated with these biochemical and microscopic features. Treatment in nonpregnant women is metronidazole. (See Chapter 110 in *Nelson Textbook of Pediatrics,* 15th ed.)

9. D. A male with a vaginal opening but no uterus or ovaries has testicular feminization syndrome. These patients classically have primary amenorrhea; they have never had any menstrual periods. (See Chapter 111 in *Nelson Textbook of Pediatrics*, 15th ed.)

10. D. Narcan is indicated in this patient with intravenous drug misuse and a heroin overdose. Nonetheless, the patient may need the ABCs of resuscitation addressed if he is cyanotic and so forth. Securing an airway while providing oxygen and artificial ventilation is the first priority—followed by Narcan, the antidote

for opiates. (See Chapter 105.1 in *Nelson Textbook of Pediatrics*, 15th ed.)

11. F. Both acute and chronic effects of organic solvent misuse produce significant morbidity and mortality. (See Chapter 105.3 in *Nelson Textbook of Pediatrics*, 15th ed.)

12. A. School performance usually deteriorates as a result of mood changes and aggressive behavior. (See Chapter 105.8 in *Nelson Textbook of Pediatrics*, 15th ed.)

13. 1. C
    2. D
    3. B
    4. A
    5. A
    6. B
    7. A
    8. C
    9. A
    10. A
    11. D
    12. C
    (See Chapter 107 in *Nelson Textbook of Pediatrics*, 15th ed.)

14. A. Fibroadenomas (and benign cysts—not a choice here) are most common in adolescents. Carcinoma is rare, and thus mammography is not usually indicated. (See Chapter 112 in *Nelson Textbook of Pediatrics*, 15th ed.)

15. 1. B
    2. A
    3. B
    4. A
    5. C
    6. C
    7. B
    8. A
    9. D
    (See Chapter 107 in *Nelson Textbook of Pediatrics*, 15th ed.)

16. A. Violence—including accidents, homicides, and suicides—accounts for 70% of all adolescent deaths. Neoplasms account for 7%. Although sexually transmitted diseases are very common, they are not often associated with mortality. (See Chapter 102 in *Nelson Textbook of Pediatrics*, 15th ed.)

17. D. Norplant is a reasonable choice, but many adolescents have trouble with its side effects (weight gain, irregular periods) and often ask to have it removed. (See Chapter 109 in *Nelson Textbook of Pediatrics*, 15th ed.)

18. D. Bacillus Calmette-Guérin (BCG) is not indicated. If she is exposed to tuberculosis,

purified protein derivative should be given. If the result is positive and the chest radiograph shows no abnormality and she has no extrapulmonary signs of tuberculosis, she should be treated with isoniazid. The other immunizations all are appropriate. (See Chapter 115 in *Nelson Textbook of Pediatrics*, 15th ed.)

19. B. Such severe wasting is compatible with anorexia nervosa. Bulimia does not produce such severe weight loss. Additional features of anorexia nervosa include bradycardia, hypothermia, amenorrhea, and hypokalemia. (See Chapter 107 in *Nelson Textbook of Pediatrics*, 15th ed.)

20. C. Von Willebrand disease is the most common coagulation defect and may be present in as many as 1% of children. Menstruation in affected patients may be complicated by hemorrhagic shock. (See Chapter 111.2 in *Nelson Textbook of Pediatrics*, 15th ed.)

14 The Immunologic System and Disorders

1. C. The child described in the question has severe aplastic anemia as defined by a platelet count of less than 20,000, absolute neutrophil count of less than 500, and anemia with a reticulocyte count of less than 1%. The mortality due to hemorrhage or infection is quite high. (See Chapter 132.1 in *Nelson Textbook of Pediatrics*, 15th ed.)

2. B. Red blood cell transfusions should be avoided in patients with aplastic anemia because of the high risk of sensitization and the risk of graft rejection after bone marrow transplantation. Furthermore, the patient described in the question should tolerate a hematocrit of 25%. (See Chapter 132.1 in *Nelson Textbook of Pediatrics*, 15th ed.)

3. B. Graft-versus-host disease (GVHD) may also produce graft-versus-leukemia disease and thus adds an advantage to the overall outcome. Acute and chronic (combined) or chronic GVHD has been associated with improved survival. (See Chapter 132.3 in *Nelson Textbook of Pediatrics*, 15th ed.)

4. B. Acute stage 2 GVHD, occurring in the first 100 days after transplantation, is relatively common and may be beneficial if a graft-versus-leukemia reaction also develops. (See Chapter 132.3 in *Nelson Textbook of Pediatrics*, 15th ed.)

5. E. Because of chronic or recurrent infections, most patients with CGD demonstrate hypergammaglobulinemia. (See Chapter 132.3 in *Nelson Textbook of Pediatrics*, 15th ed.)

6. B. Nitroblue tetrazolium (NBT) tests the neutrophils' ability to generate superoxide anion and thus kill ingested bacteria. (See Chapter 129 in *Nelson Textbook of Pediatrics*, 15th ed.)

7. C. CGD, in the patient described in the question, is X linked (seen in 50% to 55%) and is associated with an absence of cytochrome b. NBT testing reveals failure to generate intracellular superoxide anion. (See Chapter 129 in *Nelson Textbook of Pediatrics*, 15th ed.)

8. B. Interferon-γ increases superoxide anion generation in vitro and reduces the incidence of new infections. Long-term use of trimethoprim-sulfamethoxazole may also be effective in reducing infections. (See Chapter 129 in *Nelson Textbook of Pediatrics*, 15th ed.)

9. A. Leukocyte adhesion defect is associated with severe inability to recruit neutrophils to sites of infection due to a deficiency of membrane-bound ligands (carbohydrate, glycoprotein). Inability to adhere to the blood vessel wall prevents neutrophil egress but does not prevent the marked leukocytosis. (See Chapter 125 in *Nelson Textbook of Pediatrics*, 15th ed.)

10. D. Although severe life-threatening sepsis may occur, it is extremely rare in patients with cyclic neutropenia. (See Chapter 124.5 in *Nelson Textbook of Pediatrics*, 15th ed.)

11. C. Kostmann disease, an autosomal recessive severe infantile form of agranulocytosis, manifests with persistently low neutrophil counts (<200) and severe recurrent and at times lethal (by age 3 years) infection. (See Chapter 124.5 in *Nelson Textbook of Pediatrics*, 15th ed.)

12. D. Granulocyte colony-stimulating factor (G-CSF) is the treatment of choice and has dramatically improved the neutrophil count while reducing the incidence and severity of infection. (See Chapter 124.5 in *Nelson Textbook of Pediatrics*, 15th ed.)

13. D. Transient, benign neutropenia associated with various non–life-threatening viral infections is the most common cause of neutropenia in previously healthy children. Neonatal neutropenia due to alloimmune, autoimmune, or preeclamptic processes is often asymptomatic and transient. (See

Chapter 124 in *Nelson Textbook of Pediatrics*, 15th ed.)

14. D. Rheumatic fever is not associated with low complement levels, but all the other diseases listed in the question are; the deficiency is usually due to increased activation. (See Chapter 121.3 in *Nelson Textbook of Pediatrics*, 15th ed.)

15. 1. C
    2. A
    3. B
    4. E
    5. D
    (See Chapter 121 in *Nelson Textbook of Pediatrics*, 15th ed.)

16. E. Immunodeficiency with eczema and thrombocytopenia is associated with the combined risks of recurrent bleeding and serious infections plus a 12% incidence of fatal malignancy in long-term survivors. (See Chapter 119.11 in *Nelson Textbook of Pediatrics*, 15th ed.)

17. D. Bone marrow transplantation has been effective in some patients with Wiskott-Aldrich syndrome. (See Chapter 119.11 in *Nelson Textbook of Pediatrics*, 15th ed.)

18. E. Because T-lymphocyte deficiency is present at birth, most patients manifest serious infections before the age of 1 year. It should be noted that many patients have partial or incomplete DiGeorge syndrome and that these patients may have sufficient lymphocyte activity to avoid having serious infections. (See Chapter 118.1 in *Nelson Textbook of Pediatrics*, 15th ed.)

19. D. AIDS has not been reported as a complication of the use of intravenous immunoglobulin (IVIG) prepared from human donors. Donors are screened for human immunodeficiency virus and hepatitis B seropositivity, and preparative methods would inactivate both of these viruses. The remaining choices are rare but worrisome complications of IVIG therapy. Nonetheless, IVIG has been a remarkable aid in the treatment of patients with congenital antibody deficiency states. (See Chapter 117.8 in *Nelson Textbook of Pediatrics*, 15th ed.)

20. B. Agammaglobulinemia, an X-linked disorder, becomes apparent after maternally derived transplacental antibodies significantly decline in concentration at approximately 4 months of age. Affected boys have little palpable lymph tissue, have an inability to produce antibodies of all classes, and may become neutropenic. Patients with AIDS usually

have hypertrophied lymph nodes, and most have hypergammaglobulinemia. (See Chapter 117.1 in *Nelson Textbook of Pediatrics*, 15th ed.)

21. C. Long-term therapy for Bruton agammaglobulinemia includes IVIG given monthly, avoidance of live viral vaccines, and prompt treatment of bacterial infections. (See Chapter 117.1 in *Nelson Textbook of Pediatrics*, 15th ed.)

22. 1. B
    2. C
    3. E
    4. A
    5. F
    6. G
    7. D
    8. J
    9. I
    10. H
    (See Chapters 117–119 in *Nelson Textbook of Pediatrics*, 15th ed.)

23. D. Bruton disease does not present with thrombocytopenia. (See Chapter 117.1 in *Nelson Textbook of Pediatrics*, 15th ed.)

24. E. Job syndrome is also known as hyperimmunoglobulin E recurrent infection syndrome. (See Chapter 119.13 in *Nelson Textbook of Pediatrics*, 15th ed.)

25. C. The number of neutrophils and their ability to increase in numbers are normal. The white blood cells cannot reduce NBT. (See Chapter 129 in *Nelson Textbook of Pediatrics*, 15th ed.)

15 Allergic Disorders

1. A. Although allergens have been implicated in the etiology of eczema, the precise role of allergen or of IgE is unknown. (See Chapter 138 in *Nelson Textbook of Pediatrics*, 15th ed.)

2. D. If one arm is covered and the itchy skin cannot be scratched, there will be no lesions of atopic dermatitis. (See Chapter 138 in *Nelson Textbook of Pediatrics*, 15th ed.)

3. 1. B
   2. A
   3. B
   4. B
   5. A
   6. A
   7. A
   8. C
   9. D
   (See Chapter 138 in *Nelson Textbook of Pediatrics*, 15th ed.)

4. A. Epinephrine is the treatment of choice. If the blood pressure does not respond, lactated Ringer solution should be given. Benadryl, cimetidine, and prednisone are second-line therapies to be given after epinephrine and fluids. (See Chapter 142 in *Nelson Textbook of Pediatrics*, 15th ed.)

5. D. Anaphylaxis to penicillin usually occurs within 30 to 90 minutes of administration of this drug. Anaphylactic shock is often missed as a diagnosis unless there is a high index of suspicion *and* a complete history is taken. (See Chapter 140 in *Nelson Textbook of Pediatrics*, 15th ed.)

6. B. The theophylline level is 45 μg/mL. Pediazole contains erythromycin, which interferes with theophylline metabolism and thus can raise the serum level of theophylline to the toxic range (>20 μg/mL). (See Chapter 135.1 in *Nelson Textbook of Pediatrics*, 15th ed.)

7. A. Activated charcoal, given in 2- to 3-hour intervals, can effectively enhance the clearance and half-life of theophylline in the circulation. It therefore removes more theophylline than was ingested. (See Chapter 135.1 in *Nelson Textbook of Pediatrics*, 15th ed.)

8. B. Cystic fibrosis may be confused with the wheezing of asthma. Some patients with cystic fibrosis have a component of reactive airway disease. The case described in the question is atypical of asthma and more typical of cystic fibrosis because of the purulent sputum, digital clubbing, failure to thrive, and delayed puberty. (See Chapter 137 in *Nelson Textbook of Pediatrics*, 15th ed.)

9. A. *Giardia* is not an "invasive" parasite and thus does not elicit eosinophilia. Allergic eosinophilia is usually no greater than 15% to 20% of the leukocytes on peripheral smear. Higher levels suggest rheumatic, oncologic, parasitic, or toxic causes. (See Chapter 122.2 in *Nelson Textbook of Pediatrics*, 15th ed.)

10. A. Avoidance of the offending allergen is the mainstay of the management of allergy when the allergen is identified and is easily avoided. (See Chapter 145 in *Nelson Textbook of Pediatrics*, 15th ed.)

11. D. High humidity in the house encourages the survival of mites. It is recommended to keep the humidity to less than 50%. (See Chapter 135 in *Nelson Textbook of Pediatrics*, 15th ed.)

12. D. Smoking cigarettes or marijuana and eating charcoal-cooked meats, in addition

to various drugs (rifampin, anticonvulsants) and diseases (hyperthyroidism, cystic fibrosis), increase theophylline clearance and thus decrease serum levels of theophylline. (See Chapter 135.1 in *Nelson Textbook of Pediatrics*, 15th ed.)

13. C. Asthma is present but not consistently among monozygotic twins, suggesting some additional environmental factor. (See Chapter 137 in *Nelson Textbook of Pediatrics*, 15th ed.)

14. D. Reactive airways may be noted in patients who have respiratory distress syndrome (RDS) and who develop bronchopulmonary dysplasia. Uncomplicated RDS is not a risk factor for asthma. (See Chapter 137 in *Nelson Textbook of Pediatrics*, 15th ed.)

15. B. Allergy per se is not usually a risk for fatal asthma. However, unusual and excessive exposure to allergens may predispose to severe and even fatal asthma. (See Chapter 137 in *Nelson Textbook of Pediatrics*, 15th ed.)

16. D. In a tachypneic patient with asthma, poor air entry and exit (no wheeze) are very serious signs of acute life-threatening airway obstruction. It is a medical emergency. (See Chapter 137 in *Nelson Textbook of Pediatrics*, 15th ed.)

17. E. Other serious signs of severe asthma are altered mental status (confusion, agitation, sleepiness), inaudible breath sounds (silent chest), tachycardia, and tachypnea. (See Chapter 137 in *Nelson Textbook of Pediatrics*, 15th ed.)

18. E. Allergic rhinitis is often seasonal and associated with allergic conjunctivitis. Eosinophils predominate in the nasal secretions. (See Chapter 136 in *Nelson Textbook of Pediatrics,* 15th ed.)

19. A. Sinusitis is a possible complication of allergic rhinitis. A change in the nature of the nasal discharge, facial pain, and fever may all herald the onset of sinusitis. (See Chapter 136 in *Nelson Textbook of Pediatrics*, 15th ed.)

20. B. Local reactions to Hymenoptera venom in children are not managed by immunotherapy. (See Chapter 135.2 in *Nelson Textbook of Pediatrics*, 15th ed.)

21. C. The possibility of reaction to the other choices in the question is much higher than that to the dye. (See Chapter 139 in *Nelson Textbook of Pediatrics*, 15th ed.)

22. A. Immunotherapy in children is indicated only for systemic reactions. (See Chapter

143 in *Nelson Textbook of Pediatrics*, 15th ed.)

23. A. Such skin testing is specific for penicillin and cannot determine if a patient has an erythromycin allergy. The latter is a possibility. (See Chapter 142 in *Nelson Textbook of Pediatrics*, 15th ed.)

24. B. The urticarial reaction described in the question may develop into anaphylaxis; the latter requires emergency treatment. In addition, the penicillin should be stopped and a substitute nonpenicillin antibiotic chosen. (See Chapter 140 in *Nelson Textbook of Pediatrics*, 15th ed.)

25. E. Early onset is usually not a risk for death due to asthma, but many psychosocial, medical, and behavioral risk factors (e.g., choices *A* to *D*) place a child at risk for death. (See Chapter 137 in *Nelson Textbook of Pediatrics*, 15th ed.)

26. D. Asthma may indeed have a higher incidence in urban settings. (See Chapter 137 in *Nelson Textbook of Pediatrics*, 15th ed.)

27. C. Mitocidal agent treatment of carpets may have some value in reducing mite-induced allergic manifestations. (See Chapter 135 in *Nelson Textbook of Pediatrics*, 15th ed.)

28. C. Loratadine, a nonsedating, long-acting tricyclic antihistamine, has selective peripheral H_1 receptor antagonist activity. (See Chapter 135.1 in *Nelson Textbook of Pediatrics*, 15th ed.)

29. C. The erythromycin component of Pediazole inhibits hepatic theophylline metabolism, thus producing theophylline toxicity. (See Chapter 135.1 in *Nelson Textbook of Pediatrics*, 15th ed.)

30. C. The child described in the question has classic manifestations and complications of allergic rhinitis. Hismanal most definitely suppresses skin test reactivity for at least 2 weeks. (See Chapter 136 in *Nelson Textbook of Pediatrics*, 15th ed.)

16 Rheumatologic Disease

1. C. The purpura on the lower extremities suggests Henoch-Schönlein vasculitis. Meningococcemia is generalized. (See Chapter 152.1 in *Nelson Textbook of Pediatrics*, 15th ed.)

2. E. Cancel the operation until the patient described in the question is further examined and the results of the urinalysis are considered. (See Chapter 152.1 in *Nelson Textbook of Pediatrics*, 15th ed.)

3. B. Henoch-Schönlein purpura is a common

vasculitis in childhood and manifests with involvement of the skin (nonthrombocytopenic petechiae), joints (arthritis), kidneys (nephritis), and intestine (vasculitis, mucosal hemorrhage, intussusception). (See Chapter 152.1 in *Nelson Textbook of Pediatrics*, 15th ed.)

4. C. Raynaud phenomenon occurs in approximately 10% to 15% of children with SLE but is not a diagnostic criterion. Raynaud phenomenon may be idiopathic or associated with autoimmune diseases; it is more prevalent in scleroderma than in SLE. (See Chapter 157.2 in *Nelson Textbook of Pediatrics*, 15th ed.)

5. D. An echocardiogram reveals a moderate-sized pericardial effusion, the most probable cause of this boy's chest pain. An ESR is not diagnostic and may occasionally show low values in serious inflammatory, infectious, or oncologic diseases. A chest radiograph may reveal cardiomegaly due to a pericardial effusion; nonetheless, it does not distinguish between cardiomegaly from heart failure or an effusion. A bone marrow aspirate may be of value if leukemia is a consideration. (See Chapter 148 in *Nelson Textbook of Pediatrics*, 15th ed.)

6. D. An oral anti-inflammatory agent or steroids would improve this boy's pericardial effusion. (See Chapter 148 in *Nelson Textbook of Pediatrics*, 15th ed.)

7. A. Systemic-onset JRA often manifests with prolonged fevers, a salmon-pink macular rash, pericarditis, leukocytosis, anemia of chronic inflammatory disease, hepatosplenomegaly, and lymphadenopathy. Arthralgia or myalgia may be present, but arthritis does not usually develop until later in the course of the illness. SLE and rheumatic fever may also produce rheumatologic symptoms and a pericardial effusion. (See Chapter 148 in *Nelson Textbook of Pediatrics*, 15th ed.)

8. 1. C
   2. A
   3. B
   4. E
   5. D
   (See Chapter 148 in *Nelson Textbook of Pediatrics*, 15th ed.)

9. D. Rheumatoid factor, usually an IgM directed against the Fc portion of IgG, is detected in many states of enhanced immunoglobulin synthesis or immune stimulation. (See Chapter 147 in *Nelson Textbook of Pediatrics*, 15th ed.)

10. 1. F
    2. B
    3. D
    4. C
    5. A
    6. E
    (See Chapters 148–157 in *Nelson Textbook of Pediatrics*, 15th ed.)

11. B. CPK is 7500 IU/mL. (See Chapter 153 in *Nelson Textbook of Pediatrics*, 15th ed.)

12. B. Dermatomyositis classically affects preadolescent females with an insidious onset of muscle weakness. Vasculitic rashes may be present over the knuckles, the malar area, or the eyelids (violet tinged). (See Chapter 153 in *Nelson Textbook of Pediatrics*, 15th ed.)

13. D. Prednisone is the initial treatment of choice for dermatomyositis. (See Chapter 153 in *Nelson Textbook of Pediatrics*, 15th ed.)

14. A. Generalized lymphadenopathy is not a criterion for Kawasaki disease, but cervical lymphadenopathy with one node usually greater than 1.5 cm is the defined criterion. (See Chapter 152.2 in *Nelson Textbook of Pediatrics*, 15th ed.)

15. E. Myocarditis, a rare but potentially life-threatening feature of Kawasaki disease, is present early in the course of the disease. (See Chapter 152.2 in *Nelson Textbook of Pediatrics*, 15th ed.)

16. D. Nonsteroidal anti-inflammatory agents would be the appropriate medication for the patient described in the question. (See Chapter 149 in *Nelson Textbook of Pediatrics*, 15th ed.)

17. E. Reiter syndrome may follow an enteric (*Shigella, Yersinia, Campylobacter*) or a genital (*Chlamydia*) infection. Nonsteroidal antiinflammatory agents and physical therapy are important approaches to the treatment of Reiter syndrome. (See Chapter 149 in *Nelson Textbook of Pediatrics*, 15th ed.)

18. 1. D
    2. E
    3. A
    4. B
    5. F
    6. C
    7. G
    (See Chapters 155–164 in *Nelson Textbook of Pediatrics*, 15th ed.)

17 Infectious Disease

1. B. Oral rehydration is all that is needed for most immunocompetent children with

Cryptosporidium-associated diarrhea. (See Chapter 244.4 in *Nelson Textbook of Pediatrics*, 15th ed.)

2. D. *Ascaris* is not a known cause of daycare-associated diarrheal epidemics, but choices *A* to *C* are. (See Chapter 250 in *Nelson Textbook of Pediatrics*, 15th ed.)

3. A. No antiviral therapy is indicated for roseola. Antipyresis may keep the temperature from becoming excessively high but may not prevent febrile seizures because HHV-6 is often recovered in the cerebrospinal fluid (CSF) of such patients. (See Chapter 212 in *Nelson Textbook of Pediatrics*, 15th ed.)

4. D. Roseola-like symptoms unfortunately do not herald HHV-6 infection in immunosuppressed patients. (See Chapter 212 in *Nelson Textbook of Pediatrics*, 15th ed.)

5. B. Seroconversion is critical, because many children older than 1 to 2 years are already seropositive. PCR may detect recurrent, persistent, or reactivated disease. (See Chapter 212 in *Nelson Textbook of Pediatrics*, 15th ed.)

6. D. HHV-6 is the agent of roseola (erythema subitum), the childhood exanthem present in the infant described in the question. (See Chapter 212 in *Nelson Textbook of Pediatrics*, 15th ed.)

7. E. Pertussis is a "family" disease with various degrees of symptoms and colonization. (See Chapter 181 in *Nelson Textbook of Pediatrics*, 15th ed.)

8. D. It is hoped that the acellular pertussis vaccine will prove to reduce toxicity without reducing immunogenicity so that it will be available to children of all ages. (See Chapter 181 in *Nelson Textbook of Pediatrics*, 15th ed.)

9. D. The incidence of severe pertussis with prolonged coughing is often reduced or eliminated after complete vaccination. (See Chapter 181 in *Nelson Textbook of Pediatrics*, 15th ed.)

10. A. Pertussis is often transmitted to unimmunized children from adults who have waning immunity and who do not manifest the classic signs of pertussis and have adult illnesses resembling a nonspecific upper respiratory tract infection. (See Chapter 181 in *Nelson Textbook of Pediatrics*, 15th ed.)

11. A. Oral acyclovir may suppress recurrences of genital herpes simplex virus type 2 (HSV-2) lesions while the patient takes this antiviral agent. (See Chapter 211 in *Nelson Textbook of Pediatrics*, 15th ed.)

12. B. Prophylactic acyclovir prevents reactivation of latent HSV. (See Chapter 211 in *Nelson Textbook of Pediatrics*, 15th ed.)

13. E. The child has herpetic gingivostomatitis; he has autoinoculated his (sucking) thumb and has developed herpetic whitlow. (See Chapter 211 in *Nelson Textbook of Pediatrics*, 15th ed.)

14. C. The CSF profile and temporal lobe lesion are highly suggestive of HSV encephalitis. (See Chapter 211 in *Nelson Textbook of Pediatrics*, 15th ed.)

15. B. Although rare, rat-bite fever needs to be considered in the differential diagnosis of arthritis, fever, and rash. Juvenile rheumatoid arthritis seems to be more common, however. (See Chapter 201.2 in *Nelson Textbook of Pediatrics*, 15th ed.)

16. C. The infant described in the question requires a complete course of therapy for neurosyphilis. (See Chapter 201.1 in *Nelson Textbook of Pediatrics*, 15th ed.)

17. B. The infant described in the question must be treated. The mother may have reacquired syphilis at a later time in her pregnancy, because if properly treated, the VDRL result should return to normal. (See Chapter 201.1 in *Nelson Textbook of Pediatrics*, 15th ed.)

18. A. Specific testing is indicated to determine if the maternal titers are a true positive. If the infant's fluorescent treponemal antibody (FTA) result is positive, treatment is indicated. (See Chapter 201.1 in *Nelson Textbook of Pediatrics*, 15th ed.)

19. A. *Nocardia* infection is characterized by remissions and exacerbations. (See Chapter 203 in *Nelson Textbook of Pediatrics*, 15th ed.)

20. D. Pelvic actinomycosis is an unusual complication of IUD use. (See Chapter 202 in *Nelson Textbook of Pediatrics*, 15th ed.)

21. B. Cervicofacial actinomycosis, an unusual infection, in this particularly at-risk child is compatible with the history of dental caries and a firm mandibular mass. (See Chapter 202 in *Nelson Textbook of Pediatrics*, 15th ed.)

22. C. Treatment of cysticercosis with an effective antiparasitic drug first exacerbates the inflammatory response and may lead to acute hydrocephalus. If there is evidence of viable parasites in the

central nervous system (CNS), the patient may be treated after or during the shunting procedure. The boy, his household contacts, and members of the immediate family should have stool and serologic examinations. (See Chapter 245.2 in *Nelson Textbook of Pediatrics*, 15th ed.)

23. A. A patient who has only been in an urban area and has not participated in agricultural activities, has never traveled to areas endemic for hydatid transmission (e.g., in North America, areas where there are moose), nor had contact with sheep or dogs is unlikely to acquire echinococcal infection. The sensitivity of echinococcal serologic study varies from 60% to 90%. Healthy hydatid cysts may not stimulate much of an immune response. The other choices mentioned are not relevant to cystic liver disease. (See Chapter 245.3 in *Nelson Textbook of Pediatrics*, 15th ed.)

24. 1. D
    2. B
    3. A and E
    4. C
    5. D
    6. C
    7. D
    8. C
    (See Chapter 184 in *Nelson Textbook of Pediatrics*, 15th ed.)

25. C. *Aeromonas* may resemble *E. coli* and needs oxidase testing. *V. cholerae* needs thiosulfate-citrate-bile salt (TCBS) media. (See Chapters 184.1 and 185 in *Nelson Textbook of Pediatrics*, 15th ed.)

26. E. Hypoglycemia and seizures suggest a poor outcome for cholera. (See Chapter 185 in *Nelson Textbook of Pediatrics*, 15th ed.)

27. C. Chronic bacterial diarrhea is unusual, but one should consider these pathogens or an unusual host or parasitic disease (giardiasis). (See Chapter 184 in *Nelson Textbook of Pediatrics*, 15th ed.)

28. E. Chronic intracellular infection with intermittent or low-grade bacteremia characterizes *S. typhi* infection. (See Chapters 182 and 187 in *Nelson Textbook of Pediatrics*, 15th ed.)

29. D. Typhoid fever may or may not be associated with diarrhea or constipation and is a prolonged, serious illness. (See Chapter 182.2 in *Nelson Textbook of Pediatrics*, 15th ed.)

30. E. There is no indication for antimotility agents in children with acute gastroenteritis. (See Chapters 182–184 and 186 in *Nelson Textbook of Pediatrics*, 15th ed.)

31. A. Necrotic areas of bone due to osteonecrosis from local sickling may predispose patients with sickle cell anemia to salmonella osteomyelitis. (See Chapter 182.1 in *Nelson Textbook of Pediatrics*, 15th ed.)

32. E. Fecal leukocyte examination is a nonspecific test that may suggest lower colonic-rectal inflammation. (See Chapter 171 in *Nelson Textbook of Pediatrics*, 15th ed.)

33. B. Ileus, coma with a risk of aspiration, shock, and peritonitis (e.g., pneumoperitoneum) are contraindications for oral therapy. (See Chapter 171 in *Nelson Textbook of Pediatrics*, 15th ed.)

34. D. *C. jejuni* is a commonly associated pathogen in Guillain-Barré syndrome (autoimmune polyneuropathy). (See Chapter 186 in *Nelson Textbook of Pediatrics*, 15th ed.)

35. Part A. D. *H. pylori*
    Part B. D. Triple therapy is the most effective method of treating peptic ulcer disease associated with gastric *H. pylori* infection. (See Chapter 187 in *Nelson Textbook of Pediatrics*, 15th ed.)

36. C. Toxigenic pathogens typically produce profuse and profound watery diarrhea of ileal origin that is secretory in nature. The large fluid losses produce severe dehydration. (See Chapters 184 and 185 in *Nelson Textbook of Pediatrics*, 15th ed.)

37. C. *E. coli* 0157:H7 is an enterohemorrhagic pathogen and is responsible for most episodes of hemolytic-uremic syndrome. *Shigella dysenteriae* serotype 1 is occasionally responsible for the hemolytic-uremic syndrome. (See Chapter 184 in *Nelson Textbook of Pediatrics*, 15th ed.)

38. C. *Shigella* usually causes diarrhea and fever and in some, particularly young infants, seizures. (See Chapter 183 in *Nelson Textbook of Pediatrics*, 15th ed.)

39. A. Ampicillin (or Bactrim) is the antibiotic of choice for susceptible strains, not neomycin. Humans are the reservoir, especially in institutions. Bacteremia is common in infections with *Salmonella*, not *Shigella*. (See Chapter 183 in *Nelson Textbook of Pediatrics*, 15th ed.)

40. B. Adenovirus 11 or 21 probably is the

cause. (See Chapter 219 in *Nelson Textbook of Pediatrics*, 15th ed.)

41. E. The standard high-risk wound is described in the question. Hyperbaric oxygen may be of value for gas gangrene after appropriate débridement. (See Chapter 194 in *Nelson Textbook of Pediatrics*, 15th ed.)

42. A. Children born in 1965 in the United States were the last large risk group after the epidemic of 1964. (See Chapters 97.5 and 207 in *Nelson Textbook of Pediatrics*, 15th ed.)

43. G. Congenital toxoplasmosis is associated with organ dysfunction, inflammation, or undergrowth, such as thrombocytopenia, hepatitis, retinitis, cerebritis, or nephrosis, but not with true congenital anomalies. (See Chapter 244.8 in *Nelson Textbook of Pediatrics*, 15th ed.)

44. D. Cat-scratch disease is rarely encountered in African-American children. The reason for this is unknown. (See Chapter 205 in *Nelson Textbook of Pediatrics*, 15th ed.)

45. A. Bronchoalveolar lavage (BAL) is the best mechanism to identify the organism. Open lung biopsy is occasionally needed, especially in patients with diagnoses other than acquired immunodeficiency syndrome (AIDS). Patients with AIDS often have a high number of organisms in BAL fluid. (See Chapter 237 in *Nelson Textbook of Pediatrics*, 15th ed.)

46. B. Severe combined immunodeficiency (SCID), with its T-lymphocyte deficiency, predisposes to *P. carinii* pneumonia (PCP). (See Chapter 237 in *Nelson Textbook of Pediatrics*, 15th ed.)

47. A. Trimethoprim-sulfamethoxazole is very effective therapy and is also of value as prophylaxis for PCP. (See Chapter 237 in *Nelson Textbook of Pediatrics*, 15th ed.)

48. D. PCP is unfortunately an AIDS-defining illness, a complication that is potentially preventable, and a cause of significant morbidity and mortality. (See Chapter 237 in *Nelson Textbook of Pediatrics*, 15th ed.)

49. C. Amoxicillin is the treatment of choice for this early lesion of erythema chronicum migrans. (See Chapter 198 in *Nelson Textbook of Pediatrics*, 15th ed.)

50. E. Try to ascertain what the mother's understanding of Lyme disease is. Then speak further with the child to try to identify whether there are any issues about which he has substantial anxiety.

(See Chapter 198 in *Nelson Textbook of Pediatrics*, 15th ed.)

51. B. The risk of Lyme disease is very small, and observing the patient for the development of a rash is reasonable. Most patients with Lyme disease develop erythema chronicum migrans even if a tick bite is not remembered. (See Chapter 198 in *Nelson Textbook of Pediatrics*, 15th ed.)

52. B. *Sporothrix* infection can come from sources other than rose thorns. (See Chapter 236 in *Nelson Textbook of Pediatrics*, 15th ed.)

53. C. Cryptococcosis in children with HIV is particularly severe and difficult to cure completely. Children with other T-lymphocyte defects are also at risk. (See Chapter 234 in *Nelson Textbook of Pediatrics*, 15th ed.)

54. A. Primary pulmonary histoplasmosis in normal children either is asymptomatic or is an illness indistinguishable from a mild viral illness. (See Chapter 231 in *Nelson Textbook of Pediatrics*, 15th ed.)

55. E. Hyperinflation due to air trapping is not always noted in allergic bronchopulmonary aspergillosis, nor is hilar lymphadenopathy. The inflammatory response does not necessarily produce either of these lesions. (See Chapter 230 in *Nelson Textbook of Pediatrics*, 15th ed.)

56. D. Postnatal treatment of congenital toxoplasmosis is recommended and should include pyrimethamine, sulfadizine, and leucovorin. (See Chapter 244.8 in *Nelson Textbook of Pediatrics*, 15th ed.)

57. D. Immunocompetent mothers must show serologic evidence of *T. gondii* infection by specific IgG, IgM, IgA, or IgE. (See Chapter 244.8 in *Nelson Textbook of Pediatrics*, 15th ed.)

58. D. Serogroup B is the most common in this region and age group. (See Chapter 178 in *Nelson Textbook of Pediatrics*, 15th ed.)

59. B. Dogs do not carry oocysts. The other sources listed in the question are compatible with transmission of toxoplasmosis. (See Chapter 244.8 in *Nelson Textbook of Pediatrics*, 15th ed.)

60. E. Sinusitis and otitis media are not caused by *T. gondii*. (See Chapter 244.8 in *Nelson Textbook of Pediatrics*, 15th ed.)

61. B. Meningococcal meningitis is often epidemic, associated with a prior

respiratory tract infection, or sporadic. Prophylaxis with rifampin is indicated for all close contacts, including the parents and siblings. (See Chapter 178 in *Nelson Textbook of Pediatrics*, 15th ed.)

62. C. The patient described in the question most probably has meningococcemia. Nonetheless, pneumococci may occasionally produce similar manifestations, especially in patients without a spleen. (See Chapter 178 in *Nelson Textbook of Pediatrics*, 15th ed.)

63. A. In addition to gonococcal disease, Fitz-Hugh–Curtis syndrome may also be due to *Chlamydia*. (See Chapter 179 in *Nelson Textbook of Pediatrics*, 15th ed.)

64. D. Bacteremia and septic arthritis are common manifestations of disseminated gonococcal infection in neonates. (See Chapter 179 in *Nelson Textbook of Pediatrics*, 15th ed.)

65. C. Even with disseminated disease (bacteremia, arthritis meningitis), ceftriaxone is the drug of choice because of the high rate of penicillin resistance. (See Chapter 179 in *Nelson Textbook of Pediatrics*, 15th ed.)

66. C. Because of high rates of penicillin resistance, ceftriaxone is the treatment of choice for gonococcal disease. (See Chapter 179 in *Nelson Textbook of Pediatrics*, 15th ed.)

67. D. Laryngeal papillomatosis develops in the first few years after birth, has the same serotype as the virus in the maternal genital lesions, and is often difficult to treat. (See Chapter 224 in *Nelson Textbook of Pediatrics*, 15th ed.)

68. B. Histologic examination demonstrates the typical features of papillomavirus. Other tests are usually not available in most hospitals. (See Chapter 224 in *Nelson Textbook of Pediatrics*, 15th ed.)

69. A. If diphtheria is suspected, antitoxin should be given as soon as possible to prevent binding of the toxin to tissues. Once the toxin binds, tissue damage develops and is not reversed by antitoxin. (See Chapter 180 in *Nelson Textbook of Pediatrics*, 15th ed.)

70. E. Older individuals and those from foreign countries, particularly Russia, are at risk for acquiring diphtheria. (See Chapter 180 in *Nelson Textbook of Pediatrics*, 15th ed.)

71. C. Cutaneous diphtheria is seen in warm climates as an ulcer with a membrane and is readily transmitted to others. In infected patients with cutaneous disease, the illness is usually milder unless the diagnosis is delayed. (See Chapter 180 in *Nelson Textbook of Pediatrics*, 15th ed.)

72. E. Toxin production helps distinguish the pathologic organisms of *C. diphtheriae*. (See Chapter 180 in *Nelson Textbook of Pediatrics*, 15th ed.)

73. C. This method is rapid because it requires only a small quantity of colonial growth (adequate in 48 hours), and the procedure can be completed in less than 2 hours. (See Chapter 233 in *Nelson Textbook of Pediatrics*, 15th ed.)

74. A. Inasmuch as most cases of coccidioidomycosis have a benign clinical course and at present it is not known whether administration of the available antifungal agents preclude extrapulmonary dissemination, administration of such medications in all cases of coccidioidomycosis is not yet advisable. (See Chapter 233 in *Nelson Textbook of Pediatrics*, 15th ed.)

75. A. *Coccidioides* is acquired by inhalation of the arthroconidial stage found in nature (in the soil) or in the usual laboratory cultures. Although rarely arthroconidia-like structures have been detected in pulmonary cavities, human-to-human transmission does not occur despite intimate contact between infected individuals and others. Therefore, isolation of patients with coccidioidomycosis is not necessary, although careful disposition of sputum, exudates, and wound dressings is essential. (See Chapter 233 in *Nelson Textbook of Pediatrics*, 15th ed.)

76. E. The thick smear of peripheral blood should be diagnostic, especially if repeated. Laboratory manuals help identify the morphologic forms needed to distinguish the different malarial species. (See Chapter 244.7 in *Nelson Textbook of Pediatrics*, 15th ed.)

77. A. Although the parasite that causes cerebral malaria has various patterns of drug resistance, quinidine or, if not available, quinine is still the treatment of choice. (See Chapter 244.7 in *Nelson Textbook of Pediatrics*, 15th ed.)

78. D. Control of the mosquito vector and netting to keep mosquitoes away from children during the night are key features of malaria prevention. (See Chapter 244.7 in *Nelson Textbook of Pediatrics*, 15th ed.)

79. C. Malaria is the first diagnosis to be considered in this patient, who has the unfavorable prognostic features of hypoglycemia and coma. (See Chapter 244.7 in *Nelson Textbook of Pediatrics*, 15th ed.)

80. C. Psittacosis, a bird-borne chlamydial disease, produces severe pneumonia with systemic manifestations similar to *Mycoplasma* pneumonia or legionnaires' disease. (See Chapter 197 in *Nelson Textbook of Pediatrics*, 15th ed.)

81. C. Culture is of poor value, but serologic studies are the diagnostic tests of choice in the patient described in Question 80. (See Chapter 197 in *Nelson Textbook of Pediatrics*, 15th ed.)

82. D. Acute chest syndrome of sickle cell anemia, when associated with infectious pneumonia, may be due to many bacteria and viruses, including those listed in this question. (See Chapters 196 and 197 in *Nelson Textbook of Pediatrics*, 15th ed.)

83. E. Treatment of *C. pneumoniae* and *M. pneumoniae* is with erythromycin (azithromycin or clarithromycin) or, if in patients older than 10 to 12 years, doxycycline or tetracycline. Patients with sickle cell anemia are also at risk for other pathogens and may also receive cefotaxime as empiric therapy for pneumonia. (See Chapters 196 and 197 in *Nelson Textbook of Pediatrics*, 15th ed.)

84. A. Culture remains the most accurate test for *C. trachomatis* infection. (See Chapter 197 in *Nelson Textbook of Pediatrics*, 15th ed.)

85. C. Both intrapartum infection and sexual contact are possible routes of transmission of *C. trachomatis*, but a careful assessment is needed to rule out sexual abuse. (See Chapter 197 in *Nelson Textbook of Pediatrics*, 15th ed.)

86. A. Cervical infection with *C. trachomatis* may be symptomatic but is often asymptomatic; both types of infection predispose to neonatal colonization and in some to disease (conjunctivitis or pneumonia). (See Chapter 197 in *Nelson Textbook of Pediatrics*, 15th ed.)

87. D. False-positive results of tests for antibodies against *B. burgdorferi* are common and lead to considerable confusion and overtreatment. Polymerase chain reaction and newer-generation antibody tests are being developed. (See Chapter 198 in *Nelson Textbook of Pediatrics*, 15th ed.)

88. C. The risk of Lyme disease is relatively low, and a simple tick bite is not an indication for treatment. If the tick is still on the child, it must be removed by gentle traction in an upward motion. Use gloves or tweezers. (See Chapter 198 in *Nelson Textbook of Pediatrics*, 15th ed.)

89. B. Early therapy with oral antibiotics (amoxicillin, doxycycline, cefuroxime, erythromycin) can prevent future sequelae of Lyme disease. Doxycycline should not be given to children younger than 10 to 12 years. (See Chapter 198 in *Nelson Textbook of Pediatrics*, 15th ed.)

90. D. The oculoglandular (conjunctivitis, lymph node) syndrome is the most frequent atypical manifestation of cat-scratch disease. (See Chapter 205 in *Nelson Textbook of Pediatrics*, 15th ed.)

91. A. Despite limb scratches, the head and neck are the most common sites of node involvement due to cat-scratch disease in children. (See Chapter 205 in *Nelson Textbook of Pediatrics*, 15th ed.)

92. C. Fever occurs in only 30% of cases of cat-scratch disease. (See Chapter 205 in *Nelson Textbook of Pediatrics*, 15th ed.)

93. C. The lag phase after a cat scratch may be 5 to 60 days, with an average incubation of 12 days. (See Chapter 205 in *Nelson Textbook of Pediatrics*, 15th ed.)

94. C. Ninety-five percent of patients have cat contacts, whereas 75% have actual scratches. Being licked by cats, dog scratches, thorns, and other mechanisms have also been reported to be associated with cat-scratch disease. (See Chapter 205 in *Nelson Textbook of Pediatrics*, 15th ed.)

95. D. The organism that causes cat-scratch disease is most probably *Bartonella henselae*. (See Chapter 205 in *Nelson Textbook of Pediatrics*, 15th ed.)

96. A. Oral amoxicillin or tetracycline is the treatment of choice for Lyme arthritis. (See Chapter 198 in *Nelson Textbook of Pediatrics*, 15th ed.)

97. E. *Listeria monocytogenes* may contaminate dairy products (milk, cheese) and may survive, replicate, and spread in a family's refrigerator. (See Chapter 191 in *Nelson Textbook of Pediatrics*, 15th ed.)

98. D. Early-onset neonatal listeriosis is a severe bacteremic illness with a septic shocklike picture and occasionally with an erythematous maculopapular rash. (See Chapter 191 in *Nelson Textbook of Pediatrics*, 15th ed.)

99. D. Titers are of no value in the diagnosis or confirmation of neonatal listeriosis. Culture and biopsy (of skin lesions) usually reveal the organism. (See Chapter 191 in *Nelson Textbook of Pediatrics*, 15th ed.)

100. D. Ceftriaxone is ineffective for treating brucellosis in any age group. Doxycycline plus an aminoglycoside is the treatment of choice for severe disease, especially in children older than 8 to 9 years, when the risk of a tetracycline-induced tooth lesions are low. (See Chapter 190 in *Nelson Textbook of Pediatrics*, 15th ed.)

101. B. A high IgM titer with a low IgG titer is most consistent with successful brucellosis therapy, which is often prolonged (4 to 6 weeks) and requires two antibiotics (tetracycline or doxycycline and, if severe, an aminoglycoside). Trimethoprim-sulfamethoxazole may be substituted for tetracycline in children younger than 8 to 9 years. (See Chapter 190 in *Nelson Textbook of Pediatrics*, 15th ed.)

102. E. *Brucella* organisms are intracellular parasites that are often difficult to culture, as evidenced by the four *(A to D)* true statements. (See Chapter 190 in *Nelson Textbook of Pediatrics*, 15th ed.)

103. D. *B. abortus* infects cows, *B. suis* is found in hogs, *B. neotomae* is found in desert wood rats, and *B. ovis* affects sheep and hares. (See Chapter 190 in *Nelson Textbook of Pediatrics*, 15th ed.)

104. D. The vaccine against bubonic plague is not recommended for children. It is recommended for persons in at-risk occupations (exposure to infected rodents or microbiology laboratory). (See Chapter 188 in *Nelson Textbook of Pediatrics*, 15th ed.)

105. A. Many patients affected by *Y. pseudotuberculosis* do not have diarrhea, and thus a stool culture is not considered. If the involvement is a mesenteric adenitis, the stool culture results may be negative. (See Chapter 188 in *Nelson Textbook of Pediatrics*, 15th ed.)

106. C. Right lower quadrant abdominal pain from terminal ileitis or mesenteric adenitis is a common symptom of *Y. pseudotuberculosis* infection. (See Chapter 188 in *Nelson Textbook of Pediatrics*, 15th ed.)

107. B. *Y. enterocolitica*–induced diarrhea is similar to *Shigella*-induced dysentery, with fecal leukocytes, abdominal pain, and fever. (See Chapter 188 in *Nelson Textbook of Pediatrics*, 15th ed.)

108. E. *Y. enterocolitica* infection most often develops from contaminated food (animals, milk, water), from animals (dogs), or from human-to-human contact. Transfusion-related disease remains a risk but is uncommon. (See Chapter 188 in *Nelson Textbook of Pediatrics*, 15th ed.)

109. D. The serum agglutination test is reliable, but positive results cannot be obtained until patients have been ill with tularemia for 1 week. (See Chapter 189 in *Nelson Textbook of Pediatrics*, 15th ed.)

110. A. Ulceroglandular disease is noted in 80% of patients with tularemia. A primary maculopapular lesion is noted within 72 hours and then ulcerates in 4 to 5 days. Thereafter, the ulcer may require 1 month to heal, while regional lymphadenopathy develops. (See Chapter 189 in *Nelson Textbook of Pediatrics*, 15th ed.)

111. E. Tularemia, an important zoonotic infection, is most often acquired from a tick bite or directly from rabbits. Flies, fleas, mosquitoes, lice, and many animals (squirrels, beavers, birds) are additional vectors. (See Chapter 189 in *Nelson Textbook of Pediatrics*, 15th ed.)

112. B. Sensorineural hearing loss is a risk after asymptomatic congenital CMV infection. The incidence of neonatal CMV-positive urine is much greater than the incidence of symptomatic neonatal CMV inclusion disease (microcephaly, retinitis, small for gestational age, petechiae, hepatitis, intracranial calcifications, and so forth). (See Chapter 214 in *Nelson Textbook of Pediatrics*, 15th ed.)

113. B. Limb reduction defects are encountered more often after chorionic villus sampling. The mechanism remains undetermined, and the absolute risk remains very low. (See Chapter 96 in *Nelson Textbook of Pediatrics*, 15th ed.)

114. E. The risk of fetal defects resulting from maternal chickenpox during early gestation is low. Nonetheless, all pregnant women who have never had chickenpox and who are exposed to an active case should receive varicella-zoster immunoglobulin (VZIG) to try to attenuate or prevent varicella. (See Chapters 97.3 and 213 in *Nelson Textbook of Pediatrics*, 15th ed.)

115. C. Parvovirus B-19, the agent of fifth disease (erythema infectiosum), produces congenital infection of the fetal

erythrocyte precursor cells, producing transient fetal anemia. If the anemia is severe, it produces nonimmune hydrops with the possibility of intrauterine fetal demise. Intrauterine (umbilical venous) blood transfusion is curative but poses significant risk. (See Chapters 97.4 and 210 in *Nelson Textbook of Pediatrics*, 15th ed.)

116. B. Intravenous acyclovir is the treatment of choice for neonatal HSV infection. The lethargy may also signify encephalitis-meningitis due to HSV. Without treatment, neonates with HSV either die or have severe neurodevelopmental sequelae. (See Chapters 97.2 and 211 in *Nelson Textbook of Pediatrics*, 15th ed.)

117. D. Scarring dermatomal skin lesions with limb hypoplasia are seen only in varicella-zoster disease. Prenatal onset of HSV with fetal sequelae is quite rare compared with the postnatal onset of vertically acquired HSV from the maternal genital tract during labor. (See Chapters 97.3 and 213 in *Nelson Textbook of Pediatrics*, 15th ed.)

118. A. Congenital heart disease (patent ductus arteriosus) is primarily seen in congenital rubella syndrome compared with all other TORCH diseases. The problems listed in *B* to *E* may occur in CMV and rubella. (See Chapters 97.5 and 207 in *Nelson Textbook of Pediatrics*, 15th ed.)

119. D. Treatment of HIV-positive mothers can dramatically reduce the incidence of HIV infection in infants. Treatment reduces the overall risk of infection from approximately 25% to 30% to 8%. Treatment begins any time after 14 weeks of gestation and continues during labor and delivery and for another 6 weeks (in the infants). (See Chapters 97.6 and 223 in *Nelson Textbook of Pediatrics*, 15th ed.)

120. D. It is unusual to find poliovirus in the CSF during the meningitis stage. Stool cultures are more appropriate. (See Chapter 209 in *Nelson Textbook of Pediatrics*, 15th ed.)

121. D. Guillain-Barré syndrome, or autoimmune peripheral neuropathy, is symmetric and involves sensory but more so motor nerves. Polio is an anterior horn cell disease and is purely motor. (See Chapter 209 in *Nelson Textbook of Pediatrics*, 15th ed.)

122. C. This is a classic presentation for an enterovirus (hand-foot-mouth syndrome) infection, usually due to coxsackievirus

A-16. (See Chapter 209 in *Nelson Textbook of Pediatrics*, 15th ed.)

123. B. Enteroviruses retain infectivity for several days at room temperature. (See Chapter 209 in *Nelson Textbook of Pediatrics*, 15th ed.)

124. 1. D
      2. A
      3. B
      4. C
      5. E
      (See Chapter 245 in *Nelson Textbook of Pediatrics*, 15th ed.)

125. D. Approximately 1 billion people (of the more than 4.5 billion in the world's population) have hookworm infection. (See Chapter 245.9 in *Nelson Textbook of Pediatrics*, 15th ed.)

126. C. *Paragonimus westermani* is the oriental lung fluke. Although this is not the most common cause of eosinophilic CSF pleocytosis, the child's residence history, past symptoms of hemoptysis, and dietary history make the diagnosis of CNS paragonimiasis most likely. (See Chapter 245.8 in *Nelson Textbook of Pediatrics*, 15th ed.)

127. D. *Schistosoma haematobium* is not endemic to the areas visited. It also does not affect the portal circulation, preferring the ureteral and bladder veins. (See Chapter 245.11 in *Nelson Textbook of Pediatrics*, 15th ed.)

128. A. The treatment of choice of symptomatic nontuberculous mycobacterial lymphadenitis is complete excision. Fine-needle aspiration may help with the diagnosis, but excisional biopsy is the cure. (See Chapter 200 in *Nelson Textbook of Pediatrics*, 15th ed.)

129. D. *Mycobacterium avium-intracellulare* produces chronic bacteremic disease that responds poorly to therapy in children with AIDS. Some therapeutic benefit has been found with the newer erythromycin-like agents (clarithromycin-azithromycin) when used in combination with other antimycobacterial agents such as rifampin. (See Chapter 200 in *Nelson Textbook of Pediatrics*, 15th ed.)

130. C. *M. avium* complex commonly is noted as firm, nontender cervical adenitis. The borderline PPD test result is suggestive, especially in the absence of known exposure to tuberculosis. Such adenitis may be more common in southern states. (See Chapter 200 in *Nelson Textbook of Pediatrics*, 15th ed.)

131. B. *M. pneumoniae* produces an atypical pneumonia not unlike *C. pneumoniae* or *Legionella* species. The age, the season, the systemic features, and the x-ray finding suggest this diagnosis. Nonetheless, if uncertain, pneumococci may also be a possibility. With pneumococci, one might expect higher fever, a single consolidation, and a higher WBC count with a shift to the left. (See Chapter 196 in *Nelson Textbook of Pediatrics*, 15th ed.)

132. E. Osteomyelitis has not been considered a complication of *M. pneumoniae*. As noted, this organism often has diverse and protean manifestations. (See Chapter 196 in *Nelson Textbook of Pediatrics*, 15th ed.)

133. C. Bartonellosis in a nonimmune person presents with anorexia, headache, fever, diaphoresis, jaundice, pallor, and anemia (Oroya fever). The disease is endemic in Peru, and the vector is the sand fly. (See Chapter 204 in *Nelson Textbook of Pediatrics*, 15th ed.)

134. B. *Candida* species may produce fungemia, hepatosplenic granulomas, cutaneous lesions, ophthalmitis, urinary tract infection, and possibly meningitis. Aspergillosis is always a concern, is more difficult to treat, and is associated with prolonged periods of profound neutropenia and immunosuppression. (See Chapter 229 in *Nelson Textbook of Pediatrics*, 15th ed.)

135. B. *S. epidermidis* is the most common pathogen producing bacteremia in neutropenic febrile patients with hematologic malignancies. Its frequency is due in part to the presence of indwelling catheters used for nutrition, chemotherapy, and antibiotics. It is important to examine the sites of these catheters (or ports) for evidence of exit site infections and tunnel track infections. The latter are most difficult to treat. The treatment of choice for *S. epidermidis* bacteremia is intravenous vancomycin. (See Chapter 174.2 in *Nelson Textbook of Pediatrics*, 15th ed.)

136. B. Tunnel track infections are difficult to treat whatever the pathogen. In addition, candidemia associated with an indwelling line may not respond to antifungal therapy (remember to give the drug through each lumen of the catheter), necessitating catheter removal. (See Chapter 229 in *Nelson Textbook of Pediatrics*, 15th ed.)

137. B. The live measles virus is contraindicated in patients with T-cell immunodeficiency because disseminated disease may occur. Nonetheless, it is recommended that HIV-infected patients be given this vaccine because measles itself is a serious illness once they develop AIDS. (See Chapter 206 in *Nelson Textbook of Pediatrics*, 15th ed.)

138. D. These are the current World Health Organization *and* the American Academy of Pediatrics recommendations for the treatment of diarrhea. (See Chapter 171 in *Nelson Textbook of Pediatrics*, 15th ed.)

139. D. With such close exposure, the child described in the question must be considered to have active tuberculosis until proved otherwise. (See Chapter 199 in *Nelson Textbook of Pediatrics*, 15th ed.)

140. C. In addition, a PPD test should be repeated frequently during the first year of life for the child described in the question, beginning at 3 to 4 months of age. (See Chapter 199 in *Nelson Textbook of Pediatrics*, 15th ed.)

141. C. Primary pulmonary tuberculosis in childhood is usually not contagious because there are no active cavitary lesions or productive sputum. The infiltrate is an intense T-cell–monocyte reaction to the bacillus. (See Chapter 199 in *Nelson Textbook of Pediatrics*, 15th ed.)

142. D. Active isoniazid prophylaxis after such close contact is valuable in preventing serious pulmonary or extrapulmonary disease. (See Chapter 199 in *Nelson Textbook of Pediatrics*, 15th ed.)

143. B. In evaluating children for a fever of unknown origin (FUO), nail fold capillaroscopy may help determine abnormal patterns of the blood vessels (tufts, microaneurysms, looping) compatible with autoimmune connective tissue disorders. (See Chapter 167 in *Nelson Textbook of Pediatrics*, 15th ed.)

144. E. Multiorgan system involvement is typical of SIRS following activation of choices *A* to *D* in the question and includes adult respiratory distress syndrome, acute tubular necrosis, hepatic failure, cardiac failure, seizures, coma, disseminated intravascular coagulation, and others. (See Chapter 168 in *Nelson Textbook of Pediatrics*, 15th ed.)

145. B. Remember that juvenile rheumatoid arthritis may initially present without arthritis and only manifest as high spiking fever with a faint rash. Nonetheless, most cases of FUO in children are infectious and are either common and typical, atypical manifestations of typical common diseases, or less often atypical uncommon infectious diseases. (See Chapter 167 in *Nelson Textbook of Pediatrics*, 15th ed.)

146. A. A careful history and physical examination help direct the evaluation of FUO and avoid unnecessary, invasive, risky, or expensive testing. (See Chapter 167 in *Nelson Textbook of Pediatrics*, 15th ed.)

147. C. Vancomycin is the current treatment of choice for penicillin/cephalosporin-resistant pneumococci. (See Chapter 176 in *Nelson Textbook of Pediatrics*, 15th ed.)

148. B. Cases of *H. influenzae* type b meningitis, cellulitis, epiglottitis, pneumonia, and septic arthritis have virtually disappeared from children's hospitals in the United States since the development and use of the conjugate *H. influenzae* vaccine. (See Chapter 177 in *Nelson Textbook of Pediatrics*, 15th ed.)

149. E. Other than low-risk, febrile, and stable patients with sickle cell anemia, all remaining patients with any of the manifestations in choices *A* to *D* require inpatient management for presumed bacterial sepsis. The combination of splenic hypofunction and a deficiency of the properdin system of complement activation places patients with sickle cell anemia at increased risk of bacteremia from encapsulated organisms (pneumococcus, *H. influenzae*). (See Chapters 176 and 177 in *Nelson Textbook of Pediatrics*, 15th ed.)

150. E. Regardless of a child's age, the signs noted in choices *A* to *D* are very significant and suggest serious bacterial illnesses that require prompt supportive care (oxygen, fluids) and antibiotics. (See Chapter 168 in *Nelson Textbook of Pediatrics*, 15th ed.)

151. E. In the absence of diarrhea, a stool culture has a low yield except under unusual circumstances (e.g., travel history to typhoid endemic area). (See Chapter 167 in *Nelson Textbook of Pediatrics*, 15th ed.)

152. D. Ancestry rarely predisposes to urinary tract infections, whereas choices *A, B, C,* and *E* all are significant risk factors. (See Chapter 492 in *Nelson Textbook of Pediatrics*, 15th ed.)

153. D. *P. aeruginosa* is an unusual pathogen in a normal host who is not exposed to an abnormal hospital-based bacterial flora. In a chronically hospitalized critically ill or institutionalized patient *Pseudomonas* should be considered. (See Chapter 184.1 in *Nelson Textbook of Pediatrics*, 15th ed.)

154. C. Serious infections in young infants include urinary tract infection, bacteremia, meningitis, gastroenteritis, bone and soft tissue infection, and pneumonia. (See Chapter 168 in *Nelson Textbook of Pediatrics*, 15th ed.)

155. E. Murine typhus is encountered worldwide and is associated with the cat flea or more often the rat flea. It is endemic in Texas. Murine typhus is much milder than epidemic typhus. (See Chapter 240 in *Nelson Textbook of Pediatrics*, 15th ed.)

156. B. Human ehrlichiosis is a rickettsia-like multisystem illness, with or without a rash. It is endemic and probably is more common than reported. (See Chapter 242 in *Nelson Textbook of Pediatrics*, 15th ed.)

157. D. Most tick bites do not produce systemic disease. Alternatively, many patients with tick-borne infectious diseases do not remember a tick bite. (See Chapter 238 in *Nelson Textbook of Pediatrics*, 15th ed.)

158. B. Empirical antibiotic therapy should be started as soon as possible in a presumptive case of Rocky Mountain spotted fever. Titers take too long to be of value in the acute phase, and skin biopsy is helpful only if results are positive. Doxycycline or chloramphenicol is the treatment of choice. Although doxycycline is not always recommended before 8 years of age, some physicians treat any patient with doxycycline. (See Chapter 239 in *Nelson Textbook of Pediatrics*, 15th ed.)

18 The Digestive System

1. C. If an avulsed tooth is clean and the risk of aspiration is not too high, the tooth should be reimplanted in its socket and held in place on the way to the dentist. If this is not possible, the tooth should be placed in milk or water. (See Chapter 260 in *Nelson Textbook of Pediatrics*, 15th ed.)

2. B. A facial space inflammatory response to

a tooth abscess is the cause of such facial swelling until proved otherwise. (See Chapter 258 in *Nelson Textbook of Pediatrics*, 15th ed.)

3. A. The therapeutic window for fluoride and mild mottling of teeth is narrow. (See Chapter 258 in *Nelson Textbook of Pediatrics*, 15th ed.)

4. C. Teeth are present at birth in 1 in 2000 neonates. Children with natal teeth may have a positive family history or evidence of a syndrome with other malformations present. (See Chapter 253.1 in *Nelson Textbook of Pediatrics*, 15th ed.)

5. E. Appendicitis may produce infectious (wound, right lower quadrant, hepatic, sepsis) and noninfectious (systemic inflammatory response syndrome—acute respiratory distress syndrome, disseminated intravascular coagulation, and so forth) complications. Chronic complications include infertility in females and intestinal obstruction from adhesions. (See Chapter 289 in *Nelson Textbook of Pediatrics*, 15th ed.)

6. C. Direct tenderness, particularly localized to the right lower quadrant, is a valuable sign in appendicitis. This may be absent in an appendix located in the retrocecum or pelvis or early in the progression of the disease. (See Chapter 289 in *Nelson Textbook of Pediatrics*, 15th ed.)

7. B. Inflammatory bowel disease is one of the most common causes of chronic or recurrent abdominal pain in adolescents. Functional abdominal pain (irritable bowel) is in the differential diagnosis but is precluded by the presence of anemia and weight loss. (See Chapter 283 in *Nelson Textbook of Pediatrics*, 15th ed.)

8. D. Depending on the stage of the illness and its progression, very few signs or symptoms can definitively rule out appendicitis as the cause of abdominal pain. Although crampy pain and pain that begins after vomiting are atypical, they do not eliminate the diagnosis of appendicitis. A patient (parent) should never be sent home and told that the cause of abdominal pain cannot be appendicitis. This could delay seeking medical attention if the pain persists. (See Chapter 289 in *Nelson Textbook of Pediatrics*, 15th ed.)

9. B. Administration of milk help calms a child and helps dilute the alkali in the esophagus and stomach. (See Chapter 270 in *Nelson Textbook of Pediatrics*, 15th ed.)

10. D. Endoscopy is indicated to assess the severity of inflammation and necrosis. Even without oral lesions, significant esophageal involvement with future stricture formation is possible. Prednisone is of no value in preventing strictures. (See Chapter 270 in *Nelson Textbook of Pediatrics*, 15th ed.)

11. 1. E
    2. D
    3. F
    4. A
    5. B
    6. C
    (See Chapter 291 in *Nelson Textbook of Pediatrics*, 15th ed.)

12. C. Diaphragmatic hernia was confirmed by an immediate chest radiograph. The child remained hypoxic and hypercarbic despite mechanical ventilation and required extracorporeal membrane oxygenation (ECMO) before surgical repair of the defect in the diaphragm. (See Chapter 317 in *Nelson Textbook of Pediatrics*, 15th ed.)

13. B. Choices *A, B,* and *C* must be considered because each may produce similar hepatic and extrahepatic manifestations. Chronic active hepatitis of the autoimmune (lupoid hepatitis) type is often associated with other autoimmune diseases (the patient described in the question had Hashimoto thyroiditis) and is more prevalent in adolescent females. High titers of liver-kidney microsomal antibodies are present. The antinuclear antibody response is positive in a smaller percentage of patients. (See Chapter 307.2 in *Nelson Textbook of Pediatrics*, 15th ed.)

14. C. The ammonia level of the girl described in the question was exceedingly high. This child developed Reye syndrome after receiving aspirin to control her fever during an influenza virus infection. Her parents thought that it was safe for her to receive aspirin now that she was a teenager. (See Chapter 306 in *Nelson Textbook of Pediatrics*, 15th ed.)

15. C. In the patient described in the question, the hepatic abscess developed as a complication of a partially treated ruptured appendix following acute appendicitis. The over-the-counter medication was an oral antibiotic that suppressed some of the signs of appendicitis. The right lower quadrant fullness is a walled-off appendiceal abscess. This is treated with antibiotics and resected at a later date.

The hepatic abscess developed after

septic embolization into the portal vein (during the acute appendicitis) and subsequently the liver. The organisms are usually enteric anaerobes in this form of liver abscess. Treatment includes antibiotics (including metronidazole or clindamycin) and percutaneous drainage under ultrasonographic or computed tomographic (CT) guidance. (See Chapter 304 in *Nelson Textbook of Pediatrics*, 15th ed.)

16. D. Wilson disease should be suspected in any child who has acute or chronic hepatitis and is older than 5 years. This is especially true if cognitive performance is becoming impaired. Glycosuria reflects a renal tubular defect, and hemolysis may be due to copper-induced red blood cell membrane injury. (See Chapter 303.2 in *Nelson Textbook of Pediatrics*, 15th ed.)

17. D. Vitamin E deficiency has a long latency before it eventually produces ataxia, posterior (spinal cord) column signs, and peripheral neuropathy. Early treatment with water-soluble vitamin E may reverse these neurologic processes. (See Chapter 302.1 in *Nelson Textbook of Pediatrics*, 15th ed.)

18. 1. A
    2. B
    3. A
    4. B
    5. C
    (See Chapter 302 in *Nelson Textbook of Pediatrics*, 15th ed.)

19. 1. A
    2. A
    3. B
    4. C
    5. C
    6. A
    7. B
    8. B
    9. A
    10. B
    11. B
    12. A
    (See Chapters 88.3, 302, and 303 in *Nelson Textbook of Pediatrics*, 15th ed.)

20. D. (See Chapter 297 in *Nelson Textbook of Pediatrics*, 15th ed.)

21. D. All of the choices listed in the question must be in the differential diagnosis. Nonetheless, acute onset of severe pain and emesis should lead one to suspect pancreatitis. The hematemesis is most probably secondary to a Mallory-Weiss tear of the gastroesophageal mucosa due to severe retching. (See Chapter 297 in *Nelson Textbook of Pediatrics*, 15th ed.)

22. B. Pancreatitis may develop in patients with total body casts. Associated features may also include hypercalcemia and hypertension. (See Chapter 297 in *Nelson Textbook of Pediatrics*, 15th ed.)

23. D. Tracheoesophageal atresia often presents after a pregnancy with excessive amniotic fluid because fetal swallowing is interrupted. After birth, the esophageal atresia (most commonly associated with the tracheoesophageal fistula) prevents swallowing and placement of a nasogastric tube. The tube often coils around in the proximal blind-ending esophageal pouch. (See Chapter 265 in *Nelson Textbook of Pediatrics*, 15th ed.)

24. D. Hydrocephalus or any central nervous system defect is unusual in patients with tracheoesophageal fistula. Indeed, IQ is often normal. Although many patients have an isolated tracheoesophageal fistula, others may have the VATER syndrome: vertebral, anal, tracheoesophageal, and renal/radial anomalies. (See Chapter 265 in *Nelson Textbook of Pediatrics*, 15th ed.)

25. 1. E
    2. D
    3. C
    4. B
    5. A
    6. F
    7. G
    (See Chapter 286 in *Nelson Textbook of Pediatrics*, 15th ed.)

26. E. Secondary lactase deficiency frequently follows severe rotavirus infection that involves the small intestinal mucosal cells and results in villus atrophy. Refeeding with a non–lactose-containing formula until the villi regenerate and produce lactase is the appropriate treatment. (See Chapter 286.11 in *Nelson Textbook of Pediatrics*, 15th ed.)

27. D. All of the choices in the question must be included in the differential diagnosis. Pelvic inflammatory disease often presents with lower abdominal suprapubic pain, a vaginal discharge, and signs of peritoneal irritation. A ruptured ectopic pregnancy would be unlikely but not unheard of in a Tanner stage 2 girl. Mesenteric adenitis may present in a similar manner as appendicitis (pseudoappendicitis) and can be detected by abdominal ultrasonography or CT scan. This patient has the characteristic appendicitis sequence of

periumbilical pain, followed more often by nausea and less often by emesis and then followed by right lower quadrant pain. The 2-day history is typical of appendicitis, as is the apprehension about the examiner's hand during the abdominal palpation. (See Chapter 289 in *Nelson Textbook of Pediatrics*, 15th ed.)

28. 1. A
    2. A
    3. A
    4. C
    5. C
    6. A
    7. B
    (See Chapter 283 in *Nelson Textbook of Pediatrics*, 15th ed.)

29. C. The patient described in the question most likely has *Helicobacter pylori* associated with peptic ulcer disease. Without triple antimicrobial therapy, patients with *H. pylori*–associated ulcers suffer relapse. Cure is possible with such therapy. (See Chapter 282.1 in *Nelson Textbook of Pediatrics*, 15th ed.)

30. D. Intussusception should be suspected in any toddler or young child with an acute illness characterized by intermittent episodes of abdominal pain (colic) and blood in the stool. A physical examination, abdominal kidney-ureter-bladder (KUB) radiograph, or ultrasonography may show that the bowel is being pulled into the next segment of bowel. Nonetheless, the diagnostic test of choice and treatment of choice is a barium enema. Hydrostatic pressure during the enema reduces the intussusception in approximately 80% to 90% of patients. (See Chapter 279.3 in *Nelson Textbook of Pediatrics*, 15th ed.)

31. 1. A
    2. A
    3. B
    4. B
    5. A
    (See Chapter 252 in *Nelson Textbook of Pediatrics*, 15th ed.)

32. E. Pyloric stenosis is most often encountered in a first-born boy after the second or third week of life. Recurrent emesis of gastric contents results in dehydration plus loss of H^+, K^+, and Cl^-, resulting in hypokalemic metabolic alkalosis. On physical examination immediately after feeding the patient described in the question, an olive-shaped mass was felt in the epigastrium. A surgical pyloromyotomy cured the patient, who was taking oral feeding 12 hours later.

(See Chapter 275 in *Nelson Textbook of Pediatrics*, 15th ed.)

33. C. Scrubbing an avulsed tooth, especially the root, can cause permanent damage and prevent reimplantation. The remaining choices, including plugging the sink drain to avoid losing the tooth, are all correct. (See Chapter 260 in *Nelson Textbook of Pediatrics*, 15th ed.)

34. D. Pierre Robin syndrome includes mandibular hypoplasia producing micrognathia, a high arched or cleft palate, and relative macroglossia-glossoptosis. In the supine position, the relatively large tongue falls backward to the posterior pharynx and obstructs the airway. Treatment includes caring for the infant in a prone position and, if needed, a tracheostomy. (See Chapter 257 in *Nelson Textbook of Pediatrics*, 15th ed.)

35. 1. C
    2. D
    3. E
    4. B
    5. A
    (See Chapter 253 in *Nelson Textbook of Pediatrics*, 15th ed.)

36. B. When an obstruction is proximal to the ampulla of Vater, the vomitus cannot be bile stained, and because most of the vomitus has stomach (hydrochloric) acid, hypochloremic alkalosis ensues. (See Chapter 275 in *Nelson Textbook of Pediatrics*, 15th ed.)

37. D. Chronic active hepatitis is the more serious form of chronic hepatitis. (See Chapter 307.2 in *Nelson Textbook of Pediatrics*, 15th ed.)

38. C. (See Chapter 275 in *Nelson Textbook of Pediatrics*, 15th ed.)

39. A. If you suggest choice *B, C,* or *D,* the mother will either go elsewhere or call you back in an hour to say things are worse and that now her son has bloody, jellylike stools. This is not the appropriate time for a referral, nor is a surgeon the appropriate person to refer the child to. (See Chapter 279.3 in *Nelson Textbook of Pediatrics*, 15th ed.)

40. D. The history is classic for intussusception. (See Chapter 279.3 in *Nelson Textbook of Pediatrics*, 15th ed.)

41. E. Barium enema usually resolves intussusception. If it fails, if the symptoms have been present for too long a time. If a leading point or signs of obstruction, perforation, or peritonitis are found, it is

time for surgery. (See Chapter 279.3 in *Nelson Textbook of Pediatrics*, 15th ed.)

42. A. The loss of hydrogen ions in prolonged vomiting of gastric fluid leads to metabolic alkalosis. (See Chapter 275 in *Nelson Textbook of Pediatrics*, 15th ed.)

43. C. Greasy stools or an oil slick in the toilet bowl indicates the presence of gross steatorrhea (except when a child is receiving mineral oil to treat constipation). Among the causes of malabsorption, one should think of pancreatic insufficiency when fat is noticed in the stool. The most common cause of pancreatic insufficiency in childhood is cystic fibrosis. Gluten-sensitive enteropathy, giardiasis, and even carbohydrate malabsorption (sucrase-isomaltase deficiency) can be associated with mild steatorrhea, usually without gross evidence of fecal fat. In gluten-sensitive enteropathy, the malabsorption is usually mild, and failure to thrive is more typically related to anorexia. Hypothyroidism is associated with constipation; steatorrhea is rare and mild. (See Chapter 286 in *Nelson Textbook of Pediatrics*, 15th ed.)

44. D. The acute phase response to inflammation that is most likely to be encountered in Crohn disease is an elevation of the platelet count (typically >500,000/mm³). As the disease is brought under control with treatment, the count usually returns to normal. The erythrocyte sedimentation rate (ESR) can be elevated, but this is less likely than an elevated platelet count. However, the ESR may not be elevated at all, even with fulminant colitis. Therefore, a normal ESR does not rule out the possibility of Crohn disease. The white blood cell count may or may not be elevated and is not a reliable index of bowel inflammation. The ANCA test result is positive in 65% of children with ulcerative colitis but only 20% of children with Crohn disease. Serum albumin level can be reduced because of protein-losing enteropathy or poor protein intake. (See Chapter 283.2 in *Nelson Textbook of Pediatrics*, 15th ed.)

45. B. Joint tenderness, episcleritis, erythema nodosum, and fever can be associated with either Crohn disease or ulcerative colitis. Prominent perianal skin tags (i.e., 1 to 3 cm in diameter) as well as perianal fistulas are findings that usually suggest Crohn disease. (See Chapter 283.2 in *Nelson Textbook of Pediatrics*, 15th ed.)

46. A. Stool electrolyte values are useful in distinguishing osmotic from secretory diarrhea. The stool electrolyte content is approximately two times the sum of the stool sodium and potassium content; in the example given in the question, this equals 70 mEq/L. Because stool is usually isotonic (~290 mOsm/L), the difference between the stool osmolality and electrolyte content is, in this example, about 220 mOsm/L. When the difference is greater than 50 mOsm/L, an exogenous osmotically active solute must be present. This can be a malabsorbed carbohydrate such as lactose in a lactose-intolerant individual. Bile acid malabsorption, neuroblastoma, ulcerative colitis, and pseudomembranous enterocolitis all are associated with secretory diarrhea, and the electrolyte content of the stool should account for greater than 240 mOsm/L. (See Chapter 287 in *Nelson Textbook of Pediatrics*, 15th ed.)

47. B. A practitioner would want to know whether the father of the child described in the question had had familial polyposis coli. An individual with familial polyposis coli has essentially a 100% chance of developing colon cancer, usually in young adulthood. The risk is generally thought to begin to increase after about 10 years of age; individuals at risk for inheriting this autosomal dominant trait require annual endosocopic screening, recommended to begin at about this time. Peutz-Jeghers syndrome is associated with an increased risk of development of cancer, although it is more likely to be extraintestinal rather than bowel cancer. The risk of developing colon cancer with juvenile polyposis coli or with neurofibromatosis is very low. If the father had colon cancer in association with ulcerative colitis, the child would have a greater risk of developing inflammatory bowel disease than the general population but would not require further evaluation unless symptoms developed. If the father had hereditary nonpolyposis colon cancer, the child would be at risk for developing colon cancer but not until after 20 years of age and would not require screening at the present age. (See Chapter 291 in *Nelson Textbook of Pediatrics*, 15th ed.)

48. A. The newest regimen in some transplant centers is FK506 (tacrolimus) and steroids. Perhaps with more experience, the more correct answer would be this new combination. However, the only correct

choice among those listed is *A*, because *B*, *C*, and *D* are outdated and choice *E* is in error. (See Chapter 313 in *Nelson Textbook of Pediatrics*, 15th ed.)

49. D. Many viruses are difficult management problems for an immunosuppressed host. Epstein-Barr virus may lead to various complications, the most ominous being progressive lymphoma. Awareness of this complication may allow earlier reduction of immune suppression and a possibly benign course. Measurement of titers may be helpful, especially if the patient has not been previously exposed to Epstein-Barr virus. (See Chapter 313 in *Nelson Textbook of Pediatrics*, 15th ed.)

50. E. Vitamin E deficiency is a major cause of morbidity in patients with prolonged cholestasis. (It is also responsible for symptoms in abetalipoproteinemia.) Previously, the management of this deficiency was quite difficult, and parenteral therapy occasionally was necessary. Awareness of this problem is mandatory for physicians who are caring for patients with cholestasis. (See Chapter 302.1 in *Nelson Textbook of Pediatrics*, 15th ed.)

51. C. Biliary atresia is an important indication for liver transplantation. There are 300 to 400 new cases of extrahepatic biliary atresia each year in the United States. Pediatricians should be familiar with its diagnosis, initial therapy, and the role of liver transplantation in the management of this condition. (See Chapter 302.1 in *Nelson Textbook of Pediatrics*, 15th ed.)

52. C. Pancreatitis is rarely associated with the other conditions listed in the question, despite elevations of serum amylase levels. (See Chapter 297 in *Nelson Textbook of Pediatrics*, 15th ed.)

53. D. ERCP is an endoscopic-radiographic technique for visualization of the ducts of the pancreas and biliary tree. Ductal disorders such as strictures, choledochal cyst, and intraductal stones are common causes of recurrent pancreatitis. Serum amylase determination confirms the diagnosis of pancreatitis. A CT scan or ultrasonography can confirm the diagnosis of pancreatitis and diagnose complications such as pseudocyst but cannot determine the underlying causes of pancreatitis. Undiagnosed cystic fibrosis is an unlikely cause of recurrent pancreatitis. (See Chapter 297 in *Nelson Textbook of Pediatrics*, 15th ed.)

54. B. Pancreas divisum is an anatomic abnormality of the pancreas due to the failure of fusion of the dorsal and ventral pancreatic ductal systems. Functionally, the pancreas is normal. The other three entities listed in the question all are characterized by exocrine pancreatic failure. (See Chapter 293.1 in *Nelson Textbook of Pediatrics*, 15th ed.)

55. C. The bentiromide test is based on the ability of chymotrypsin to digest a synthetic peptide and release *P*-aminobenzoic acid, which is then absorbed and excreted in the urine. This test result is abnormal in pancreatic insufficiency, regardless of the cause, because there is inadequate chymotrypsin for digestion of this peptide. (See Chapter 294 in *Nelson Textbook of Pediatrics*, 15th ed.)

56. C. Remember that a mass in the labium of a female may be a gonad (testis, ovum-testis, ovary). (See Chapter 292 in *Nelson Textbook of Pediatrics*, 15th ed.)

57. E. Choices *A* to *D* must be considered in the differential diagnosis but are usually discernible by the history and the findings on physical examination. (See Chapter 292 in *Nelson Textbook of Pediatrics*, 15th ed.)

58. C. In the absence of incarceration, a hernia may be operated on an elective basis, depending on the general condition of the patient. The elective basis is usually soon after the diagnosis is made, to avoid the complications of incarceration or strangulation. (See Chapter 292 in *Nelson Textbook of Pediatrics*, 15th ed.)

59. C. Failure of the processus vaginalis to obliterate is the most common pathology producing hernias in males. (See Chapter 292 in *Nelson Textbook of Pediatrics*, 15th ed.)

60. B. Indirect inguinal hernias are the most common. (See Chapter 292 in *Nelson Textbook of Pediatrics*, 15th ed.)

61. C. Sacral agenesis may reduce the ability for continence in the future. (See Chapter 281 in *Nelson Textbook of Pediatrics*, 15th ed.)

62. B. Many patients with a rectourethral fistula may pass meconium through the urethra. (See Chapter 281 in *Nelson Textbook of Pediatrics*, 15th ed.)

63. B. Many patients with a vestibular fistula pass meconium through the fistula. (See Chapter 281 in *Nelson Textbook of Pediatrics*, 15th ed.)

64. C. The first consideration in a neonate with an anorectal malformation is the need for a colostomy. The next is the risk for urologic

problems, and the third is the possibility of other malformations. (See Chapter 281 in *Nelson Textbook of Pediatrics*, 15th ed.)

65. B. Cystic fibrosis and other disorders associated with malabsorption or chronic diarrhea are risk factors for rectal prolapse. (See Chapter 290.4 in *Nelson Textbook of Pediatrics*, 15th ed.)

66. B. Crohn disease and prior anorectal abscesses are diseases associated with perianal fistula formation. (See Chapter 290.2 in *Nelson Textbook of Pediatrics*, 15th ed.)

67. A. Idiopathic perianal abscess most often occurs in the first 2 years of life. The abscess contains a mixed bacterial flora such as gram-negative enteric organisms, *Staphylococcus aureus*, and anaerobic bacteria. (See Chapter 290.2 in *Nelson Textbook of Pediatrics*, 15th ed.)

68. C. Stool softeners, bran, and so on are of value in treating anal fissures. (See Chapter 290.1 in *Nelson Textbook of Pediatrics*, 15th ed.)

69. A. Unfortunately, despite improvement with antacids or H$_2$-blocking agents, *H. pylori*–positive patients frequently suffer a relapse with these treatments. (See Chapter 282.1 in *Nelson Textbook of Pediatrics*, 15th ed.)

70. D. The patient described in the question may have a tracheoesophageal fistula as part of the VATER syndrome (vertebral, anal, tracheoesophageal, radial-renal). Congenital heart disease is also an associated anomaly. Intelligence is normal, and central nervous system malformations are rare or nonexistent. (See Chapter 265 in *Nelson Textbook of Pediatrics*, 15th ed.)

71. E. Hearing aid batteries are highly corrosive and must be removed if swallowed. The location in the boy described in the question also suggests that it will not pass into his stomach. (See Chapter 273 in *Nelson Textbook of Pediatrics*, 15th ed.)

72. E. The patient described in the question has achalasia, which is traditionally managed surgically. A few patients have responded to intraesophageal injection of botulinum toxin. (See Chapter 267 in *Nelson Textbook of Pediatrics*, 15th ed.)

73. E. Stress ulcers are frequently gastric and unrelated to *H. pylori*. (See Chapter 282.2 in *Nelson Textbook of Pediatrics*, 15th ed.)

74. C. The pneumococcus is a common pathogen in any condition causing ascites (nephrosis, cirrhosis). Next in frequency is *Escherichia coli*. (See Chapters 315 and 316 in *Nelson Textbook of Pediatrics*, 15th ed.)

75. B. Leukocytosis, acidosis, and positive Gram stain or culture results help confirm the diagnosis of primary peritonitis, usually caused by the pneumococcus or less often *E. coli*. (See Chapter 316.1 in *Nelson Textbook of Pediatrics*, 15th ed.)

76. B. A low-fat diet potentially enriched with medium-chain triglycerides, which do not require lymphatic-chylous transport and are absorbed directly into the circulation, is appropriate for the treatment of an infant with postsurgical chylous ascites. (See Chapter 315.1 in *Nelson Textbook of Pediatrics*, 15th ed.)

77. D. Ascitic fluid with a milky appearance suggests chylous ascites or effusion but is helpful only if the child has recently received a milk feeding. (See Chapter 315.1 in *Nelson Textbook of Pediatrics*, 15th ed.)

19 The Respiratory System

1. D. Choanal atresia is complete obstruction of the nasal passages, usually due to bony obliteration of the nasal airway. Mouth breathing during crying bypasses the obstruction, but in quiet states, an affected newborn may become an obligate nasal breather. Treatment requires an oral airway and nasal surgery. (See Chapter 325 in *Nelson Textbook of Pediatrics*, 15th ed.)

2. C. Asplenia is not usually associated with choanal atresia. Other anomalies may constitute the CHARGE syndrome: coloboma, heart disease, atresia choanae, retarded growth (or CNS anomalies), genital anomalies, and ear anomalies (or deafness). (See Chapter 325 in *Nelson Textbook of Pediatrics*, 15th ed.)

3. B. Laryngeotracheomalacia, a congenital weakness of the larynx and trachea, often causes positional airway obstruction that worsens with upper airway infections. The child described in the question has an acute upper respiratory tract infection exacerbating the congenital lesion. (See Chapter 331.2 in *Nelson Textbook of Pediatrics*, 15th ed.)

4. B. Pulmonary sequestration should be suggested by recurrent episodes of pneumonia in a location that does not change with time. Lower lobes are frequently involved. The sequestered lung receives its blood supply from the aorta, not the pulmonary artery. This can be determined by Doppler ultrasonography or

by aortography. (See Chapter 331.4 in *Nelson Textbook of Pediatrics*, 15th ed.)

5. 1. A
   2. C
   3. A
   4. B
   5. C
   6. B
   7. B
   8. A
   9. A
   10. B
   (See Chapter 327 in *Nelson Textbook of Pediatrics*, 15th ed.)

6. D. Foreign body aspiration into the trachea or bronchi is often heralded by the abrupt onset of cough, choking, and wheezing. The age group at highest risk is small children younger than 3 years. Either bronchus may contain the foreign body. (See Chapter 333 in *Nelson Textbook of Pediatrics*, 15th ed.)

7. D. For the child described in the question, administer oxygen and provide supportive care. Further emesis may cause aspiration pneumonia, as might gastric lavage. (See Chapter 340.2 in *Nelson Textbook of Pediatrics*, 15th ed.)

8. D. Allergic bronchopulmonary aspergillosis occurs when *Aspergillus* organisms colonize the bronchi and produce an inflammatory reaction that resembles or exacerbates asthma or even cystic fibrosis. The treatment of choice is prednisone. (See Chapter 344 in *Nelson Textbook of Pediatrics*, 15th ed.)

9. D. Goodpasture syndrome, although uncommon, does occur in children and presents with renal impairment and hemoptysis. Circulating antibasement membrane antibodies are usually present. (See Chapter 349 in *Nelson Textbook of Pediatrics*, 15th ed.)

10. D. Pulmonary embolism must be considered with the sudden onset of chest pain, dyspnea, and cyanosis. A normal-appearing chest radiograph with significant hypoxia is classic for a pulmonary embolism. (See Chapter 356 in *Nelson Textbook of Pediatrics*, 15th ed.)

11. E. Pulmonary alveolar proteinosis, in both the neonatal and adult forms, rarely causes hemoptysis. The neonatal form produces severe hypoxia, respiratory failure, and death despite extracorporeal membrane oxygenation (ECMO). Lung transplantation is the only treatment available for the neonatal form. (See Chapter 356.1 in *Nelson Textbook of Pediatrics*, 15th ed.)

12. D. Other intestinal obstruction is possible and includes neonatal meconium ileus, congenital ileal atresia, neonatal mucus plug syndrome, meconium ileus equivalent (from insufficient use of pancreatic enzyme replacement), intussusception, inguinal hernias, and appendiceal obstruction. (See Chapter 363 in *Nelson Textbook of Pediatrics*, 15th ed.)

13. E. *Pseudomonas aeruginosa* bacteremia is uncommon despite the active and persistent pulmonary infection with this significant bacterial agent. (See Chapter 363 in *Nelson Textbook of Pediatrics*, 15th ed.)

14. C. Chest physiotherapy may be dangerous during an acute episode of hemoptysis and is usually discontinued. (See Chapter 363 in *Nelson Textbook of Pediatrics*, 15th ed.)

15. D. Sweat chloride should be determined in a child with recurrent pneumonia, diarrhea, and poor growth. Other indications for a sweat chloride test include hemoptysis, a family history of cystic fibrosis, male azoospermia, pansinusitis, hypochloremic alkalosis, meconium ileus or plug, rectal prolapse, biliary cirrhosis, hypoproteinemia, or deficiencies of vitamins E, K, D, or A. (See Chapter 363 in *Nelson Textbook of Pediatrics*, 15th ed.)

16. D. Peritonsillar abscess often follows or complicates pharyngitis. As the tonsillar abscess develops, trismus, deviation of the uvula away from the abscess, and intense pain ensue. Treatment is with penicillin and aspiration of the abscess cavity. (See Chapter 327.7 in *Nelson Textbook of Pediatrics*, 15th ed.)

17. A. Penicillin is the treatment of choice for dental space infections with secondary facial space inflammation. In the patient described in the question, the left canine (cuspid) tooth was tender and abscessed. After penicillin therapy, the tooth was extracted. (See Chapter 258 in *Nelson Textbook of Pediatrics*, 15th ed.)

18. C. Empyema and chylothorax are not sudden in onset, and staphylococcal pneumonia is not likely in adolescents. (See Chapter 366 in *Nelson Textbook of Pediatrics*, 15th ed.)

19. E. (See Chapter 362 in *Nelson Textbook of Pediatrics*, 15th ed.)

20. B and C. (See Chapter 362 in *Nelson Textbook of Pediatrics*, 15th ed.)

21. D. This case sounds like an allergic reactive airway disease, perhaps even a first attack of asthma. Coughing is one manifestation

of asthma even in the absence of wheezing. The family history, lack of evidence of chronic disease, nocturnal symptoms, and wheezes all point to that diagnosis. (See Chapter 137 in *Nelson Textbook of Pediatrics*, 15th ed.)

22. B. (See Chapter 333 in *Nelson Textbook of Pediatrics*, 15th ed.)

23. B. (See Chapter 333 in *Nelson Textbook of Pediatrics*, 15th ed.)

24. C. (See Chapter 333 in *Nelson Textbook of Pediatrics*, 15th ed.)

25. C. With a toxic child, admission is reasonable, and blood culture offers the best chance of diagnosis. Ceftriaxone is a reasonable drug of choice. The recurrence, however, is the tip-off that something else is going on, and in this age group a foreign body is common—thus the need for bronchoscopy. (See Chapter 333 in *Nelson Textbook of Pediatrics*, 15th ed.)

26. A. Neonatal pulmonary alveolar proteinosis is a distinct entity from adolescent-adult–onset alveolar proteinosis. (See Chapter 350 in *Nelson Textbook of Pediatrics*, 15th ed.)

27. D. Patients with the neonatal form of pulmonary alveolar proteinosis have been treated with ECMO of varying duration with a temporizing improvement in oxygenation. (See Chapter 350 in *Nelson Textbook of Pediatrics*, 15th ed.)

28. B. Lung transplantation is the only known available therapy for neonatal alveolar proteinosis. (See Chapter 350 in *Nelson Textbook of Pediatrics*, 15th ed.)

29. A. Defects in the gene encoding the surfactant associated protein SP-B are the cause of the neonatal form of lethal alveolar proteinosis. (See Chapter 350 in *Nelson Textbook of Pediatrics*, 15th ed.)

30. B. Bronchoscopy is the approach of choice to visualize and remove a bronchial foreign body. (See Chapter 333 in *Nelson Textbook of Pediatrics*, 15th ed.)

31. E. The etiology of spasmodic croup is poorly understood or is multifactorial. (See Chapter 332 in *Nelson Textbook of Pediatrics*, 15th ed.)

32. E. α_1-Antitrypsin deficiency rarely causes lung disease during childhood and has never been associated with reflux. (See Chapter 354.4 in *Nelson Textbook of Pediatrics*, 15th ed.)

20 The Cardiovascular System

1. C. The murmur may represent a patent ductus arteriosus (PDA). If the PDA closes, marked cyanosis would supervene and result in acidosis, shock, and death. Prostaglandin E_1 (PGE$_1$) maintains patency of the ductus arteriosus between the pulmonary artery and the aorta. (See Chapters 82.2, 87.3, and 386.8 in *Nelson Textbook of Pediatrics*, 15th ed.)

2. D. Pulmonary atresia is manifested by a small right ventricle, decreased pulmonary vascular markings, early and marked cyanosis without heart failure, and ductal dependence to maintain some pulmonary blood flow. (See Chapter 387.4 in *Nelson Textbook of Pediatrics*, 15th ed.)

3. C. The child described in the question is suffering from tetralogy of Fallot with exercise-induced cyanosis. The more serious episode is a cyanotic, blue, or "tet" spell and may be due to decreased systemic vascular resistance, increased pulmonary artery pressure, or right ventricular outflow tract obstruction. The murmur of tetralogy (the pulmonary stenosis) often disappears or lessens during a spell. (See Chapter 387.2 in *Nelson Textbook of Pediatrics*, 15th ed.)

4. A. Epinephrine is potentially dangerous because it may exacerbate inotropy and contractile forces, which may obstruct the right ventricular infundibulum. Indeed, propranolol has been used to treat "tet" spells. (See Chapter 387.2 in *Nelson Textbook of Pediatrics,* 15th ed.)

5. G. No surgical approach has been found for total correction of tricuspid atresia. The modified Fontan operation is the choice for surgical management. Depending on the pulmonary blood flow, choices *B, E,* or *F* may develop before surgery. (See Chapter 387.5 in *Nelson Textbook of Pediatrics*, 15th ed.)

6. D. VSDs are not noted in patients with Ebstein anomaly. (See Chapter 387.8 in *Nelson Textbook of Pediatrics*, 15th ed.)

7. A. Total anomalous venous return with obstruction of the venous return presents with severe and immediate refractory cyanosis and a white-out (respiratory distress [RDS]-like, pulmonary edema-like) pattern on chest radiographs. The diagnosis is confirmed by echocardiography or cardiac catheterization. (See Chapter 387.14 in *Nelson Textbook of Pediatrics*, 15th ed.)

8. B. Poor pulses, reduced left ventricular forces on ECG, cardiogenic shock, and severe cyanosis are typical of hypoplastic left

heart syndrome. (See Chapter 387.17 in *Nelson Textbook of Pediatrics*, 15th ed.)

9. 1. A
   2. C
   3. A
   4. A
   5. C
   6. B
   7. A
   8. B
   9. D
   (See Chapter 387.18 in *Nelson Textbook of Pediatrics*, 15th ed.)

10. C. (See Chapter 388.1 in *Nelson Textbook of Pediatrics*, 15th ed.)

11. B. Placing an iced saline bag over a neonate's face is the vagal maneuver of choice to break supraventricular tachycardia (SVT). (See Chapter 388.1 in *Nelson Textbook of Pediatrics*, 15th ed.)

12. C. Adenosine is the treatment of choice to break SVT in most age groups. Verapamil in neonates has been associated with cardiac arrest owing to its negative inotropic effects. DC cardioversion is indicated only in hemodynamically unstable patients. (See Chapter 388.1 in *Nelson Textbook of Pediatrics*, 15th ed.)

13. C. Atrial septal defects (ASDs) have low flow, a minimal jetlike stream, and little turbulence. (See Chapter 390 in *Nelson Textbook of Pediatrics*, 15th ed.)

14. 1. C
   2. D
   3. A
   4. E
   5. B
   6. G
   7. F
   (See Chapter 380 in *Nelson Textbook of Pediatrics*, 15th ed.)

15. A. Central nervous system (CNS) lesions are more often associated with right-to-left shunts. Intraoperative CNS lesions are possible in all types of congenital heart disease. (See Chapters 386.1–386.11 in *Nelson Textbook of Pediatrics*, 15th ed.)

16. 1. C
   2. A
   3. B
   4. E
   5. F
   6. D
   7. H
   8. G
   9. I
   (See Chapter 380 in *Nelson Textbook of Pediatrics*, 15th ed.)

17. C. A small, restrictive VSD is quite common. The vast majority create a loud murmur and palpable thrill but often close spontaneously before 5 years of age. (See Chapter 386.6 in *Nelson Textbook of Pediatrics*, 15th ed.)

18. C. A large VSD with a large left-to-right shunt produces significant heart failure. The age of onset usually corresponds to the time when the normally high fetal pulmonary vascular resistance declines in the first 1 to 3 months of life. With decreasing pulmonary artery pressure, the left-to-right shunt increases. (See Chapter 386.6 in *Nelson Textbook of Pediatrics*, 15th ed.)

19. A. Six months after the time of repair, patients with a previous PDA or ASD–ostium secundum without a patch no longer need antibiotic prophylaxis for endocarditis. (See Chapter 386.8 in *Nelson Textbook of Pediatrics*, 15th ed.)

20. C. Balloon valvuloplasty has greatly improved the management of stenotic lesions of the pulmonic and aortic valves. (See Chapter 386.12 in *Nelson Textbook of Pediatrics*, 15th ed.)

21. D. The lower extremity blood pressure of the patient described in the question was 90/70 mm Hg, confirming the diagnosis of coarctation of the aorta. One must be careful before treating upper extremity hypertension in a child with a coarctation. (See Chapter 386.17 in *Nelson Textbook of Pediatrics*, 15th ed.)

22. D. Migraines are unusual in the situation described in the question. Severe headache should suggest hypertension due to recurrent coarctation or essential hypertension with or without intracranial subarachnoid hemorrhage. (See Chapter 386.17 in *Nelson Textbook of Pediatrics*, 15th ed.)

23. A. The child described in the question is having angina-like episodes. The ECG reveals lateral wall myocardial infarction (wide Q waves in leads I, V_5, and V_6) and elevated ST segments in V_5 and V_6. (See Chapter 386.27 in *Nelson Textbook of Pediatrics*, 15th ed.)

24. B. Failure to thrive is much more common than obesity in children with Eisenmenger syndrome. (See Chapter 386.28 in *Nelson Textbook of Pediatrics*, 15th ed.)

25. A. Paradoxic pulse is also noted in asthma. (See Chapter 397.1 in *Nelson Textbook of Pediatrics*, 15th ed.)

26. B. An apical heave occurs with left

ventricular hypertrophy. (See Chapter 380 in *Nelson Textbook of Pediatrics*, 15th ed.)

27. C. Choice *B* would be a venous hum, and *D* an innocent pulmonic murmur. A Still murmur is most common between 3 and 7 years of age, so *E* is incorrect, and it is innocent, so *A* is also wrong. (See Chapter 380 in *Nelson Textbook of Pediatrics*, 15th ed.)

28. B. VSDs are most common in infants and children. (See Chapter 386.6 in *Nelson Textbook of Pediatrics*, 15th ed.)

29. A. Of all the aortic stenosis syndromes, the supravalvular type is rare but is the only type associated with the features mentioned in the question. (See Chapter 386.16 in *Nelson Textbook of Pediatrics*, 15th ed.)

30. A. Mitral insufficiency occurs first. Mitral or aortic stenosis (also aortic insufficiency) may follow after a number of years. Tricuspid insufficiency is uncommon. (See Chapter 391 in *Nelson Textbook of Pediatrics*, 15th ed.)

31. C. Rib notching is caused by increased collateral arteries trying to supply the lower trunk and extremities and bypass the aortic coarctation. (See Chapter 386.17 in *Nelson Textbook of Pediatrics*, 15th ed.)

32. D. The critical laboratory test in the diagnosis of subacute bacterial endocarditis is the blood culture. All others are secondary. Blood cultures should be of sufficient volume and incubated for sufficient time to detect low-grade bacteremia and fastidious slow-growing organisms. (See Chapter 390 in *Nelson Textbook of Pediatrics*, 15th ed.)

33. B. Weight loss, diet, and exercise may significantly lower the blood pressure of hypertensive obese adolescents. (See Chapter 404 in *Nelson Textbook of Pediatrics*, 15th ed.)

34. A. ACE inhibitors are very effective in all cases of non–catecholamine-induced hypertension but particularly those caused by activation of the renin-angiotensin-aldosterone system. (See Chapter 404 in *Nelson Textbook of Pediatrics*, 15th ed.)

35. E. Primary renal pathology (anomalies, reflux, and so on) are most often associated with hypertension in young children. (See Chapter 404 in *Nelson Textbook of Pediatrics*, 15th ed.)

36. C. Anxiety (white-coat hypertension) may frequently increase the blood pressure on a first visit. Blood pressure should be determined several times on that and subsequent visits to diagnose hypertension.

(See Chapter 404 in *Nelson Textbook of Pediatrics*, 15th ed.)

21 Diseases of the Blood

1. A. A complete blood count (CBC) reveals a hemoglobin value of 12 g/dL, a white blood cell (WBC) count of 11,000, and a platelet count of 5000. (See Chapter 439.4 in *Nelson Textbook of Pediatrics*, 15th ed.)

2. D. Idiopathic thrombocytopenia (ITP) or autoimmune thrombocytopenia is an acute process that often follows an upper respiratory tract infection. Leukemia is always a worrisome possibility but is extremely unusual in the absence of anemia, leukopenia or blasts, lymphadenopathy, or hepatosplenomegaly. (See Chapter 439.4 in *Nelson Textbook of Pediatrics*, 15th ed.)

3. B. The boy described in the question has hemophilia A. His factor VIII level was 4%, which is in the moderate severity category. (See Chapter 432.1 in *Nelson Textbook of Pediatrics*, 15th ed.)

4. D. (See Chapter 432.1 in *Nelson Textbook of Pediatrics*, 15th ed.)

5. B. Factor VIII antibodies (IgG) develop in 10% to 15% of patients with hemophilia and are not related to the number of replacement therapies. (See Chapter 432.1 in *Nelson Textbook of Pediatrics*, 15th ed.)

6. C. Immunosuppression alone is ineffective, but perhaps combined with immune tolerance and intravenous immunoglobulin therapy, it may be of value. (See Chapter 432.1 in *Nelson Textbook of Pediatrics*, 15th ed.)

7. 1. B
   2. C
   3. A
   4. D
   5. F
   6. E
   (See Chapters 406–418, 423, and 449 in *Nelson Textbook of Pediatrics*, 15th ed.)

8. D. Methemoglobinemia presents with intense cyanosis, desaturated hemoglobin, chocolate-colored blood, but a normal PaO_2. Treatment for significant methemoglobinemia includes methylene blue. Methemoglobinemia can be measured in the blood sample; subsequent studies are needed to determine if this is a defect in the hemoglobin (hemoglobin M) or more likely in the NADH cytochrome b5 reductase system. (See Chapter 419.7 in *Nelson Textbook of Pediatrics*, 15th ed.)

9. B. Sickle cell anemia is associated with at least two defects of host defense: splenic hypofunction and a defect in opsonization by the properdin system. Both defects predispose to bacteremia and meningitis due to encapsulated organisms, in particular pneumococci. Without antibiotic prophylaxis, 1 in 25 children with sickle cell anemia will develop pneumococcal meningitis. (See Chapter 419 in *Nelson Textbook of Pediatrics*, 15th ed.)

10. D. (See Chapter 419 in *Nelson Textbook of Pediatrics*, 15th ed.)

11. D. Intravenous vancomycin is now indicated because patients may have a penicillin (cephalosporin)-resistant pneumococcal infection. In some institutions where resistant pneumococci are prevalent, infectious disease consultants recommend *beginning* therapy with a combination of vancomycin *and* ceftriaxone. (See Chapter 179 in *Nelson Textbook of Pediatrics*, 15th ed.)

12. E. Aplastic crisis is due to parvovirus B19. (See Chapter 419 in *Nelson Textbook of Pediatrics*, 15th ed.)

13. D. Spherocytosis is an autosomal dominant (or recessive) disease with hemolysis, neonatal hyperbilirubinemia, and splenomegaly. As in many chronic hemolytic anemias, a family history of splenectomy (to reduce splenic destruction of red blood cells [RBCs]) or cholecystectomy (for bilirubinate gallstones) is helpful. (See Chapter 415 in *Nelson Textbook of Pediatrics*, 15th ed.)

14. 1. D
    2. E
    3. F
    4. A
    5. G
    6. B
    7. C
    (See Chapters 415–422 in *Nelson Textbook of Pediatrics*, 15th ed.)

15. C. Iron deficiency anemia is the most common type of anemia in toddlers and is associated with poor iron intake (cow's milk) and with gastrointestinal blood loss (cow's milk allergic colitis). The very low MCV, suggestive of thalassemia, is also characteristic of iron deficiency. (See Chapter 413 in *Nelson Textbook of Pediatrics*, 15th ed.)

16. D. Folate deficiency, a megaloblastic anemia, is common in infants fed goat's milk, which is severely deficient in folate. (See

Chapter 412.1 in *Nelson Textbook of Pediatrics*, 15th ed.)

17. B. Iron deficiency may be common in children with chronic diseases treated with anti-inflammatory agents, which cause gastrointestinal blood loss. If the iron deficiency is significant, erythropoietin is unable to stimulate erythropoiesis. (See Chapter 413 in *Nelson Textbook of Pediatrics*, 15th ed.)

18. C. The CBC reveals a hemoglobin value of 6 g/dL with a reticulocyte count of 1.0%. The platelet and WBC counts are normal. (See Chapter 405 in *Nelson Textbook of Pediatrics*, 15th ed.)

19. A. Congenital hypoplastic anemia (Diamond-Blackfan syndrome) usually presents between 2 and 3 months of age, a time when other causes of anemia (iron deficiency, transient erythroblastopenia of childhood) are unusual. (See Chapter 406 in *Nelson Textbook of Pediatrics*, 15th ed.)

20. 1. A
    2. B
    3. A
    4. B
    5. C
    6. A
    7. C
    8. B
    (See Chapter 405 in *Nelson Textbook of Pediatrics*, 15th ed.)

21. 1. A
    2. D
    3. B
    4. A
    5. B
    6. A
    7. A
    8. D
    9. C
    (See Chapters 406 and 408 in *Nelson Textbook of Pediatrics*, 15th ed.)

22. D. Physiologic anemia occurs at 3 months of age. (See Chapter 411 in *Nelson Textbook of Pediatrics*, 15th ed.)

23. A. This is a classic case of iron deficiency anemia, undoubtedly nutritional in origin. Pica is a common symptom and makes lead poisoning a possible diagnosis but not the most likely diagnosis. (See Chapter 413 in *Nelson Textbook of Pediatrics*, 15th ed.)

24. B. Reticulocytosis peaks at 5 to 7 days. (See Chapter 413 in *Nelson Textbook of Pediatrics*, 15th ed.)

25. C. Stores of iron need to be repleted, and 4 to

8 weeks is required. (See Chapter 413 in *Nelson Textbook of Pediatrics*, 15th ed.)

26. A, B, and E. Sickle cell anemia is not usually seen in Caucasians, and urinary tract infection is highly unlikely in an otherwise healthy boy. (See Chapter 405 in *Nelson Textbook of Pediatrics*, 15th ed.)

27. 1. B. Purpura, but with normal counts
    2. B. Adhesiveness is impaired
    3. A. Idiopathic thrombocytopenic purpura, obviously
    4. A. Also eczema and immune deficiency
    5. C. Thrombocytosis is common
    6. A. Platelets are consumed along with the factors
    7. A. The name gives the answer again
    8. A. On the basis of trapping of the platelets in the cavernous hemangioma
    (See Chapter 439 in *Nelson Textbook of Pediatrics*, 15th ed.)

28. C. It is hoped that as screening tests for all hepatitis viruses improve, the incidence will become even lower. Nonetheless, posttransfusion hepatitis carries significant morbidities and should be avoided if possible by reducing the use of blood products. (See Chapter 430 in *Nelson Textbook of Pediatrics*, 15th ed.)

29. B. Fresh frozen plasma is a good source of protein C. The child described in *B* probably has a homozygotic deficiency of this anticoagulant protein. (See Chapter 429 in *Nelson Textbook of Pediatrics*, 15th ed.)

30. C. Thrombocytopenia in "sick" neonates, due to any condition, places these neonates at risk for severe intracranial bleeding. The risk may be greatest in isoimmune thrombocytopenia, however, even in the absence of comorbidities such as respiratory distress syndrome. (See Chapter 427 in *Nelson Textbook of Pediatrics*, 15th ed.)

31. A. With such a low hemoglobin level, together with significant pulmonary disease and risk of hypoxia, this child's oxygen delivery (oxygen-carrying capacity and cardiac output) is significantly reduced. (See Chapter 426 in *Nelson Textbook of Pediatrics*, 15th ed.)

32. C. In the child described in the question, suspect an infectious lymphadenitis, most often due to draining infection from the oral cavity and due to streptococci, staphylococci, or anaerobes. (See Chapter 444 in *Nelson Textbook of Pediatrics*, 15th ed.)

33. C. A firm, rubbery consistency suggests malignancy. All the other choices suggest infection/inflammation. (See Chapter 444 in *Nelson Textbook of Pediatrics*, 15th ed.)

34. B. Posteroanterior and lateral chest radiographs are an important screening method to determine the presence of hilar or other intrathoracic nodes. Suspect malignancy! (See Chapter 444 in *Nelson Textbook of Pediatrics*, 15th ed.)

35. A. A mild to moderate degree of splenic hypofunction is present in premature infants. (See Chapter 442 in *Nelson Textbook of Pediatrics*, 15th ed.)

36. D. Neonatal exchange transfusion through the umbilical vein may produce omphalitis and septic phlebitis of the portal system. Extrahepatic portal obstruction may then produce hypersplenism. Omphalitis in the absence of exchange transfusion is also a risk. (See Chapter 441 in *Nelson Textbook of Pediatrics*, 15th ed.)

37. E. The risk of infection with pneumococci is greatly increased and may last for the life of the patient. Prophylaxis with penicillin is recommended. (See Chapter 442 in *Nelson Textbook of Pediatrics*, 15th ed.)

38. B. The mild to moderately affected patient described in the question will benefit from partial splenectomy. This procedure may not be available in all institutions. Therefore, the balance between anemia and total splenectomy must be weighed. (See Chapter 442 in *Nelson Textbook of Pediatrics*, 15th ed.)

39. C. Abdominal ultrasonography is a good screening test that presents little risk and no radiation exposure. (See Chapter 441 in *Nelson Textbook of Pediatrics*, 15th ed.)

40. 1. C
    2. B
    3. B
    4. A
    5. A
    6. C
    7. B
    8. A
    (See Chapter 405 in *Nelson Textbook of Pediatrics*, 15th ed.)

41. E. The values listed in the question are normal, thus emphasizing the need to know age-adjusted normal values for hemoglobin *and* MCV. (See Chapter 405 in *Nelson Textbook of Pediatrics*, 15th ed.)

42. A. Intrauterine hypoxia associated with intrauterine growth retardation produces fetal and hence neonatal polycythemia. Additional fetal causes of polycythemia include diabetes in the mother, Down

syndrome, hyperthyroidism, and adrenogenital syndrome. (See Part XXI, Section 4 in *Nelson Textbook of Pediatrics*, 15th ed.)

43. B. Familial-genetic defects in hemoglobin (higher than usual affinity for oxygen) may produce compensatory polycythemia. (See Chapter 419.6 in *Nelson Textbook of Pediatrics*, 15th ed.)

44. E. Additional features include an elevated serum indirect bilirubin and lactate dehydrogenase level, abnormal findings on a blood smear, positive Coombs test results, and a reduced haptoglobin value. (See Part XXI, Section 3 in *Nelson Textbook of Pediatrics*, 15th ed.)

45. D. Sickle cell anemia is usually normocytic and without spherocytes but obviously with sickled cells. (See Chapter 419 in *Nelson Textbook of Pediatrics*, 15th ed.)

46. D. Oxidant drug–induced hemolysis with anemia and hemoglobinuria is common in G6PD-deficient patients. (See Chapter 420.3 in *Nelson Textbook of Pediatrics*, 15th ed.)

47. B. The enzyme assay is of value, but results may be falsely normal immediately after a hemolytic episode because younger cells may have normal G6PD levels. (See Chapter 420.3 in *Nelson Textbook of Pediatrics*, 15th ed.)

48. B. No treatment is required unless the anemia worsens, and a transfusion is then needed. Forced diuresis is needed to prevent hemoglobinuric renal failure. (See Chapter 420.3 in *Nelson Textbook of Pediatrics*, 15th ed.)

49. E. Immune-mediated hemolysis often produces spherocytes. (See Chapter 421 in *Nelson Textbook of Pediatrics*, 15th ed.)

50. D. The Coombs tests detect antibody directed against RBCs. Further analysis determines the IgM or IgG nature of the autoantibodies. (See Chapter 421 in *Nelson Textbook of Pediatrics*, 15th ed.)

51. D. Many would begin prednisone as the initial treatment of choice for autoimmune hemolytic anemia. (See Chapter 421 in *Nelson Textbook of Pediatrics*, 15th ed.)

52. C. Parvovirus B19 (agent in erythema infectiosum-fifth disease) is the most common identifiable cause of aplastic crisis. (See Chapter 407 in *Nelson Textbook of Pediatrics*, 15th ed.)

53. E. If the reticulocyte count is low, autoimmune antibodies may be destroying the reticulocytes too. (See Part XXI, Section 3 in *Nelson Textbook of Pediatrics*, 15th ed.)

54. D. Both elevated values for hemoglobin A_2 and fetal hemoglobin are compatible with this diagnosis. (See Chapter 419.9 in *Nelson Textbook of Pediatrics*, 15th ed.)

55. E. Methemoglobinemia has many causes, as evidenced by the three answers to this question. (See Chapter 419 in *Nelson Textbook of Pediatrics*, 15th ed.)

56. C. The patient described in the question is at very low risk for sickling unless exposed to severe hypoxia. (See Chapter 419.2 in *Nelson Textbook of Pediatrics*, 15th ed.)

57. A. The risk of pneumococcal sepsis and meningitis is much higher in patients with sickle cell anemia. This risk is significantly reduced by prophylactic antibiotics begun as soon as possible. (See Chapter 419 in *Nelson Textbook of Pediatrics*, 15th ed.)

58. E. α-Thalassemia, hemoglobin E, and β-thalassemia produce microcytosis and hemolysis, especially in patients from Southeast Asia. (See Chapter 419 in *Nelson Textbook of Pediatrics*, 15th ed.)

59. C. Factor VIII is not needed for platelet adhesion, but von Willebrand factor is. (See Chapter 432.1 in *Nelson Textbook of Pediatrics*, 15th ed.)

60. D. Factor VII is an important coagulation factor of the extrinsic or tissue coagulation pathway. This factor is called stable factor. (See Chapter 432.4 in *Nelson Textbook of Pediatrics*, 15th ed.)

61. C. Malabsorption of fat-soluble vitamins may occur with nutrient fat malabsorption. The patient described in the question may also have or develop vitamin D, E, or A deficiencies. (See Chapter 435 in *Nelson Textbook of Pediatrics*, 15th ed.)

62. C. Hemophilia A is characterized by factor VIII deficiency of various degrees of severity. The patient described in the question has mild disease (6 to 30 units/dL). (See Chapter 432.1 in *Nelson Textbook of Pediatrics*, 15th ed.)

63. A, C, and D. These are all important historical clues to the diagnosis of coagulopathies. (See Chapter 431 in *Nelson Textbook of Pediatrics*, 15th ed.)

64. A, B, C, and D. Only factor X is preserved. (See Chapter 438 in *Nelson Textbook of Pediatrics*, 15th ed.)

65. B. The prothrombin time is usually the first value to be prolonged in vitamin K deficiency and is never abnormal in classic hemophilia (factor VIII deficiency). (See

Chapter 431 in *Nelson Textbook of Pediatrics*, 15th ed.)

66. 1. C
    2. D
    3. B
    4. C
    (See Chapter 432 in *Nelson Textbook of Pediatrics*, 15th ed.)
67. C. The bleeding time tests the platelet vascular endothelium interaction, and results are abnormal in conditions with thrombocytopenia, platelet dysfunction, or abnormal endothelium. (See Chapter 431 in *Nelson Textbook of Pediatrics*, 15th ed.)
68. B. Phase one of coagulation is best studied with the PTT. Factor VIII deficiency (classic hemophilia) is suggested if this test result is prolonged while other coagulation test results are normal. Confirmation requires specific quantification of factor VIII levels. (See Chapter 431 in *Nelson Textbook of Pediatrics*, 15th ed.)

22 Neoplastic Diseases and Tumors

1. D. Leukemic relapse often recurs in the bone marrow. The central nervous system (CNS) (headache, cranial neuropathies) and testis (painless swelling) are the two most common extramedullary sites. (See Chapter 449 in *Nelson Textbook of Pediatrics*, 15th ed.)
2. C. Chest radiography is important for two reasons, first to document mediastinal involvement and second to determine if these lymph nodes threaten the patency of the airway. (See Chapter 450 in *Nelson Textbook of Pediatrics*, 15th ed.)
3. D. At this time, a lymph node biopsy can confirm the suspicion of Hodgkin disease. Thereafter, CT scans and bone marrow biopsy are useful in staging the extent of the lymph node and extranodal involvement. (See Chapter 450.1 in *Nelson Textbook of Pediatrics*, 15th ed.)
4. A. Secondary acute myelogenous leukemia (AML) may develop in a significant number of survivors of Hodgkin disease. The secondary AML may develop between 5 and 15 years later. Secondary solid tumors (breast cancer) may also occur. (See Chapter 450.1 in *Nelson Textbook of Pediatrics*, 15th ed.)
5. 1. C
   2. A
   3. B
   4. A
   5. A

6. A
7. D
8. B
9. B
10. A
11. B
    (See Chapters 451 and 452 in *Nelson Textbook of Pediatrics*, 15th ed.)
6. D. Orbital rhabdomyosarcoma is a common site for rhabdomyosarcoma, which produces local signs as it grows and displaces normal tissues. (See Chapter 453.1 in *Nelson Textbook of Pediatrics*, 15th ed.)
7. 1. A
   2. C
   3. B
   4. C
   5. A
   6. B
   7. D
   8. A
   9. C
   10. B
   (See Chapter 454 in *Nelson Textbook of Pediatrics*, 15th ed.)
8. E. Cases such as the one described in the question raise a suspicion of retinoblastoma and warrant immediate attention and visualization. A CT examination may also identify this ocular tumor. (See Chapter 455 in *Nelson Textbook of Pediatrics*, 15th ed.)
9. 1. C
   2. D
   3. C
   4. C
   5. A
   6. B
   (See Chapters 451, 456, and 457.1 in *Nelson Textbook of Pediatrics*, 15th ed.)
10. C. Panhypopituitarism may follow cranial irradiation and result in growth failure and delayed puberty. Cranial irradiation may also produce cognitive defects, and spinal radiation may produce scoliosis or may limit vertebral growth and the final height of the patient. (See Chapter 449 in *Nelson Textbook of Pediatrics*, 15th ed.)
11. D. Pneumococcal sepsis has developed in this survivor of Hodgkin disease because a splenectomy was performed at the time of the original diagnosis for staging purposes. The patient initially received prophylactic penicillin, and before the splenectomy he received the pneumococcal vaccine. At age 18 years, he stopped receiving penicillin

prophylaxis. (See Chapter 450.1 in *Nelson Textbook of Pediatrics*, 15th ed.)

12. B. Neuroblastoma involving the cervical sympathetic nervous system may present with Horner syndrome. (See Chapter 451 in *Nelson Textbook of Pediatrics*, 15th ed.)

13. D. The patient described in the question has had a cerebral hemorrhage, most likely due to the marked thrombocytopenia. A CT scan revealed the hemorrhage in the cortex. In all childhood cancer centers, severe thrombocytopenia is treated with platelet transfusion before signs of bleeding develop. (See Chapter 449.1 in *Nelson Textbook of Pediatrics*, 15th ed.)

14. D. Tumor lysis syndrome is most likely with a very high WBC count and acute lymphocytic leukemia, which is usually sensitive to chemotherapy. The serum uric acid level was 15.0, and uric acid crystals were noted in the urine sediment. (See Chapter 449 in *Nelson Textbook of Pediatrics*, 15th ed.)

15. 1. B
    2. D
    3. A
    4. C
    5. E
    (See Chapter 448.1 in *Nelson Textbook of Pediatrics*, 15th ed.)

16. 1. D
    2. A
    3. B
    4. C
    5. F
    6. D
    7. E
    (See Chapter 447 in *Nelson Textbook of Pediatrics*, 15th ed.)

17. 1. D
    2. E
    3. A
    4. B
    5. F
    6. G
    7. C
    (See Chapter 446 in *Nelson Textbook of Pediatrics*, 15th ed.)

18. 1. F
    2. A
    3. B
    4. C
    5. G
    6. D
    7. E
    (See Chapters 445–447 in *Nelson Textbook of Pediatrics*, 15th ed.)

19. B. Ewing sarcoma typically occurs in older children and presents in the midportion of long bones or in flat bones. The tumor often causes lytic lesions in bone. A stained biopsy section of the tumor typically reveals a large number of small round cells that stain for glycogen, and tumor cytogenics typically reveal an 11;22 translocation, which results in fusion of the *EWS* gene with the *FLI* gene and an abnormal, tumor-specific transcript. (See Chapter 454.2 in *Nelson Textbook of Pediatrics*, 15th ed.)

20. B. Classic presentations for neuroblastoma in a child younger than 3 years include a large abdominal mass with or without periorbital ecchymoses due to tumor metastasis (i.e., raccoon eyes) or a tumor in the upper mediastinum compressing the recurrent laryngeal nerve and cervical sympathetic chain, causing a Horner syndrome. Although other tumors could cause the latter presentation, the vast majority of such cases are due to neuroblastoma. (See Chapter 451 in *Nelson Textbook of Pediatrics*, 15th ed.)

21. E. Bone pain and swollen lymph nodes suggest infiltration by malignant cells in the setting of pancytopenia (i.e., decreased neutrophils, red blood cells, and platelets). Therefore, acute leukemia is a likely diagnosis. Acute lymphoblastic leukemia (ALL) is more likely (85% for ALL vs. 15% for AML in childhood). (See Chapter 449.1 in *Nelson Textbook of Pediatrics*, 15th ed.)

22. C. Carcinomas are common in elderly adults, but ALL and sarcomas (i.e., rhabdomyosarcoma, Ewing sarcoma, osteosarcoma) predominate in children. (See Chapter 449.1 in *Nelson Textbook of Pediatrics*, 15th ed.)

23. A. Actinomycin D, vincristine, and, for advanced-stage or unfavorable histology tumors, Adriamycin with or without cyclophosphamide have systematically been used to treat Wilms tumor presenting with various degrees of tumor spread. Antimetabolites such as 6-mercaptopurine, cytosine arabinoside, and methotrexate are used for lymphoblastic leukemia. Allopurinol prevents conversion of xanthines to uric acid as tumor cells break down, thus often preventing uric acid nephropathy. Because tumor cell breakdown is not dramatic in Wilms tumor, allopurinol is not needed. (See Chapter 452.1 in *Nelson Textbook of Pediatrics*, 15th ed.)

24. B. Increasing leukocyte count consisting of lymphoblasts is consistently associated with shorter survival in pediatric ALL. The high WBC count indicates a high tumor burden. The likelihood of a mutation that leads to drug resistance is increased as the number of tumor cells increases (i.e., the increased risk of treatment failure). (See Chapter 452.1 in *Nelson Textbook of Pediatrics*, 15th ed.)

23 Nephrology

1. A. IgA is the predominant immunoglobulin deposited in the glomeruli of patients with Berger nephropathy. (See Chapter 464 in *Nelson Textbook of Pediatrics*, 15th ed.)

2. C. The name gives the answer away. (See Chapter 472 in *Nelson Textbook of Pediatrics*, 15th ed.)

3. D. The abdominal mass in the patient described in the question is likely to be hydronephrosis. (See Chapter 494 in *Nelson Textbook of Pediatrics*, 15th ed.)

4. D. Living related donor transplant (LRD-T) is the treatment of choice for children with ESRD. Hemodialysis maintained for prolonged periods (years) is poorly tolerated by young children, whose physical, intellectual, and emotional maturation becomes seriously impaired. The use of LRD-T does not guarantee that the grafted organ will function adequately, but the odds are that it will work better and longer than a cadaveric organ and that chances of severe, intractable rejection reaction will not occur as frequently as in a cadaveric organ. Major complications can still happen in the form of technical complications, infection, and recurrence of the original disease in the graft. Despite these hurdles, the key issue is that LRD-T survival has proved superior to the cadaveric, 80% by 3 to 4 years versus 55% to 60%, respectively. (See Chapter 490 in *Nelson Textbook of Pediatrics*, 15th ed.)

5. E. Whether a transplanted kidney comes from a cadaver or an LRD, rejection reaction (RR) remains the major cause of graft loss. Hyperacute rejection due to preformed antibodies has been almost completely eliminated in renal transplantation. However, acute, progressive or accelerated, and chronic RR develop in 89%, 12%, and 62% of renal transplants in children, respectively. Most acute rejections are treatable with return of graft function; more severe and aggressive RR is occasionally uncontrollable. Chronic rejection of a graft that has functioned through the expected survival period is also progressive. Despite extensive transplantation networks and active organ procurement, the availability of cadaveric kidneys at present is limited, primarily because of insufficient kidney donation. (See Chapter 490 in *Nelson Textbook of Pediatrics*, 15th ed.)

6. C. Causes of ESRD vary with the patient's age. In younger children, congenital, obstructive, and metabolic diseases predominate over glomerulonephrites. Diabetes mellitus is responsible for 25% to 30% of ESRD in adults. This predicament is infrequent in young children because more than 10 years elapse before type I (insulin-dependent) diabetes mellitus leads to renal disease. Two to 4 years after this, ESRD occurs and dialysis and transplantation are necessary. In older children, the glomerulonephrites predominate. (See Chapter 489 in *Nelson Textbook of Pediatrics*, 15th ed.)

7. C. In the clinical setting described in the question, symptoms and signs and laboratory abnormalities are compatible with acute RR until proved otherwise. The diagnosis should be promptly documented with renal ultrasonography, graft flow studies, and angiogram and percutaneous graft biopsy if unclear. Whether the RR is primary or induced by a viral infection (cytomegalovirus [CMV], Epstein-Barr virus, *Mycoplasma*, and so on) can be determined by serologic, viral culture, and cyclosporine A trough level studies (because higher than necessary plasma concentrations of this immunosuppressive may produce renal arteriolar damage); recurrence of the disease in the graft, RR, acute tubular necrosis, cyclosporine A toxicity, and viral cellular inclusions can be detected and differentiated histopathologically. More than 60% of acute RR episodes can be reversed by appropriate antiinflammatory (prednisone, methylprednisolone) treatment. However, CMV-related RR requires a diametrically opposite therapy (i.e., a significant decrease in immunosuppression and aggressive antiviral medications [acyclovir, ganciclovir, and anti-CMV immunoglobulin]). This therapeutic dilemma may be ameliorated by avoiding the transplantation of a CMV-positive kidney into a CMV-negative patient. Because of the scarcity of kidneys in

general and the high prevalence of CMV asymptomatic infection, it is standard practice to treat CMV-negative recipients of CMV-positive grafts prophylactically with ganciclovir. All the other choices listed in the question are possible, but clinical and laboratory data and, when necessary, graft biopsy allow a clear differentiation. (See Chapter 490 in *Nelson Textbook of Pediatrics*, 15th ed.)

8. 1. A
   2. B
   3. C
   4. A
   5. D
   (See Chapters 465–471 and 481 in *Nelson Textbook of Pediatrics*, 15th ed.)

9. 1. A
   2. C
   3. B
   4. A
   5. B
   6. D
   (See Chapters 465–471 and 481 in *Nelson Textbook of Pediatrics*, 15th ed.)

10. A. Acute tubular necrosis (ATN) in the patient described in the question is probably secondary to diarrhea, fever, vomiting, and the associated dehydration. Intravascular volume loss, usually severe enough to produce hypotension, is a common factor predisposing to the development of ATN. (See Chapter 489.1 in *Nelson Textbook of Pediatrics*, 15th ed.)

11. C. Hypoalbuminemia, proteinuria, edema, and hyperlipidemia constitute the nephrotic syndrome. Hypertension, azotemia, edema, or hematuria would suggest nephritis but may also be encountered in minimal lesion nephrotic syndrome. This patient has nephrotic syndrome, not nephritis. (See Chapter 481 in *Nelson Textbook of Pediatrics*, 15th ed.)

12. D. Calcium carbonate is of value in reversing the elevated phosphate level in this patient with chronic renal insufficiency. (See Chapter 489.2 in *Nelson Textbook of Pediatrics*, 15th ed.)

13. A. The patient described in the question may have some form of renal dysplasia. The high potassium level and acidosis suggest a renal cause of this growth failure. (See Chapter 475 in *Nelson Textbook of Pediatrics,* 15th ed.)

24 Urologic Disorders in Infants and Children

1. B. Oligohydramnios occurring at 24 weeks' gestation is suggestive of renal agenesis. A high-level detailed fetal ultrasonogram revealed bilateral renal agenesis and no bladder. The infant died after birth as a result of the pulmonary complications of renal agenesis and oligohydramnios, which result in pulmonary hypoplasia. (See Chapter 491 in *Nelson Textbook of Pediatrics*, 15th ed.)

2. F. Primarily encountered in renal agenesis or dysplasia, the Potter phenotype (flattened face, broad nose, low-set ears, receding chin, clubfoot) is due to severe oligohydramnios. (See Chapter 491 in *Nelson Textbook of Pediatrics*, 15th ed.)

3. E. Chronic use of antibiotics is not a risk factor for urinary tract infection. All the other choices listed in the question are significant risks. (See Chapter 492 in *Nelson Textbook of Pediatrics*, 15th ed.)

4. A. In most infants with fever without a focus, one should suspect a urinary tract infection and obtain both a urine culture and a urinalysis. A catheterized specimen is the method of choice for obtaining urine for culture. (See Chapter 492 in *Nelson Textbook of Pediatrics*, 15th ed.)

5. A. Renal ultrasonography can help define most anomalies and hydronephrosis or a renal abscess. Approximately 3 weeks later, a VCUG should be obtained to identify the presence of a vesicoureteral reflux. (See Chapter 492 in *Nelson Textbook of Pediatrics*, 15th ed.)

6. A. A DMSA radionuclide scan helps to define photopenic images, which are accurate representations of chronic renal scarring. (See Chapter 493 in *Nelson Textbook of Pediatrics*, 15th ed.)

7. F. Sexual activity frequently causes cystitis in females, but this local infection does not produce significant reflux. (See Chapter 493 in *Nelson Textbook of Pediatrics*, 15th ed.)

8. D. Renal ultrasonography should be repeated at a later date. The relative oliguria of a 1-day-old neonate may reduce ureter urine flow, thus reducing the degree of obstruction. With better hydration and more urine flow, the relative obstruction may then produce hydronephrosis. Some repeat ultrasonography 1 week after birth. (See Chapter 494 in *Nelson Textbook of Pediatrics*, 15th ed.)

9. A. Renal masses are the most common lesions in neonates. Hydronephrosis and multicystic-dysplastic lesions are the most common renal masses. (See Chapter 494 in *Nelson Textbook of Pediatrics*, 15th ed.)

10. D. Urethral obstruction is the cause of prune belly syndrome and may be transient or permanent. Nonetheless, urethral atresia is an unusual finding. (See Chapter 494 in *Nelson Textbook of Pediatrics*, 15th ed.)

11. E. Always ask for and listen to complaints about the urinary stream in infant boys to detect serious problems early. Fetuses with severe obstruction may develop oligohydramnios and bilateral hydronephrosis. (See Chapter 494 in *Nelson Textbook of Pediatrics*, 15th ed.)

12. B. Abdominal ultrasonography is a helpful initial screening test to visualize the pancreas, kidneys, and other intra-abdominal, retroperitoneal, or pelvic structures. (See Chapter 494 in *Nelson Textbook of Pediatrics*, 15th ed.)

13. E. Torsions and epididymitis are painful. Hydroceles are smooth. (See Chapter 499 in *Nelson Textbook of Pediatrics*, 15th ed.)

14. B. Corrective surgery performed between 12 and 18 months of age represents a safe balance between anesthetic risk, allowance of time for the testes to descend, and the risks of leaving a testis in the abdomen. (See Chapter 499 in *Nelson Textbook of Pediatrics*, 15th ed.)

15. C. High intravesical pressure predisposes to reflux and infection. (See Chapter 497 in *Nelson Textbook of Pediatrics*, 15th ed.)

16. E. The complications listed in the question are related to the severity and duration of the obstruction and to the surgical technique (incontinence). (See Chapter 494 in *Nelson Textbook of Pediatrics*, 15th ed.)

17. C. Some neonates have transient false-negative findings on an ultrasonogram because of poor urine flow at birth. Once the infant is hydrated, the obstruction becomes more apparent. (See Chapter 494 in *Nelson Textbook of Pediatrics*, 15th ed.)

18. A. Ultrasonography helps determine many but not all anatomic abnormalities. A VCUG must eventually be performed to determine if reflux is present. (See Chapter 492 in *Nelson Textbook of Pediatrics*, 15th ed.)

25 Gynecologic Problems of Childhood

1. C. Patients with spontaneous galactorrhea should be screened by determining their prolactin level. (See Chapter 505 in *Nelson Textbook of Pediatrics*, 15th ed.)

2. A. Magnetic resonance imaging (MRI) or computed tomography (CT) of the cranium demonstrates a pituitary prolactinoma. Hypothyroidism also produces hyperprolactinemia and galactorrhea. The treatment of some small prolactinomas includes bromocriptine (Parlodel). Larger or persistently symptomatic lesions require surgery. (See Chapter 505 in *Nelson Textbook of Pediatrics,* 15th ed.)

3. A. Von Willebrand disease is associated with excessive menstrual bleeding but in the absence of vaginal trauma should not produce vaginal bleeding in a prepubertal girl. (See Chapter 504 in *Nelson Textbook of Pediatrics,* 15th ed.)

4. C. The presentation described in the question is quite typical of chronic lichen sclerosus. A biopsy may be needed to confirm the diagnosis. (See Chapter 503 in *Nelson Textbook of Pediatrics,* 15th ed.)

5. 1. B
   2. C
   3. D
   4. E
   5. A
   (See Chapter 503 in *Nelson Textbook of Pediatrics,* 15th ed.)

6. A. Nonspecific vaginitis most often occurs in prepubertal girls who wear tight-fitting clothing (leotards) or are exposed to vaginal irritants (soaps) or have poor hygiene. It is often due to coliform bacteria or group A streptococcus. (See Chapter 503 in *Nelson Textbook of Pediatrics,* 15th ed.)

7. E. Metronidazole is not indicated for this form of nonspecific vaginitis. If the process is recurrent, amoxicillin may be of value, in addition to the suggestions in choices *A* to *D*. (See Chapter 503 in *Nelson Textbook of Pediatrics,* 15th ed.)

8. A. Altered luteinizing hormone release of central origin or by altered ovarian feedback is present in polycystic ovary syndrome. (See Chapter 506 in *Nelson Textbook of Pediatrics,* 15th ed.)

9. C. (See Chapter 503 in *Nelson Textbook of Pediatrics,* 15th ed.)

10. B. Colposcopic examination can determine the extent of cervical intraepithelial neoplasia and the need for further evaluation and treatment such as conization and so on. (See Chapter 507 in *Nelson Textbook of Pediatrics,* 15th ed.)

11. E. The lesions of pityriasis versicolor are relatively common and are not sexually transmitted or indicative of abuse. (See Chapter 503 in *Nelson Textbook of Pediatrics,* 15th ed.)

12. D. (See Chapter 503 in *Nelson Textbook of Pediatrics,* 15th ed.)
13. C. *E. coli* and anaerobes and occasionally group A streptococcus are associated with nonspecific vaginitis. (See Chapter 503 in *Nelson Textbook of Pediatrics,* 15th ed.)

26 The Endocrine System

1. 1. C
   2. D
   3. A
   4. B
   5. E
   (See Chapter 528 in *Nelson Textbook of Pediatrics,* 15th ed.)
2. D. Type I autoimmune polyendocrinopathy, also known as autoimmune polyendocrinopathy candidiasis, ectodermal dystrophy (APECED), is associated with hypoparathyroidism, hypothyroidism, and Addison disease. (See Chapter 528 in *Nelson Textbook of Pediatrics,* 15th ed.)
3. E. The karyotype of the neonate described in the question will reveal that the genotype is XX, and ultrasonography will reveal normal female internal genital organs. In the most common variety of congenital adrenal hyperplasia, the serum 17-OH progesterone levels are markedly elevated (classic 21-hydroxylase deficiency). Approximately 75% of patients with 21-OH deficiency develop salt wasting in the first 1 to 2 weeks after birth. Such patients suffer emesis, diarrhea, hyponatremia, hyperkalemia, acidosis, and shock. (See Chapter 529 in *Nelson Textbook of Pediatrics,* 15th ed.)
4. E. Autoimmune polyendocrinopathy with chronic candidiasis is associated with Addison disease, not Cushing syndrome. (See Chapter 530 in *Nelson Textbook of Pediatrics,* 15th ed.)
5. 1. D
   2. D
   3. C
   4. D
   5. A
   6. B
   7. B
   8. D
   (See Chapter 531 in *Nelson Textbook of Pediatrics,* 15th ed.)
6. E. All of the choices listed in the question are critical in avoiding the dangers of hypertensive crisis during the surgical manipulation of pheochromocytoma. (See

Chapter 533 in *Nelson Textbook of Pediatrics,* 15th ed.)
7. C. Meconium peritonitis due to in utero intestinal perforation should not affect the adrenal glands located in the retroperitoneal space. (See Chapter 534 in *Nelson Textbook of Pediatrics,* 15th ed.)
8. B. Hypergonadotropic hypogonadism may result from testicular damage any time after the end of the first trimester. Absent or small testes and low serum testosterone levels are additional findings. (See Chapter 535.1 in *Nelson Textbook of Pediatrics,* 15th ed.)
9. D. Delayed and incomplete puberty are the usual pubertal problems in males with Klinefelter syndrome. (See Chapter 535.1 in *Nelson Textbook of Pediatrics,* 15th ed.)
10. A. The problem described in the question is transient and compatible with the physiology of puberty in normal males. Indeed, as many as 60% of boys have some degree of pubertal gynecomastia. Some cases are familial. (See Chapter 537 in *Nelson Textbook of Pediatrics,* 15th ed.)
11. D. Polycystic ovaries (Stein-Leventhal syndrome) are associated with obesity, hirsutism, secondary amenorrhea, and bilateral ovarian cysts. The cause is unknown. (See Chapter 538.1 in *Nelson Textbook of Pediatrics,* 15th ed.)
12. E. Congenital adrenal hyperplasia due to 11-hydroxylase deficiency produces female pseudohermaphroditism; males have normal-appearing genitalia in the neonatal period. (See Chapter 540.2 in *Nelson Textbook of Pediatrics,* 15th ed.)
13. 1. A
    2. B
    3. B
    4. A
    5. B
    6. A
    7. C
    8. A
    9. C
    10. D
    (See Part XXVI, Section 6 in *Nelson Textbook of Pediatrics,* 15th ed.)
14. B. The sex ratio is fairly equal in type I diabetes. (See Part XXVI, Section 6 in *Nelson Textbook of Pediatrics,* 15th ed.)
15. D. Increased intracranial pressure following aggressive fluid replacement and rapid lowering of the hyperosmolar state permits the development of an osmolar gradient between the now relatively hypo-osmolar plasma and the hyperosmolar intracellular

neurons in the central nervous system. Fluid is drawn into the neurons, resulting in cerebral edema. This is often fatal and may be avoidable by slowly lowering the osmolality of the plasma. (See Part XXVI, Section 6 in *Nelson Textbook of Pediatrics,* 15th ed.)

16. F. End-organ problems (choices *B, C, D,* and *E*) are preventable with tight glucose control. Unfortunately, this may result in recurrent episodes of hypoglycemia, which may compromise cognitive development or compliance among automobile-driving adolescents. (See Part XXVI, Section 6 in *Nelson Textbook of Pediatrics,* 15th ed.)

17. C. The DiGeorge syndrome is associated with hypoparathyroidism and hypocalcemia. Some patients with partial DiGeorge syndrome have normal calcium homeostasis. (See Chapter 525 in *Nelson Textbook of Pediatrics,* 15th ed.)

18. E. In pseudohypoparathyroidism, parathyroid hormone cannot stimulate its receptor. Exogenous parathyroid hormone does not alter the hypocalcemia. Therefore, patients are essentially hypoparathyroid. (See Chapter 526 in *Nelson Textbook of Pediatrics,* 15th ed.)

19. B. For the patient described in the question, the serum total calcium is 6.0 mg/dL, the phosphorus level is 8.5 mg/dL, and the albumin is normal. (See Chapter 525 in *Nelson Textbook of Pediatrics,* 15th ed.)

20. C. Acquired hypoparathyroidism with hypocalcemia may present with these symptoms in addition to seizures, cataracts, or other autoimmune disorders (alopecia areata, hepatitis, Addison disease, lymphocytic thyroiditis). (See Chapter 525 in *Nelson Textbook of Pediatrics,* 15th ed.)

21. C. Hyperparathyroidism is not an associated risk for acquired hypothyroidism. (See Chapter 520 in *Nelson Textbook of Pediatrics,* 15th ed.)

22. A. Hypotension does not result from the use of propylthiouracil or Tapazole but may occasionally complicate therapy with propranolol. (See Chapter 523.1 in *Nelson Textbook of Pediatrics,* 15th ed.)

23. B. Patients with hyperthyroidism have heat intolerance because of their hypermetabolism. (See Chapter 523.1 in *Nelson Textbook of Pediatrics,* 15th ed.)

24. E. Retinal lesions are quite rare in Graves disease, whereas choices *A* to *D* are common. (See Chapter 523.1 in *Nelson Textbook of Pediatrics,* 15th ed.)

25. A. The patient described in the question probably has early Hashimoto (lymphocytic) thyroiditis. Antibodies to both these thyroid antigens are present in 95% of individuals. Choice *E* is also useful; TSH level is moderately elevated despite normal (compensated) T_4 levels. (See Chapter 521 in *Nelson Textbook of Pediatrics,* 15th ed.)

26. A. Most patients with congenital hypothyroidism are unable to produce T_4 but do produce excessive TSH in an attempt to stimulate the thyroid gland to produce more T_4. (See Chapter 520 in *Nelson Textbook of Pediatrics,* 15th ed.)

27. E. Most patients with congenital hypothyroidism have aplasia or hypoplasia of the thyroid gland and thus do not have a goiter. (See Chapter 520 in *Nelson Textbook of Pediatrics,* 15th ed.)

28. C. In patients with McCune-Albright syndrome, the insulin stimulation pathway is unaffected. However, because of a missense mutation in the gene for the α-subunit of the G protein, which stimulates cyclic AMP, there is activation of the ACTH, TSH, LH, and FSH receptors. (See Chapter 517.5 in *Nelson Textbook of Pediatrics,* 15th ed.)

29. A. By maintaining a constant level of GnRH, the pulsatile release of FSH and LH is inhibited, thus effectively treating central precocious puberty. (See Chapter 517.1 in *Nelson Textbook of Pediatrics,* 15th ed.)

30. A. In precocious pseudopuberty in females, secretion of LH and FSH is not noted to be pulsatile, as it would be in true puberty or true precocious puberty. (See Chapter 517 in *Nelson Textbook of Pediatrics,* 15th ed.)

31. D. True precocious puberty should follow the "normal" (albeit early) sequence of pubertal development. Menstruation is a late development. (See Chapter 517.1 in *Nelson Textbook of Pediatrics,* 15th ed.)

32. D. In the patient described in the question, inappropriate ADH secretion is most likely as revealed by hyponatremia, no signs of dehydration, and excessively high urine sodium excretion. (See Chapter 514 in *Nelson Textbook of Pediatrics,* 15th ed.)

33. F. In hypertonic dehydration, the high ADH levels are appropriate but may contribute to reduced urine output during the early stages of fluid resuscitation. (See Chapter 514 in *Nelson Textbook of Pediatrics,* 15th ed.)

34. B. Neonates with diabetes insipidus often present with intense thirst and polyuria. Frequent feedings normally given to neonates may prevent hypernatremic

dehydration, which may nonetheless be precipitated by fasting, anorexia associated with viral illnesses, or longer intervals between feedings. (See Chapter 513 in *Nelson Textbook of Pediatrics,* 15th ed.)

35. F. *Mycobacterium tuberculosis* may produce diabetes insipidus; atypical mycobacteria do not. (See Chapter 513 in *Nelson Textbook of Pediatrics,* 15th ed.)

36. C. Russell-Silver syndrome may be associated with abnormalities of GH secretion, and growth may be enhanced temporarily by exogenous GH. Nonetheless, the lesion is unknown and is not a pituitary adenoma. (See Chapter 512 in *Nelson Textbook of Pediatrics,* 15th ed.)

37. E. Choices *A* to *D* in the question are true, but the mechanism of this growth delay is not known. Constitutional growth delay is not genetic short stature, because these children may attain normal adult stature. (See Chapter 512 in *Nelson Textbook of Pediatrics,* 15th ed.)

38. E. Recombinant human GH is free of the risk of Creutzfeldt-Jakob disease. Patients previously treated with cadaveric pituitary extracts are at risk for this prion disease. (See Chapter 512 in *Nelson Textbook of Pediatrics,* 15th ed.)

39. E. Nesidioblastosis, a hyperinsulinemic state, is not associated with panhypopituitarism. Developmental, genetic, and destructive lesions of the hypothalamic-pituitary region are risk factors. (See Chapter 512 in *Nelson Textbook of Pediatrics,* 15th ed.)

40. D. Hydrocephalus is rarely if ever directly related to panhypopituitarism. Hydrocephalus due to a tumor or granulomatous process may also involve the pituitary fossa indirectly. This is rare in neonates. (See Chapter 512 in *Nelson Textbook of Pediatrics,* 15th ed.)

41. A. Cranial irradiation of this magnitude can produce pituitary hypofunction, which most often is due to GH deficiency but occasionally is associated with TSH and ACTH deficiencies. (See Chapter 512 in *Nelson Textbook of Pediatrics,* 15th ed.)

42. A. IGF-1 levels are low in GH-deficient children. (See Chapter 512 in *Nelson Textbook of Pediatrics,* 15th ed.)

43. E. Exogenous GH is of no value in Laron syndrome owing to the deficient GH receptor. IGF-1 treatment may be of value because it bypasses the deficient GH-binding process. (See Chapter 512 in *Nelson Textbook of Pediatrics,* 15th ed.)

44. D. Stimulating tests include exercise or the administration of L-dopa, insulin, arginine, clonidine, or glucagon. Some recommend more than one test to reduce the number of false positives. (See Chapter 512 in *Nelson Textbook of Pediatrics,* 15th ed.)

45. A. Reassurance about lack of menarche is appropriate at age 14. Workup should be begun after 16 years of age. (See Chapter 516 in *Nelson Textbook of Pediatrics,* 15th ed.)

46. C. (See Chapter 512 in *Nelson Textbook of Pediatrics,* 15th ed.)

47. B. Children with a constitutional delay in growth have adequate growth potential. If chronologic age and skeletal maturation were similar, genetic short stature would be present. (See Chapter 512 in *Nelson Textbook of Pediatrics,* 15th ed.)

48. D. The Graefe sign is upper eyelid lag, the Moebius sign is an inability to converge, and the Stellwag sign is retraction of the eyelid. (See Chapter 523.1 in *Nelson Textbook of Pediatrics,* 15th ed.)

49. A. (See Chapter 528 in *Nelson Textbook of Pediatrics,* 15th ed.)

50. A and B. This is a case of Addison disease, and replacement therapy with both DOCA and hydrocortisone is necessary. (See Chapter 528 in *Nelson Textbook of Pediatrics,* 15th ed.)

51. D. Deficiency of 21β-hydroxylase accounts for 95% of all cases of congenital adrenal hyperplasia. (See Chapter 529.1 in *Nelson Textbook of Pediatrics,* 15th ed.)

27 The Nervous System

1. B. Metachromatic leukodystrophy is a familial degenerative disease affecting both the central nervous system (CNS) and peripheral nervous system white matter, hence the loss of deep tendon reflexes with CNS symptoms. (See Chapter 552.1 in *Nelson Textbook of Pediatrics,* 15th ed.)

2. C. The patient described in the question has juvenile myoclonic epilepsy with the later development of generalized seizures. The treatment of choice is valproic acid. (See Chapter 543.2 in *Nelson Textbook of Pediatrics,* 15th ed.)

3. E. The young girl described in the question has tetralogy of Fallot and a brain abscess partly resulting from the right-to-left cardiac shunt. Predisposing factors for brain abscesses in other patients include chronic otic and sinus infections. (See Chapter 554 in *Nelson Textbook of Pediatrics,* 15th ed.)

4. B. Video/EEG recordings help differentiate pseudoseizures by demonstrating normal cortical activity in the presence of at times bizarre or typical-appearing motor activity. (See Chapter 541 in *Nelson Textbook of Pediatrics,* 15th ed.)

5. D. Ruptured arteriovenous malformation is suggested by chronicity, preeruptive or (leak) symptoms, and bruit. Although migraine—even hemiplegic migraine—is possible, the severity of symptoms in such a young patient precludes migraine. (See Chapter 553.3 in *Nelson Textbook of Pediatrics,* 15th ed.)

6. C. Chiari crisis is a downward herniation of the medulla and cerebellar tonsils, which compress nerves as they exit the foramen magnum. Compression of the vagus produces vocal cord paralysis. Chiari malformation type II is associated with spina bifida and hydrocephalus. (See Chapter 542.11 in *Nelson Textbook of Pediatrics,* 15th ed.)

7. 1. B
   2. C
   3. B
   4. A
   5. B
   6. D
   (See Chapter 542.11 in *Nelson Textbook of Pediatrics,* 15th ed.)

8. 1. A
   2. C
   3. D
   4. A
   5. B
   (See Chapter 542.7 in *Nelson Textbook of Pediatrics,* 15th ed.)

9. D. Head MRI demonstrates a Chiari type I malformation that is not associated with hydrocephalus but does produce progressive downward displacement of the cerebellar tonsils into the foramen magnum. (See Chapter 542.11 in *Nelson Textbook of Pediatrics,* 15th ed.)

10. E. Congenital cytomegalovirus (CMV) usually causes microcephalus, not macrocephalus. Expansion of the bone marrow (hemolytic anemias), storage diseases (lysosomal, leukodystrophies), excessive cerebrospinal fluid (CSF) (hydrocephalus) and blood (subdurals), plus familial factors contribute to megalocephaly. (See Chapter 542.11 in *Nelson Textbook of Pediatrics,* 15th ed.)

11. B. Shunt infections usually occur within a few weeks of the shunt placement. Headache and abdominal pain relate to the infected CSF in the ventricles that drains into the abdomen from the distal end of the shunt. The most common pathogen is *Staphylococcus epidermidis.* (See Chapter 542.11 in *Nelson Textbook of Pediatrics,* 15th ed.)

12. D. Magnetic resonance imaging (MRI) will reveal a specific area of cerebral vascular occlusion (infarction), possibly from placental, ductal, or other sites. (See Chapter 553.4 in *Nelson Textbook of Pediatrics,* 15th ed.)

13. D. Paroxysmal nocturnal hemoglobinuria is associated with a hypercoagulable state but does not present in the neonatal period. (See Chapter 553 in *Nelson Textbook of Pediatrics,* 15th ed.)

14. C. Simple partial seizures classically are short and often repetitive, and they do not alter consciousness. The patient's EEG reveals unilateral spikes and sharp waves over the right hemisphere. (See Chapter 543.1 in *Nelson Textbook of Pediatrics,* 15th ed.)

15. D. A family history of febrile seizures is sometimes helpful but does not help in determining the presence or absence of a febrile seizure in an individual patient. Many children with typical febrile seizures have no family history of such seizures. In the patient described in the question, the young age, the seizure duration, the recurrence of seizures, and the lethargy strongly suggest another diagnosis such as meningitis. (See Chapter 543.3 in *Nelson Textbook of Pediatrics,* 15th ed.)

16. E. Spina bifida with or without hydrocephalus but without other CNS lesions does not usually produce seizures. All the other diagnoses listed in the question are associated with neonatal seizures. (See Chapter 543.5 in *Nelson Textbook of Pediatrics,* 15th ed.)

17. D. Benign paroxysmal vertigo is a relatively common condition that mimics seizures but has a benign nature that requires reassurance and no specific treatment. If attacks become clustered, treatment with dimenhydrinate is indicated. (See Chapter 544 in *Nelson Textbook of Pediatrics,* 15th ed.)

18. E. Migraines are usually benign and respond to rest and simple analgesics. Hemicrania, a visual aura, relief with rest, and a positive family history (not mentioned in this case but present in most patients), together with normal findings on physical examination, are helpful clues. (See Chapter 545 in *Nelson Textbook of Pediatrics,* 15th ed.)

19. 1. E
    2. C
    3. A
    4. B
    5. A
    6. B
    7. C
    8. D
    9. A
    10. A
    (See Chapter 546 in *Nelson Textbook of Pediatrics,* 15th ed.)
20. 1. D
    2. C
    3. D
    4. A
    5. B
    6. B
    7. C
    8. D
    9. E
    10. C
    (See Chapter 548 in *Nelson Textbook of Pediatrics,* 15th ed.)
21. C. Acetaminophen overdose does not directly involve the cerebellum or cortex unless at a later stage if hepatic failure ensues. Nonetheless, acutely, patients suffer from nausea, emesis, and abdominal pain. (See Chapter 547.1 in *Nelson Textbook of Pediatrics,* 15th ed.)
22. D. A lumbar puncture is needed to measure the titer for measles antibodies in the CSF. The diagnosis is subacute sclerosing panencephalitis, a slow measles virus infection of the CNS. (See Chapter 552 in *Nelson Textbook of Pediatrics,* 15th ed.)
23. B. MRI is most useful in confirming the diagnosis of a possible demyelinating disease such as multiple sclerosis. MRI demonstrates small 3- to 4-mm plaques compatible with this disease. (See Chapter 552.5 in *Nelson Textbook of Pediatrics,* 15th ed.)
24. 1. B
    2. D
    3. A
    4. E
    5. F
    6. B
    7. F
    8. C
    9. F
    10. C
    11. D
    12. A
    (See Chapter 552 in *Nelson Textbook of Pediatrics,* 15th ed.)

25. B. Craniopharyngiomas often present with visual disturbances due to involvement of the optic chiasm, endocrine disorders due to pressure on the pituitary, and signs of increased intracranial pressure (ICP). (See Chapter 555 in *Nelson Textbook of Pediatrics,* 15th ed.)
26. C. A CT or MRI scan would reveal a cystic cerebellar astrocytoma. Positional and progressive headache, with or without head tilt, is a significant manifestation of a brain tumor. The poor visualization of the retina is probably due to marked papilledema obscuring the optic disk. (See Chapter 555 in *Nelson Textbook of Pediatrics,* 15th ed.)
27. C. Birth asphyxia is not associated with a brain abscess in the absence of penetrating trauma (fetal scalp electrode or pH lancet) or meningitis, particularly with *Citrobacter.* (See Chapter 554 in *Nelson Textbook of Pediatrics,* 15th ed.)
28. D. The patient described in the question had a CT scan that revealed a frontal brain abscess due to anaerobic mouth flora from chronic tooth decay. As an aside, a patient with a history suspicious of a chronic CNS infection (e.g., more than 2 to 3 days) should have a head CT before a lumbar puncture. If a lumbar puncture is performed with a brain abscess, ICP may be increased (as in this patient) and cerebral herniation and death may ensue. If infection is suspected but a CT scan is indicated, the patient should be empirically treated for meningitis after a blood culture is obtained but before a lumbar puncture is performed. (See Chapter 554 in *Nelson Textbook of Pediatrics,* 15th ed.)
29. D. Aspirin in normal hosts does not produce CNS bleeding. Aspirin should not be given to children, except under unusual circumstances, owing to its strong relationship with Reye syndrome. (See Chapter 553.3 in *Nelson Textbook of Pediatrics,* 15th ed.)
30. D. Arteriovenous malformation, like an aneurysm, may rupture, producing hemiplegia or coma. Blood in the subarachnoid space produces nuchal rigidity and may be detected by a CT scan or a carefully performed lumbar puncture. (See Chapter 553.3 in *Nelson Textbook of Pediatrics,* 15th ed.)
31. E. Maple syrup urine disease produces progressive (or intermittent) crises of emesis, lethargy, coma, and seizures. Thromboembolic phenomena are rare. (See

Chapter 553 in *Nelson Textbook of Pediatrics,* 15th ed.)

32. B. Petit mal seizures start after 3 years of age and may end by puberty. Girls are affected more often than boys. (See Chapter 543.2 in *Nelson Textbook of Pediatrics,* 15th ed.)

33. 1. D
    2. B
    3. A
    4. B
    5. D
    6. B
    7. B
       The differential diagnosis of coma is important clinically. (See Chapter 549 in *Nelson Textbook of Pediatrics,* 15th ed.)

34. D. Multiple sclerosis is relatively rare in children (<1% of cases appear before 14 years of age), but with pediatricians caring for more adolescents, the symptoms are worth knowing. (See Chapter 552.5 in *Nelson Textbook of Pediatrics,* 15th ed.)

28 Neuromuscular Disorders

1. B. Guillain-Barré syndrome is an ascending peripheral polyneuropathy that is predominantly motor but may have mild sensory symptoms (paresthesias). An upper respiratory tract infection or diarrhea (often due to *Campylobacter*) often precedes the onset of paralysis. (See Chapter 567 in *Nelson Textbook of Pediatrics,* 15th ed.)

2. E. Pulmonary function tests, such as measurement of negative inspiratory force, are helpful in detecting impending respiratory failure due to intercostal or phrenic nerve involvement. Reductions in inspiratory force often precede abnormalities of the arterial blood gases (hypercarbia, hypoxia) and should be monitored frequently in any patient with acute progressive muscle weakness. (See Chapter 567 in *Nelson Textbook of Pediatrics,* 15th ed.)

3. B. Spinal muscular atrophy of the infant type (Werdnig-Hoffmann syndrome) is due to progressive loss of anterior horn cells. Profound and progressive hypotonia, ascending weakness, and loss of reflexes are characteristically associated with marked muscle fasciculations. The fasciculations are best noted on the tongue because fatty replacement over peripheral muscles makes this sign difficult to perceive. (See Chapter 563.2 in *Nelson Textbook of Pediatrics,* 15th ed.)

4. E. Ticks (wood or dog) may produce a motor-

sensory neuropathy indistinguishable from Guillain-Barré syndrome. On removal of the tick (often on the scalp), the paralysis rapidly resolves. (See Chapter 563 in *Nelson Textbook of Pediatrics,* 15th ed.)

5. 1. A
   2. B
   3. D
   4. C
   5. A
   (See Chapters 559–568 in *Nelson Textbook of Pediatrics,* 15th ed.)

6. B. Congenital myotubular myopathy classically affects males, with onset before birth, thus leading to fetal and neonatal weakness with insufficient respiratory effort at birth and the need for rapid resuscitation. In contrast to Pompe disease, the cardiac muscles are not involved, and in contrast to muscular dystrophy, the serum creatine phosphokinase (CPK) level is not elevated. Tongue atrophy is common, but in contrast to Werdnig-Hoffmann disease, patients have no tongue fasciculations. (See Chapter 559.1 in *Nelson Textbook of Pediatrics,* 15th ed.)

7. D. The patient described in the question has one of the congenital myopathies (central core disease), which are characterized by intense muscle contractions when patients are exposed to a general anesthetic agent (halothane). The patient has malignant hyperthermia. (See Chapter 562.2 in *Nelson Textbook of Pediatrics,* 15th ed.)

8. E. Dantrolene is the treatment of choice for malignant hyperthermia. In addition, one should discontinue the initiating anesthetic agent, provide appropriate mechanical ventilation and fluid resuscitation, and treat the combined acidosis. Rhabdomyolysis must be managed with a forced diuresis to prevent myoglobinuric renal tubular damage leading to acute tubular necrosis and acute renal failure. (See Chapter 562.2 in *Nelson Textbook of Pediatrics,* 15th ed.)

9. C. The serum CPK level is 20,000 IU/L, but the other screening tests would have normal results or would be unnecessary (lumbar puncture), except for the Stanford-Binet, which would reveal an IQ of 75. (See Chapter 560 in *Nelson Textbook of Pediatrics,* 15th ed.)

10. D. Muscular dystrophy (Duchenne, more often) presents with normal motor milestones in the first 6 to 12 months, with progressive muscle weakness (proximal greater than distal) and markedly high levels of serum CPK. The definitive

diagnosis is based on molecular biology tools to determine the gene defect on the X chromosome or the absence of dystrophin in a typical muscle biopsy specimen. (See Chapter 560 in *Nelson Textbook of Pediatrics,* 15th ed.)

11. D. Myotonic muscular dystrophy often becomes more pronounced in the offspring of an affected mother (genetic anticipation). The molecular defect is expansion of tripeptide repeats, which apparently accelerates during transmission from a transmitting woman to her offspring. The congenital form is often lethal. (See Chapter 560.3 in *Nelson Textbook of Pediatrics,* 15th ed.)

12. 1. D
    2. F
    3. A
    4. B
    5. C
    6. G
    7. E
       (See Chapters 561 and 562 in *Nelson Textbook of Pediatrics,* 15th ed.)

13. E. Myasthenia gravis is characterized by progressive muscle weakness that is exacerbated by repetitive muscle use. The facial and extraocular muscles are classically involved. (See Chapter 563.1 in *Nelson Textbook of Pediatrics,* 15th ed.)

14. B. Edrophonium (Tensilon) is a short-acting cholinesterase-inhibiting drug that increases the amount of acetylcholine present at the motor end plate. After intravenous administration of edrophonium, ptosis and ophthalmoplegia improve within seconds but revert to the previous state within minutes. (See Chapter 563.1 in *Nelson Textbook of Pediatrics,* 15th ed.)

15. C. Endotracheal intubation or effective bag-and-mask ventilation is needed in any infant with poor respiratory effort regardless of the cause. Even if an antidote (Narcan for morphine, edrophonium for congenital myasthenia gravis) is available, one first must protect the airway. In addition, edrophonium's action is too short in neonates; some use neostigmine. (See Chapter 563.1 in *Nelson Textbook of Pediatrics,* 15th ed.)

16. D. Myasthenia gravis in adults is due to an IgG autoantibody against the acetylcholine receptor. Because IgG antibodies are transported across the placenta to a woman's fetus, autoantibodies of this class of immunoglobulin may produce a similar but usually transient disease in her neonate.

Similar diseases include Graves disease, systemic lupus erythematosus, and idiopathic thrombocytopenic purpura. (See Chapter 563.1 in *Nelson Textbook of Pediatrics,* 15th ed.)

17. C. Duchenne muscular dystrophy is also called pseudohypertrophic muscular dystrophy. (See Chapter 560.1 in *Nelson Textbook of Pediatrics,* 15th ed.)

29 Disorders of the Eye

1. 1. B
   2. C
   3. A
   4. E (congenital miosis)
   5. D
      (See Chapter 573 in *Nelson Textbook of Pediatrics,* 15th ed.)

2. B. "White eye" has an extensive and significant differential diagnosis. The cat's eye reflex is a finding or a historical observation by a parent that deserves immediate attention. (See Chapter 573 in *Nelson Textbook of Pediatrics,* 15th ed.)

3. A. A careful examination by biomicroscopy and direct ophthalmoscopy is indicated before other steps to determine whether the lesion is in the lens, vitreous, choroid, optic nerve, or retina. (See Chapter 573 in *Nelson Textbook of Pediatrics,* 15th ed.)

4. F. Coats disease is a rare problem in childhood; it does not produce leukocoria. (See Chapter 573 in *Nelson Textbook of Pediatrics,* 15th ed.)

5. A. Such actions as those described in the question attempt to avoid the double vision due to a cranial nerve palsy (sixth in this patient) or proptosis. Covering the involved eye eliminates the double vision. Diplopia is mainly a problem of abnormalities of binocular vision. Monocular diplopia is noted in dislocation of the lens or macular defects. (See Chapter 572 in *Nelson Textbook of Pediatrics,* 15th ed.)

6. B. Brain tumors produce elevated intracranial pressure with a nonlocalizing lateral rectus (sixth cranial nerve) palsy due to the pressure effect on this nerve. Squinting, new-onset strabismus, and head tilt are red flags suggestive of a brain tumor. (See Chapter 572 in *Nelson Textbook of Pediatrics,* 15th ed.)

7. A. Amblyopia is a vision loss that is not due to a specific organic lesion but is rather due to deprivation or disuse of the retina. Even after delayed removal of a cataract or correction of strabismus, the previously

unused retina tunes out the image. (See Chapter 572 in *Nelson Textbook of Pediatrics,* 15th ed.)

8. D. Myopia is unusual in infants and in preschool children. (See Chapter 571 in *Nelson Textbook of Pediatrics,* 15th ed.)

9. 1. C
   2. A
   3. D
   4. B
   5. F
   6. E
   (See Chapter 574 in *Nelson Textbook of Pediatrics,* 15th ed.)

10. 1. A
    2. B
    3. D
    4. A
    5. A
    6. B
    7. A
    8. B
    9. B
    10. C
    (See Chapter 582 in *Nelson Textbook of Pediatrics,* 15th ed.)

11. E. Acute iridocyclitis is present in the patient described in the question, as evidenced by photophobia and ciliary flush (perilimbal erythema). (See Chapter 580 in *Nelson Textbook of Pediatrics,* 15th ed.)

12. D. Pauciarticular juvenile rheumatoid arthritis (JRA) is the main variant of JRA associated with acute and chronic iritis. Untreated, this could lead to significant vision loss. (See Chapter 580 in *Nelson Textbook of Pediatrics,* 15th ed.)

13. C. Although TORCH infections produce many ocular findings of the cornea, lens, and retina, aniridia is not an association. (See Chapter 573 in *Nelson Textbook of Pediatrics,* 15th ed.)

14. G. Hyperoxia in preterm neonates usually causes retinopathy of prematurity, which may occasionally be associated with cataracts. Oxygen does not directly cause cataracts. (See Chapter 579 in *Nelson Textbook of Pediatrics,* 15th ed.)

15. D. Lid lag in hyperthyroidism is not ptosis. In addition, the globe may be proptotic. (See Chapter 575 in *Nelson Textbook of Pediatrics,* 15th ed.)

16. D. Wilms tumor is associated with aniridia, not with ptosis. (See Chapter 575 in *Nelson Textbook of Pediatrics,* 15th ed.)

17. E. The acquired triad of nystagmus, head nodding, and torticollis, in its classic form, is self-limited and benign. Nonetheless,

children with brain tumors may have signs resembling components of spasmus nutans. (See Chapter 574 in *Nelson Textbook of Pediatrics,* 15th ed.)

18. B. Aniridia is associated with Wilms tumor, which is best diagnosed with a renal ultrasonogram. (See Chapter 573 in *Nelson Textbook of Pediatrics,* 15th ed.)

19. C. Surgery is indicated to prevent amblyopia. (See Chapter 574 in *Nelson Textbook of Pediatrics,* 15th ed.)

20. A. The infant described in the question most probably has a blocked nasolacrimal duct. Massage and hygiene are sufficient, because many become unobstructed with time. (See Chapter 576 in *Nelson Textbook of Pediatrics,* 15th ed.)

21. D. The infant described in the question most likely has a congenital lesion of the uveal tract. Megalocornea with clouding of the cornea, photophobia, and tearing are common presentations. (See Chapter 583 in *Nelson Textbook of Pediatrics,* 15th ed.)

22. D. Rhabdomyosarcoma of the face, orbit, sinus, and so on often presents early because of the space-occupying and displacement effects of tumor growth. (See Chapter 575 in *Nelson Textbook of Pediatrics,* 15th ed.)

23. 1. B
    2. D
    3. E
    4. F
    5. A
    6. D
    7. C
    8. A
    (See Chapters 578, 581, 583, and 584 in *Nelson Textbook of Pediatrics,* 15th ed.)

24. B. Leukocoria is also seen in retinal detachment, persistent hyperplastic primary vitreous, visceral larva migrans, bacterial panophthalmitis, cataract, coloboma of the choroid, and retinopathy of prematurity. (See Chapter 573 in *Nelson Textbook of Pediatrics,* 15th ed.)

30 The Ear

1. F. Any mechanism that physically impairs the transmission of sound through the external or middle ear produces a conductive hearing loss. (See Chapter 587 in *Nelson Textbook of Pediatrics,* 15th ed.)

2. E. Autosomal recessive deafness represents 70% to 80% of cases of genetic congenital sensorineural hearing impairment but usually does not have other anomalies as

the syndromes listed in choices *A* to *D*. (See Chapter 587 in *Nelson Textbook of Pediatrics,* 15th ed.)

3. D. Hypocalcemia alone is not a risk factor for hearing loss. Choices *A* to *C, E,* and *F* list major risk factors for neonatal-onset hearing loss. (See Chapter 587 in *Nelson Textbook of Pediatrics,* 15th ed.)

4. E. Epilepsy is not a risk factor for hearing loss. (See Chapter 587 in *Nelson Textbook of Pediatrics,* 15th ed.)

5. D. Missed unvoiced consonant sounds occur even with slight hearing loss. (See Chapter 587 in *Nelson Textbook of Pediatrics,* 15th ed.)

6. C. Pneumococci are unusual causes of otitis externa, whereas the pathogens listed in choices *A, B, D,* and *E* occur under different circumstances. (See Chapter 589 in *Nelson Textbook of Pediatrics,* 15th ed.)

7. D. Inflammation of the external canal may occur after otitis media with perforation, but the reverse is not true in that external otitis does not cause perforation of the tympanic membrane. (See Chapter 589 in *Nelson Textbook of Pediatrics,* 15th ed.)

8. 1. B
   2. A
   3. A
   4. C
   5. D
   6. B
   7. B
   (See Chapters 589 and 590.6 in *Nelson Textbook of Pediatrics,* 15th ed.)

9. E. Otitis media occurs more often in winter and early spring than in summer. (See Chapter 590 in *Nelson Textbook of Pediatrics,* 15th ed.)

10. A. Fever is present in only 30% to 50% of patients with otitis media. (See Chapter 590 in *Nelson Textbook of Pediatrics,* 15th ed.)

11. C. Within 1 to 2 days of treatment, symptoms of acute otitis media should improve or abate. Continued manifestations suggest resistant organisms, sites of other infection (meningitis), or a suppurative complication (mastoiditis, epidural abscess). (See Chapter 590 in *Nelson Textbook of Pediatrics,* 15th ed.)

12. B. In cases of middle ear effusion persisting for 4 weeks after otitis media, most recommend another course of oral antimicrobial therapy, usually with a drug different from that used to treat the initial episode of acute otitis media. (See Chapter

590.2 in *Nelson Textbook of Pediatrics,* 15th ed.)

13. D. Sinusitis is rarely associated and is not a complication of otitis media despite similar pathogens. Recurrent sinopulmonary and otic infections should suggest an immune deficit or a dysmotile cilia syndrome. (See Chapter 590.6 in *Nelson Textbook of Pediatrics,* 15th ed.)

14. D. *H. influenzae* type b does not usually produce otitis media. With the advent of the conjugated *H. influenzae* type b vaccine, we are fortunate that we now rarely see meningitis, epiglottitis, arthritis, or cellulitis due to this pathogen. Otitis media is associated with nontypable *H. influenzae* and is not affected by this vaccine! (See Chapter 590.1 in *Nelson Textbook of Pediatrics,* 15th ed.)

31 The Skin

1. D. Kerion is a severe inflammatory response that is manifested as a boggy granulomatous lesion due to cutaneous fungi such as tinea tonsurans, *Microsporum canis,* or *Microsporum gypseum.* Treatment is oral griseofulvin, not surgery or aspiration. (See Chapter 616 in *Nelson Textbook of Pediatrics,* 15th ed.)

2. C. Children with staphylococcal scalded skin syndrome may also demonstrate pharyngitis, conjunctivitis, and cracking lips. Toxic epidermal necrolysis is similar but has a deeper cleavage plane in the epidermis and is usually associated with drugs. (See Chapter 615 in *Nelson Textbook of Pediatrics,* 15th ed.)

3. C. Alopecia areata is a rapid and complete loss of hair in round or ovoid patches. The cause is unknown. (See Chapter 612 in *Nelson Textbook of Pediatrics,* 15th ed.)

4. B. Pityriasis rosea manifests with an annular solitary herald patch of 1 to 10 cm plus an extensive maculopapular erythematous rash distributed symmetrically in the skin lines. (See Chapter 607 in *Nelson Textbook of Pediatrics,* 15th ed.)

5. 1. A
   2. E
   3. D
   4. B
   5. C
   6. G
   7. F
   (See Chapter 595 in *Nelson Textbook of Pediatrics,* 15th ed.)

6. A. This lesion is more common among

African-Americans. (See Chapter 597 in *Nelson Textbook of Pediatrics,* 15th ed.)

7. B. Pustular melanosis is a transient, benign lesion. (See Chapter 597 in *Nelson Textbook of Pediatrics,* 15th ed.)

8. D. Cutis aplasia often appears on the scalp, near the midline, but may also appear in a symmetric pattern on the face, trunk, or limbs. (See Chapter 598 in *Nelson Textbook of Pediatrics,* 15th ed.)

9. D. The flashlamp pulsed dye laser effectively destroys the dilated capillary network without scarring or discoloration. It is a remarkable advance in the treatment of port-wine stains. (See Chapter 600 in *Nelson Textbook of Pediatrics,* 15th ed.)

10. E. Giant pigmented nevi are difficult-to-manage lesions that affect males and females with equal frequency. (See Chapter 601 in *Nelson Textbook of Pediatrics,* 15th ed.)

11. C. Ephelides are freckles; these are not more common in Peutz-Jeghers syndrome. (See Chapter 602 in *Nelson Textbook of Pediatrics,* 15th ed.)

12. A. Incontinentia pigmenti is X linked dominant and is lethal in males during fetal life. (See Chapter 602 in *Nelson Textbook of Pediatrics,* 15th ed.)

13. E. Eighth-nerve deafness due to acoustic neuromas is noted in neurofibromatosis type 2. The lesion illustrated in the question is tuberous sclerosis. (See Chapter 603 in *Nelson Textbook of Pediatrics,* 15th ed.)

14. A. There is no agreed upon indication for systemic steroids in Stevens-Johnson syndrome. (See Chapter 604 in *Nelson Textbook of Pediatrics,* 15th ed.)

15. C. The Köbner response commonly occurs in patients with psoriasis. (See Chapter 607 in *Nelson Textbook of Pediatrics,* 15th ed.)

16. B. Pityriasis rosea is not hypopigmented, and the other lesions listed in the question itch. (See Chapter 607 in *Nelson Textbook of Pediatrics,* 15th ed.)

17. E. Pityriasis rosea may last from 2 weeks to 3 months. (See Chapter 607 in *Nelson Textbook of Pediatrics,* 15th ed.)

32 Bones and Joints

1. C. (See Chapter 626.4 in *Nelson Textbook of Pediatrics,* 15th ed.)
2. A. The patient described in Question 1 has a classic history of Osgood-Schlatter disease, best managed by decreased activity of the involved joint. (See Chapter 626.4 in *Nelson Textbook of Pediatrics,* 15th ed.)

3. A. The vertical talus is the most severe and serious form of flatfoot. (See Chapter 623.4 in *Nelson Textbook of Pediatrics,* 15th ed.)

4. D. Traction is crucial to stretch the contracted hip muscles before operation. (See Chapter 627.1 in *Nelson Textbook of Pediatrics,* 15th ed.)

5. D. Legg-Calvé-Perthes disease occurs at a younger age. The pain is referred to the knee. (See Chapter 627.3 in *Nelson Textbook of Pediatrics,* 15th ed.)

6. D. (See Chapter 630.3 in *Nelson Textbook of Pediatrics,* 15th ed.)

7. B and D. This is a classic history of dislocation of the radial head. Supination of the forearm is curative, and counseling parents not to pull small children by the arm is important. (See Chapter 630.3 in *Nelson Textbook of Pediatrics,* 15th ed.)

8. E. Infantile cortical hyperostosis is also called Caffey disease, after the radiologist who first described it. (See Chapter 644 in *Nelson Textbook of Pediatrics,* 15th ed.)

9. 1. C
   2. D
   3. A
   4. B
   5. E
   (See Chapter 622 in *Nelson Textbook of Pediatrics,* 15th ed.)

10. B. (See Chapter 172 in *Nelson Textbook of Pediatrics,* 15th ed.)

11. B and D. *Pseudomonas* probably comes from the sneaker, and *S. aureus* from the skin. (See Chapter 172 in *Nelson Textbook of Pediatrics,* 15th ed.)

12. C. Incision and drainage with debridement of necrotic infected material is one of the most important aspects of treatment. After the material is cultured and Gram stained, the patient is started on a combination of intravenous nafcillin and gentamicin. (See Chapter 172 in *Nelson Textbook of Pediatrics,* 15th ed.)

13. D. Normal in utero positioning produces tibial torsion, which may also be associated with metatarsus adductus. (See Chapter 624.5 in *Nelson Textbook of Pediatrics,* 15th ed.)

14. 1. D
    2. A
    3. B
    4. E
    5. C
    (See Chapters 623 and 624 in *Nelson Textbook of Pediatrics,* 15th ed.)

15. C. Developmental dysplasia of the hip is present in 10% of children with metatarsus adductus. (See Chapter 623.1 in *Nelson Textbook of Pediatrics,* 15th ed.)

16. E. Prematurity is not a typical risk factor. All the other choices are associated with developmental dysplasia of the hip. (See Chapter 627.1 in *Nelson Textbook of Pediatrics,* 15th ed.)

17. C. Toxic synovitis or transient monoarticular synovitis frequently follows a nonspecific viral-like illness and does not have features suggestive of septic arthritis—osteomyelitis of the femoral head. Features suggestive of a septic process include fever, toxicity, limited range of motion, an externally rotated and partially flexed posture of the involved leg (antalgic posture), leukocytosis, a high ESR, and positive findings on bone scans. Toxic synovitis usually resolves spontaneously in 1 to 3 weeks and responds to rest and nonsteroidal antiinflammatory agents. (See Chapter 627.2 in *Nelson Textbook of Pediatrics,* 15th ed.)

18. 1. A
    2. B
    3. B
    4. A
    5. D
    6. B
    7. C
    8. A
    9. B
    10. A
    (See Chapter 627 in *Nelson Textbook of Pediatrics,* 15th ed.)

19. D. A right curve is typical of scoliosis and is usually *not* painful. A left curve is worrisome and may suggest an underlying spinal cord, vertebral, or neuromuscular disorder. (See Chapter 628.5 in *Nelson Textbook of Pediatrics,* 15th ed.)

20. B. All children and their parents should be counseled about the risk of injuries. Boys with a single testicle can be offered the option of wearing a protective cup. (See Chapter 633 in *Nelson Textbook of Pediatrics,* 15th ed.)

21. 1. C
    2. D
    3. A
    4. B
    5. F
    6. E
    (See Chapters 634–645 in *Nelson Textbook of Pediatrics,* 15th ed.)

22. 1. D
    2. A
    3. B
    4. C
    5. F
    6. E
    (See Chapters 634–645 in *Nelson Textbook of Pediatrics,* 15th ed.)

23. C. The normal alkaline phosphatase level of the child described in the question is a clue. In nutritional rickets, an elevation of the alkaline phosphatase level is the first abnormality. (See Chapter 648 in *Nelson Textbook of Pediatrics,* 15th ed.)

24. 1. C
    2. A
    3. B
    4. E
    5. D
    (See Chapters 648–656 in *Nelson Textbook of Pediatrics,* 15th ed.)

25. D. This pool is available for mobilization in times of poor calcium intake or increased losses. (See Chapter 647 in *Nelson Textbook of Pediatrics,* 15th ed.)

26. 1. B
    2. D
    3. A
    4. E
    5. C
    (See Chapters 648–656 in *Nelson Textbook of Pediatrics,* 15th ed.)

27. A. At this time, therapy to lower the body burden of cystine is essential. This could prevent future damage to the eyes and other organs. (See Chapter 483.3 in *Nelson Textbook of Pediatrics,* 15th ed.)

28. C. The differential diagnosis of Fanconi syndrome is extensive and includes drugs and toxins. (See Chapter 483.2 in *Nelson Textbook of Pediatrics,* 15th ed.)

33 Unclassified Diseases

1. D. Gastroesophageal reflux as a risk for SIDS has not been related to sleeping position. Although the fear of aspiration in a supine position is a theoretic concept, it has not been observed in practice in normal infants without pathologic reflux. (See Chapter 657 in *Nelson Textbook of Pediatrics,* 15th ed.)

2. C. Small-for-gestational-age infants and premature neonates have an increased risk of SIDS, not large infants. If an infant who is large for gestational age has a SIDS-like episode, suspect hypoglycemia or subdural hematoma (due to birth trauma). (See

Chapter 657 in *Nelson Textbook of Pediatrics,* 15th ed.)

3. D. Apnea such as that described in the question is not associated with a DPT immunization, nor is SIDS. (See Chapter 657 in *Nelson Textbook of Pediatrics,* 15th ed.)

4. E. Although some of the choices may be epidemiologic risk factors, many children with SIDS have no identifiable epidemiologic risk factors, making prediction of SIDS quite difficult. (See Chapter 657 in *Nelson Textbook of Pediatrics,* 15th ed.)

5. C. Increased levels of hypoxanthine may actually be present in the vitreous humor, suggesting prior hypoxia. (See Chapter 657 in *Nelson Textbook of Pediatrics,* 15th ed.)

6. B. Although there are many causes of "sudden" death in infants, SIDS remains a disease of unknown and probable central nervous system origin. (See Chapter 657 in *Nelson Textbook of Pediatrics,* 15th ed.)

7. C. Hutchinson-Gilford progeria syndrome is a rare disease of unknown cause. It is associated with premature aging and early atherosclerotic, cardiac, or cerebrovascular disease. (See Chapter 659 in *Nelson Textbook of Pediatrics,* 15th ed.)

8. C. Etoposide is considered the treatment of choice for the systemic disseminated form of Langerhans cell histiocytosis. (See Chapter 660 in *Nelson Textbook of Pediatrics,* 15th ed.)

9. C. Multisystem familial erythrophagocytic lymphohistiocytosis is often lethal and is characterized by pancytopenia, hemophagocytosis, hyperlipidemia, aseptic meningitis, coagulopathy, and multiorgan system dysfunction. (See Chapter 660 in *Nelson Textbook of Pediatrics,* 15th ed.)

10. A. Langerhans cell histiocytosis is probably due to a monoclonal expansion of this cell type. (See Chapter 660 in *Nelson Textbook of Pediatrics,* 15th ed.)

11. B. Although choices *A, C,* and *E* are suggestive, definitive diagnosis of sarcoidosis depends on the presence of noncaseating granulomas together with the clinical manifestations. (See Chapter 658 in *Nelson Textbook of Pediatrics,* 15th ed.)

12. D. A slit lamp can help determine the presence of uveitis. (See Chapter 658 in *Nelson Textbook of Pediatrics,* 15th ed.)

13. B. Electron microscopy is essential in determining the presence of the diagnostic

Birbeck granules. (See Chapter 660 in *Nelson Textbook of Pediatrics,* 15th ed.)

34 Environmental Health Hazards

1. D. No congenital neoplasias have been reported, nor has leukemia developed in fetuses exposed to atomic blast radiation. (See Chapter 662 in *Nelson Textbook of Pediatrics,* 15th ed.)

2. 1. B
   2. A
   3. D
   4. C
   5. E
   (See Chapter 663 in *Nelson Textbook of Pediatrics,* 15th ed.)

3. D. Milk is an unusual source of mercury. (See Chapter 664 in *Nelson Textbook of Pediatrics,* 15th ed.)

4. B. Pulmonary, renal, and gastrointestinal manifestations are the usual consequences of acute exposure to mercury vapor. (See Chapter 664 in *Nelson Textbook of Pediatrics,* 15th ed.)

5. D. Cerebral edema is often noted with blood lead levels exceeding 100 μg/dL. Encephalopathy due to lead may be lethal or associated with significant neurodevelopmental sequelae. (See Chapter 665 in *Nelson Textbook of Pediatrics,* 15th ed.)

6. A. Anemia is usually but not always due to the iron deficiency that is associated with lead intoxication. (See Chapter 665 in *Nelson Textbook of Pediatrics,* 15th ed.)

7. E. Choices *A, B,* and *C,* are dangerous and may induce pulmonary aspiration if emesis occurs. Steroids are of no value and may predispose to infection. Supportive therapy is indicated and includes oxygen and fluids. (See Chapter 666.4 in *Nelson Textbook of Pediatrics,* 15th ed.)

8. 1. C
   2. A
   3. B
   4. E
   5. D
   6. G
   7. F
   (See Chapter 666 in *Nelson Textbook of Pediatrics,* 15th ed.)

9. E. Intravenous deferoxamine and standard supportive therapy are indicated for severe iron toxicity. (See Chapter 666.5 in *Nelson Textbook of Pediatrics,* 15th ed.)

10. A. Sodium bicarbonate, especially with frequent premature ventricular contractions

and a wide QRS in this patient with signs of drug ingestion, is indicated to stabilize the myocardium. (See Chapter 666.1 in *Nelson Textbook of Pediatrics,* 15th ed.)

11. E. Activated charcoal is the preferred method of preventing absorption and probably of extracting this drug from the circulation. (See Chapter 666.1 in *Nelson Textbook of Pediatrics,* 15th ed.)

12. C. Tricyclic antidepressants cause anticholinergic-like symptoms plus arrhythmias, prolongation of the QRS, and depressed levels of consciousness. (See Chapter 666.6 in *Nelson Textbook of Pediatrics,* 15th ed.)

13. 1. A
   2. C
   3. A
   4. C
   5. A
   6. A
   7. A
   8. B
   9. B
  10. D
  11. B
  12. B
(See Chapter 668 in *Nelson Textbook of Pediatrics,* 15th ed.)

14. 1. B
   2. A
   3. D
   4. C
   5. E
(See Chapter 666.9 in *Nelson Textbook of Pediatrics,* 15th ed.)

15. C. To alleviate tick paralysis, one need only remove the tick. Those sensitive to bees (systemic manifestations) should undergo immune therapy (hyposensitization), because there is no antivenin. (See Chapter 668 in *Nelson Textbook of Pediatrics,* 15th ed.)

16. E. A Public Health Service review of the benefits and possible adverse effects of fluoride in 1991 showed no relation to osteosarcoma. Studies have been adequate, and there is no basis for thinking that congenital malformations can be induced. The review did attribute a small increase in fluorosis of the teeth to the administration of fluoride in toothpaste or by dentists in addition to that in the water supply. Young children should be taught to use toothpaste sparingly and not to swallow it. (See Chapter 258 in *Nelson Textbook of Pediatrics,* 15th ed.)

17. D. A child with ataxia-telangiectasia, because of its hereditary DNA repair defect, is unable to repair acute radiation damage. Conventional doses of radiotherapy to treat lymphomas (to which AT predisposes) have caused acute radiation sickness, and at least three children have died. It is important to diagnose ataxia-telangiectasia in young patients with lymphoma to avoid radiotherapy. The other choices listed in the question are not associated with severe acute radiation reaction. (See Chapter 662 in *Nelson Textbook of Pediatrics,* 15th ed.)

18. C. Adenocarcinoma of the vagina has occurred in 1 in 1000 daughters of women given diethylstilbestrol before the 13th week of gestation. Hepatoma in the child has not been linked to progestational compounds administered during pregnancy, nasopharyngeal carcinoma has not been associated with maternal use of immunosuppressive drugs, and maternal cocaine use has not been found to cause cancer in offspring. Cigarette smoking does not cause mesothelioma in adults. (It potentiates the effect of asbestos in causing bronchogenic carcinoma, not mesothelioma, in adults.) (See Chapters 507 and 663 in *Nelson Textbook of Pediatrics,* 15th ed.)

19. D. Almost all human carcinogens and teratogens have been first identified by an alert practitioner. Animal experimentation almost always follows the observation in humans. Thalidomide caused phocomelia in humans but did not affect the animals tested before the drug was marketed abroad. Other species have since developed phocomelia after the drug was given. Diethylstilbestrol causes clear cell adenocarcinoma of the vagina or cervix in young women whose mothers were treated with the drug early in pregnancy. No such effect was predicted from animal experimentation. (See Chapters 662 and 663 in *Nelson Textbook of Pediatrics,* 15th ed.)

20. B. About 40 children heavily exposed to dioxin from a runaway reaction in a factory (Seveso, Italy) in 1976 developed chloracne. None of the other choices in the question have been related to the exposure. (See Chapter 663 in *Nelson Textbook of Pediatrics,* 15th ed.)

21. E. Radon in soil varies from house to house; thus, neighborhood exposure levels are not reliable indicators and would not be known in any event. In most cases, homes can be sealed against soil-emitting

radiation that enters through cracks in the basement or lowest floor. Although the risk of low-dose radon exposure is controversial, testing may be required for sale of the house or to inform the concerned home owner about the level. Results of past tests will be outdated if new cracks or leaks have developed in the basement. (See Chapter 662 in *Nelson Textbook of Pediatrics,* 15th ed.)

22. A. Although some studies suggested an association (not a causal relationship) of electromagnetic fields with leukemia or brain cancer in children whose homes were near power lines, expert committees in the United States and the United Kingdom have evaluated all the data and found no conclusive evidence of a cancer risk. There are no studies of spontaneous abortions (notoriously difficult to ascertain) or birth defects. Electromagnetic fields can affect animal behavior, but effects on human behavior have not been identified. (See Chapter 662 in *Nelson Textbook of Pediatrics,* 15th ed.)

23. A. Potassium iodide protects the thyroid against radiation, and the sooner it is given the better. At Three-Mile Island, a serious problem was the inability to obtain eyedroppers to administer the drug by mouth, and potassium iodide administration was the first measure taken. Thyroid function tests are performed much later. Results of the CBC will probably be normal. Signs of acute radiation sickness will not appear for several days and probably will not result at all from this fallout exposure. (See Chapter 662 in *Nelson Textbook of Pediatrics,* 15th ed.)

24. B. The increased frequency of small head size begins at 10 to 19 rad. For leukemia, it begins at 20 to 49 rad and for severe mental retardation at 60 rad. Aplastic anemia is too rare to be measured, and somatic cell mutations cannot be detected at exposures less than 20 rad. (See Chapter 662 in *Nelson Textbook of Pediatrics,* 15th ed.)

25. D. The boy described in the question most

likely disturbed the nest of a black widow spider and now has systemic and local manifestations of envenomation. (See Chapter 668 in *Nelson Textbook of Pediatrics,* 15th ed.)

26. E. Antivenin is not necessary for *Hymenoptera* bites or stings, but immune prophylaxis may be indicated for systemic reactions. (See Chapter 668 in *Nelson Textbook of Pediatrics,* 15th ed.)

27. D. The first approach to poisonous snakebites should try to limit lymphatic spread and venous absorption. (See Chapter 668 in *Nelson Textbook of Pediatrics,* 15th ed.)

28. C. Sprouted green potatoes produce solanine intoxication within 7 to 19 hours of ingestion. Signs of intoxication are vomiting, diarrhea, abdominal pain, and possible shock and coma. (See Chapter 667 in *Nelson Textbook of Pediatrics,* 15th ed.)

29. C. Immediately dilute the ingested drain cleaner with water or milk. The ability to predict who will develop esophageal disease is poor; thus, most recommend esophagoscopy within 12 to 24 hours of such an ingestion. Steroids are of little value in the presence of esophageal lesions and do not prevent stricture formation. (See Chapter 666.7 in *Nelson Textbook of Pediatrics,* 15th ed.)

30. D. Aspirin overdose should be considered in any toxic, febrile, tachypneic, and confused patient. Nonetheless, this pattern is usually first thought of as suggesting sepsis, which must be ruled out. The metabolic acidosis (with or without a respiratory alkalosis) is suggestive of aspirin toxicity, whereas acidosis alone is suggestive of sepsis or an ingestion. (See Chapter 666.3 in *Nelson Textbook of Pediatrics,* 15th ed.)

31. C. The patient described in the question has ingested a potentially significant amount of acetaminophen. Charcoal may reduce absorption, and the ultimate predictor of toxicity (the 4-hour serum level) will determine the need for *N*-acetylcysteine therapy. (See Chapter 666.2 in *Nelson Textbook of Pediatrics,* 15th ed.)